Field Hospitals

Field Hospitals

A Comprehensive Guide to Preparation and Operation

Edited by

Elhanan Bar-On
Sheba Medical Center, Tel Hashomer, Israel

Kobi Peleg
Tel-Aviv University, Disaster Medicine Department

Yitshak Kreiss
Sheba Medical Center, Tel Hashomer, Israel

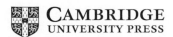

CAMBRIDGE
UNIVERSITY PRESS

University Printing House, Cambridge CB2 8BS, United Kingdom

One Liberty Plaza, 20th Floor, New York, NY 10006, USA

477 Williamstown Road, Port Melbourne, VIC 3207, Australia

314–321, 3rd Floor, Plot 3, Splendor Forum, Jasola District Centre, New Delhi – 110025, India

79 Anson Road, #06–04/06, Singapore 079906

Cambridge University Press is part of the University of Cambridge.

It furthers the University's mission by disseminating knowledge in the pursuit of
education, learning, and research at the highest international levels of excellence.

www.cambridge.org
Information on this title: www.cambridge.org/9781107141322
DOI: 10.1017/9781316493489

© Cambridge University Press 2020

First published 2020

Printed in the United Kingdom by TJ International Ltd, Padstow Cornwall

A catalogue record for this publication is available from the British Library.

Library of Congress Cataloging-in-Publication-Data

Names: Bar-On, Elhanan, editor. | Peleg, Kobi, editor. | Kreiss, Yitshak, editor.
Title: Field hospitals : a comprehensive guide to preparation and operation / edited by
Elhanan Bar-On, Kobi Peleg, Yitshak Kreiss.
Description: Cambridge, United Kingdom ; New York, NY : Cambridge University Press, 2019. |
Includes bibliographical references and index.
Identifiers: LCCN 2019019714 | ISBN 9781107141322 (hardback : alk. paper)
Subjects: | MESH: Mobile Health Units – organization & administration | Delivery of Health Care | Disasters
Classification: LCC RA975.D57 | NLM WX 190 | DDC 362.11–dc23
LC record available at https://lccn.loc.gov/2019019714

ISBN 978-1-107-14132-2 Hardback

....

Contents

Section 5 Additional Contextual Considerations

Colour plate section can be found between pages 180 and 181

Contributors

Avi Abargel, MD, MHA, MA
National Security and Homefront Defense Academic Studies
Beit Berl College, Israel

Nimrod Adi, MD
Director of Intensive Care Unit, Division of Anesthesiology, Pain and Critical Care, Tel Aviv Sourasky Medical Center, Israel

Tarif Bader, MD, MHA, MA
Surgeon General, Israel Defense Forces
The Department of Military Medicine,
The School of Medicine, Hebrew University, Jerusalem, Israel

Elhanan Bar-On, MD, MPH
Director, The Israel Center for Disaster Medicine and Humanitarian Response
Chaim Sheba Medical Center, Tel HaShomer, Israel
Associate Professor of Orthopedic Surgery, Sackler Faculty of Medicine, Tel Aviv University

Seema Biswas, PhD, FRCS
Department of Surgery, Ziv Medical Center, Safed, Galilee, Israel

Moran Bodas, MPH, PhD
Senior Researcher, Israel National Center for Trauma and Emergency Medicine Research, Gertner Institute for Epidemiology and Health Policy
Faculty Member, Department of Emergency Management and Disaster Medicine, School of Public Health, Sackler Faculty of Medicine, Tel Aviv University

Frederick M Burkle, Jr, MD, MPH, DTM, FAAP, FACEP
Professor (Ret.), Senior Fellow and Scientist, Harvard Humanitarian Initiative, Harvard University and TH Chan School of Public Health, Cambridge, Massachusetts, USA
Senior International Public Policy Scholar, Woodrow Wilson International Center for Scholars, Washington DC, USA
Institute of Medicine, National Academy of Sciences (elected 2007)
Captain, Medical Corps, USNR (Ret.)

Claire Clement
Former International Law Adviser, British Red Cross

Shir Dar, MD, MHA
Ob-gyn, Kaplan Medical Center, Rehovot, Israel

Eran Dolev, MD
Professor (Em.), The Tel Hai College, Upper Galilee, Israel
Brigadier General (Ret.) Former Surgeon General, Israel Defense Forces

Lionel Dumont, MD
Centre for Humanitarian Medicine and Disaster Management (World Health Organization Collaborative Centre), Division of Tropical and Humanitarian Medicine
Division of Anaesthesiology, Geneva University Hospitals, Switzerland

Vladislav Dvoyris, DMD, MBA
Medical Officer (Res.) Israel Defense Forces Medical Corps

Louis N Finelli, DO (COL, MC, USA)
Armed Forces Medical Examiner
Armed Forces Medical Examiner System, Dover AFB, Dover, Delaware

Eyal Fruchter, MD
Chair, Psychiatric Division, Rambam Medical Campus, Haifa, Israel

Ralph E. Gebhard, MD
Professor of Anesthesiology, Professor of Orthopedics and Rehabilitation

Chief, Division of Acute Pain Medicine and Regional Anesthesiology, University of Miami-Miller School of Medicine, Miami, Florida, USA

S David Gertz, MD, PhD, LTC (Res.)
Director, Military Medicine Track ("Tzameret") and Institute for Research in Military Medicine
Advisor to the Israel Defense Forces Surgeon General for Victim Identification
Brandman Foundation Professor of Cardiac and Pulmonary Diseases
Professor of Anatomy and Cell Biology, Faculty of Medicine
The Hebrew University and Israel Defense Forces Medical Corps, Jerusalem, Israel

Karen Ginat, MD
Former Head of Mental Health Department, Israel Defense Forces Medical Corps

Elon Glassberg, MD, MHA
Israel Defense Forces Medical Corps
Bar-Ilan University Faculty of Medicine, Safed, Israel
The Uniformed Services University of the Health Sciences, Bethesda, Maryland, USA

Ilan Green, MD, MHA
Director, Family Medicine Department, Israel Defense Forces Medical Corps

Olivier Hagon, MD
Centre for Humanitarian Medicine and Disaster Management (World Health Organization Collaborative Centre), Division of Tropical and Humanitarian Medicine, Geneva University Hospitals, Switzerland

Tami Halperin, PhD
Former Head of Clinical Medical Laboratories, The Center of Medical Services, Israel Defense Forces Medical Corps

Dan Hanfling, MD
Contributing Scholar, Johns Hopkins Bloomberg School of Public Health, Center for Health Security
Clinical Professor, George Washington University, Department of Emergency Medicine
Medical Team Manager, Virginia Task Force 1, National Urban Search and Rescue Response System

Yoel Har-Even, B Nurs., M Neuro Sc. MHA, LTC (Res.)
Chief of Staff and Director of Resource Development, Office of the Director General, Chaim Sheba Medical Center, Tel HaShomer, Israel

Former Deputy Surgeon General, Israel Defense Forces Medical Corps

Patrick Herard, MD
Surgical Orthopedic Advisor, Médecins Sans Frontières, Paris, France

Ariel Hirschhorn, DMD
Department of Oral and Maxillofacial Surgery, Chaim Sheba Medical Center, Tel HaShomer, Israel

Nisim Ifrach, MD
Department of Critical Care, Sapir Medical Center, Meir Hospital, Kfar Saba, Israel

Asima Iqbal, MD
Department of Anesthesia, Mount Sinai Hospital, Medical Center Chicago, Illinois, USA

Jean-Daniel Junod, RNA
Centre for Humanitarian Medicine and Disaster Management (World Health Organization Collaborative Centre), Division of Anaesthesiology, Geneva University Hospitals, Switzerland

Arjun Katoch
Disaster Management Advisor; Member, United Nations Disaster Assessment and Coordination
Former Chief, Field Coordination Support Section, Emergency Services Branch
United Nations Office for Coordination of Humanitarian Affairs
Member, Advisory Committee to National Disaster Management Authority, Govt. of India Senior Fellow, Delhi Policy Group
Colonel (Ret.), The Parachute Regiment, Indian Army.

Alan Kay, FRCS, FRCS (Plast) Col. L/RAMC
Consultant Plastic Surgeon, Royal Centre for Defence Medicine, Birmingham, UK

Mohamed Koronfel, MD
Department of Anesthesiology, Cleveland Clinic Foundation, Cleveland, Ohio, USA

Yitshak Kreiss, MD, MHA, MPA, Brig. Gen. (Res.)
Director General, Chaim Sheba Medical Center, Tel HaShomer, Israel
Former Surgeon General, Israel Defense Forces

Chen Kugel, MD, LTC (Res.)
Director, Israel National Institute of Forensic Medicine, Israel Ministry of Health

Advisor to the Israel Defense Forces Surgeon General for Forensic Medicine

Guy Lakovski, BSc, M Eng. M.E. Mech. Eng.
Head of Biomedical Engineering Division, Hadassah University Hospital, Jerusalem, Israel
Former Head of Biomedical Engineering Branch, Israel Defense Forces Medical Corps

Haim Lavon, MD, MHA
Otolaryngology: Head and Neck Surgery, Pvt., Mazkeret Batya, Israel

Gadi Levy, MD, MHA
Head, Radiology Informatics, Tel Aviv Sourasky Medical Center, Tel Aviv, Israel
Senior Radiology Consultant, Maccabi Health Services National Imaging Center, Tel Aviv, Israel
Former Head, Information Technologies Branch, Israel Defense Forces Medical Corps

Boris Lushniak, MD, MPH
Dean and Professor, University of Maryland School of Public Health,
College Park, Maryland, USA

Pietro D Marghella, DHSC, MSc, MA, MPH, CEM
Professorial Lecturer, The Milken Institute of Public Health, The George Washington University, Washington DC, USA

Tal Marom, MD
Department of Otolaryngology: Head and Neck Surgery, Samson Assuta Ashdod University Hospital
Ben-Gurion University Faculty of Health Sciences

Bronte Martin, MNurs, GDipNSc (Emerg), CritCCert, BNurs, DipGov & ADipPersOps, MRCNA
Director of Nursing, National Critical Care Trauma Response Centre, Darwin, Northern Territory, Australia
Mission and Clinical Lead, Australian Medical Assistance Team
WGCDR, Royal Australian Air Force
World Health Organization Emergency Medical Teams Initiative, United Nations Disaster Assessment Coordination

Ami Mayo, MD
Department of Critical Care, Assuta Medical Center, Ashdod, Israel

Ofer Merin, MD, MHA
Director General, Shaare Zedek Medical Center, Jerusalem, Israel

Ian Miskin, MD
Consultant in Infectious Diseases, Clalit Health Services, Jerusalem District
Hadassah-Hebrew University Medical School, Jerusalem, Israel

Åsa Molde, MD
Former Chief Surgeon, International Committee of the Red Cross

Melanie Morrow, BPharm, MClinPharm, FSHPA
Specialist Clinical Pharmacist, National Critical Care and Trauma Response Centre, Darwin, Northern Territory, Australia

Maximilian P Nerlander, MD
Physician and Medical Epidemiologist, Department of Public Health Sciences, Karolinska Institutet, Sweden

Ian Norton, MB BAO BCh, FACEM, AFRCSI, DTM, DIH
Manager, Emergency Medical Teams, Emergency Management and Operations, World Health Organization, Geneva, Switzerland

Inga Osmers, MD, MA
Head of Berlin Medical Unit, Médecins Sans Frontières, Switzerland

Kobi Peleg, PhD, MPH
National Center for Trauma & Emergency Medicine Research, The Gertner Institute for Health Policy and Epidemiology
Professor, Tel-Aviv University, Disaster Medicine Department

Anthony D Redmond, MD, OBE
Professor (EM), Humanitarian and Conflict Response Institute, University of Manchester, UK
Chair, UK-Med
President, World Association for Disaster and Emergency Medicine

Paul Reed, MD
US Public Health Service
Deputy Director, National Center for Disaster
Medicine and Public Health, Uniformed Services
University, Bethesda, Maryland, USA

Johan von Schreeb, MD, PhD
Specialist in General Surgery, Centre for Research on
Health Care in Disasters, Global Health – Health
System and Policy
Associate Professor, Department of Public Health
Sciences, Karolinska Institutet, Stockholm, Sweden

Eliezer Schwartz, MD, DTMH, FISTM
The Institute of Geographic Medicine and Tropical
Diseases, The Chaim Sheba Medical Center, Tel
HaShomer, Israel
The Sackler Faculty of Medicine, Tel Aviv University,
Israel

Michel Somekh, MHA
Chief Radiographer, Medical Technology, Health
Information and Research Directorate, Israel
Ministry of Health
Former Head of Imaging Division, Israel Defense
Forces Medical Corps

Dekel Stavi, MD
Department of Critical Care,
Sapir Medical Center, Meir Hospital, Kfar-Saba, Israel

Avraham Steinberg, MD, MHA
Pediatric Neurologist, Director, Medical Ethics Unit
and Chairman, Institutional Review Board,
Shaare Zedek Medical Center, Jerusalem, Israel

Kelly Suter, RN, BSN, MSN, MSBioethics

Ladd A Tremaine, MD (COL, MC, USA)
Armed Forces Medical Examiner (Immediate Past)
Armed Forces Medical Examiner System, Dover AFB,
Dover, Delaware, USA

Terry Trewin, AFSM
World Health Organization, Global Mentor EMT
Initiative
OIC Capability Development and Special Operations
Northern Territory Fire and Rescue Service,
Technical Logistics Lead Australian Medical
Assistance Team

Erez Tsumi, MD, MHA
Ophthalmologist and Ophthalmic Surgeon, Deputy
Director of the Department of Ophthalmology,
Soroka University Medical Center, Ben-Gurion
University, Be'er Sheva, Israel

Harald Veen, MD
Trauma Surgeon
Consultant, World Health Organization
Former Chief Surgeon, International Committee of
the Red Cross

Shlomo Vinker, MD, MHA
Vice Dean and Chairman, Department of Family
Medicine, Sackler Faculty of Medicine, Tel Aviv
University
General Medical Director, Leumit Health Services,
Israel

Rebecca Weir, MN, CCC, BSc – Nursing
Director of Clinical Services, Nursing and Midwifery
Northeast Health, Wangaratta, Victoria, Australia
Clinical Lead, Australian Medical Assistance Team,
EMST Senior Coordinator, MIMMS GIC Instructor

Dror Yifrah, MBA
Central District Chief Information Officer
Macabi Health Services, Tel Aviv, Israel
Former Chief Information Officer, Israel Defense
Forces Medical Corps

Preface

Elhanan Bar-On, Kobi Peleg, and Yitshak Kreiss

Field hospitals are deployed in a wide range of scenarios, including natural and man-made disasters. Earthquakes, tsunamis, storms, floods, drought, famine, epidemics, armed conflicts, and refugee crises each have their unique characteristics. These events can cause massive destruction, with many deaths, severe injuries, and displaced people. They can occur in developed countries, in remote conflict zones, or in countries where the medical systems struggle to deliver basic health care during normal times and may be overwhelmed during a disaster, lacking the resources to treat a large number of injuries and fill the concomitant medical needs. This has prompted the deployment of many emergency medical teams (EMTs) to disaster areas. These EMTs vary from small mobile units through fixed ambulatory clinics to field hospitals of various sizes and capabilities. They can be dispatched by military or civilian governmental agencies and by nongovernmental organizations (NGOs). EMTs working in a field hospital in a disaster zone or austere environment operate under circumstances markedly different from their everyday experience. There is a large imbalance between the huge needs and the limited capabilities to meet them. The operation of field hospitals under these circumstances requires adaptation to the unique environment. This is necessary in both organizational and clinical protocols, as well as in ethical considerations, to maintain standards of care and deliver optimal treatment to individual patients while considering that sometimes compromises need to be made to do the greatest good for the greatest number. Staff in field hospitals may face barriers with unfamiliar language and culture, posing both therapeutic and ethical dilemmas not normally encountered in routine circumstances. Some deployed personnel may have had prior experience in a disaster situation, but for many this could be their first encounter.

This book was compiled as a guide to teams operating field hospitals in a wide range of scenarios. It is based on the vast field experience of the authors, all having deployed such field hospitals in a large variety of organizations and countries, and in differing crisis situations. The book addresses the administrative and organizational aspects of a field hospital, as well as the conception and operating method of a field hospital as part of the overall health complex in the disaster area. It outlines the characteristics of clinical medical and nursing care delivery, and the auxiliary and logistic services essential for successful operation of a field hospital, as well as the ethical and legal aspects of such deployments. The emphasis is on highlighting the characteristics of functioning within the unique environment of a field hospital and the adaptation to extreme and austere conditions, while maintaining the highest standards of care possible in these difficult circumstances.

We hope this accumulated experience will help EMTs operating field hospitals of all types in a wide range of disaster and emergency situations around the globe in their endeavor to save lives and improve health, by delivering the best care possible to the many thousands of people in the world affected by these devastating events.

History of Military Field Hospitals

Eran Dolev

Introduction

A "field hospital" is a mobile medical unit, which temporarily takes care of casualties on site before they can be safely transported to more permanent hospital facilities. Traditionally, field hospitals were military units located close to battlefields and included physicians and surgeons who could cope with most of the medical conditions.

In the ancient world, the ability of the medical profession to cope with health problems was limited. The concept of hospitalization – caring for sick and wounded people in a special medical institution – was unknown, neither to the civilian society, nor to the military. During the battles of early empires or even in the Hellenistic world, military medicine was represented only by physicians, whose main task was to extract arrows or other foreign bodies from tissues. There was no medical service of the military organization, including no form of hospital.

Rome

The first time in the history of the Western world that hospitalization (meaning the organized care of sick and wounded patients) is noted was in the Roman army. In the eyes of the Roman-army commanders, care of the wounded was considered as a military necessity, not only because it allowed better chances to overcome the medical problem but mainly as a solution for coping with demoralization of the troops[1].

During the epoch of republican Rome, battles were fought near to home. At that time, the Roman army had no medical arrangements for the care of the sick and wounded soldiers beyond wound dressing. The more serious cases were left at patrician houses for care and recuperation. When the Roman legions began to fight at remote battlefields and in unfriendly territories, casualties could not be left to be cared for by the local population anymore.

It was the Emperor Augustus in the first century AD who understood the importance of providing medical care for his troops by an organized medical service. The solution was the establishment of a system of hospitals – valetudinaria – located along major Roman routes and at crucial occupied areas in various provinces. Some historians consider these military hospitals as "the greatest Roman innovation in medicine[2]."

Valetudinaria were the answer to the medical problems of the remote legions. They were an integral part of legion camps and forts all over Europe. They were, most probably, built to accommodate the sick, but injured soldiers were also treated there. Surgical instruments found in archeological excavations of valetudinaria proved that surgical work was performed in them[2].

During the imperial period, it became standard practice to include a hospital in any legion camp or fort. These were always ready to accommodate and treat as many as 2.5–10% of the legion[2]. The professional head of the hospital was a medical officer who reported to the camp commander. The hospital team included physicians, surgeons, and medics.

The valetudinarium was constructed as a square structure, built of stone, and was 90 m × 50 m in dimension. It was divided into four quadrangles, which enclosed an inner courtyard. These included the patients' wards. The valetudinarium could accommodate 200–220 patients in 38 rooms. The entrance hall led to a large hall, most probably a reception room, and to treatment rooms, baths, the kitchen, and the medical depot[2].

No records of the many valetudinaria have survived. Thus, the professional work that was done in these hospitals cannot be estimated. However, the assumption that these kinds of medical facilities served as the first field hospitals in the Western tradition is quite solid.

Byzantium

Many aspects of Rome's legacy were transferred to its Eastern successor: the Byzantine Empire. The military tradition was one of these aspects, including the medical services of the military organization. Thus, for many years the Byzantines continued to use the traditional Roman military hospital: the valetudinarium.

When Emperor Maurice (582–602) changed the nature of the Byzantine army by integrating infantry soldiers and mounted horsemen, the nature of the medical service in the field was also changed. In every regiment of 300–400 soldiers (numerus), a new medical unit was established. This unit included one physician and one surgeon, and 8–18 medics and stretcher bearers.

The Byzantines were the first in the Western civilization to establish general hospitals. These hospitals served both the military and the general population. They also considered the preservation of military ability as being crucial. However, they never attempted to establish hospitals for their armies in the field. The great medical centers that served the military community, according to the best professional standards of the time, were located only in the cities. Wounded and sick soldiers were treated at these hospitals[3].

Crusaders' Kingdom of Jerusalem

The Crusaders' Kingdom of Jerusalem was in an intermittent state of war with the neighboring Muslim states for almost two hundred years. Its unique innovation was the creation of the military orders. The first among them, the Order of the Knights of Saint John of Jerusalem (The Hospitallers), was established to care for sick and poor Christian pilgrims in the Holy Land and later to protect the Crusaders' Kingdom. The greatest achievement of the Order was the foundation of the hospital in Jerusalem. The concept of a "hospital" was unknown in Europe at that time and it is assumed that the hospital in Jerusalem reflected direct Byzantine influence[4]. The hospital served the population as a general hospital, but it also maintained its military obligations.

After the battle of Tel Gezer[5] in 1175, where Saladin was defeated by the Crusaders, 750 Christian battle casualties were evacuated from the battlefield and were admitted to the hospital in Jerusalem. This event demonstrated two facts: the first was the hospital was able to cope with a huge number of casualties without being overwhelmed. The second was that there were no field hospitals in the Crusaders' Kingdom[6].

Medieval Times

No medical service can be detected in European and other military organizations during the Middle Ages. A wounded soldier was bandaged by a comrade or by a medic and, in some cases, a foreign body was extracted from the soldier's tissues by a physician. No further medical or surgical treatment was expected to be given as hospitals usually did not exist. In many battles, there may have been a surgeon accompanying a king or a prince, but there was no medical service for the troops. However, some developments are noticed: at the start of the Hundred Years' War, at the Battle of Crécy in 1346, Edward III of England was accompanied by the surgeon John de Arden, but there was no medical personnel for the troops. Almost 70 years later, at Agincourt, 1415, Henry V was accompanied by the surgeon Nicholas Colnet, while Thomas Marstede was appointed army surgeon with 12 assistant surgeons: all were paid to look after the soldiers[1].

The first evidence of a field hospital during military operation can be found in the chronicles of the siege of Granada – the last stand of the Muslims in Spain – in 1484. As far as we know, the establishment of a field hospital for the sake of the sick and wounded soldiers was Queen Isabella's own idea:

> For the care of the sick and wounded, the queen sent always to the camp six large tents and their furniture, together with physicians, surgeons, medicines and attendants; and commanded that they should charge nothing, for she would pay for all. In the camps, these tents with their appointments were called the "Queen's Hospital" (Hernando del Fulgar)[1].
>
> That nothing might be lacking, the most devout army was followed by about four hundred ambulances, covered with awnings, which was called the Queen's Hospital; in these, at the Queen's expense, and in lavish outlay, was found everything necessary to the art of medicine and of surgery for the treatment of the sick or the wounded from the ranks; those attending and ministering to this duty being matrons of the most honest and trustworthy character; no prostitutes, no panderers, no perjury, no games of chance were permitted in the army, lest anyone might find opportunity to behave dishonourably or improperly (Pedro Bosca)[1].

Queen Isabella's grandson, King Charles V, followed his grandmother's example: in his armies, the sick and wounded soldiers were evacuated from the battlefield to the baggage trains and put into tents, a kind of field hospital. There, they were attended by physicians or surgeons.

Renaissance and the Religious Wars in Europe

During the fifteenth and sixteenth centuries, gunpowder weapons replaced sharp-edged weapons and became important developments in military medicine. While in the fifteenth century the professional consensus was that all wounds produced by projectiles were poisoned, this notion was challenged during the sixteenth century. It was Bartolomeo Maggi (1477–1552) who was probably the first not to accept the theory of the poisonous nature of gunshots. He was also the first to advocate that amputation due to gangrene should be performed through the living flesh. At the same time, the military surgeon Ambroise Paré (1510–1590) changed the attitude to the treatment of wounds caused by firearms (1545) and reintroduced the use of ligature, which allowed better outcome of amputations.

All these developments and innovations occurred at the level of the individual surgeon, treating wounded soldiers at the battlefield. At that time no link was established between professional innovations and organizational changes leading to a better performance of medical services at the battlefield. It should also be mentioned that the great discoveries in the field of medicine – such as Harvey's discovery of the circulation of the blood and the microscope of van Leeuwenhoek and others – had no impact on the practice of medicine and surgery in general, and on military medicine in particular during the seventeenth century.

The religious wars took place during the sixteenth and seventeenth centuries in Europe. They manifested themselves in a variety of conflicts, from local disputes to full-scale long and devastating wars, such as the Thirty Years' War (1618–1648). From professional medical and surgical points of view, no significant advances occurred during this epoch. However, some steps were taken in the direction of better organization of military medicine in the field:

The rulers of France took several actions in order to improve the state of the wounded at the battle fields. The first step was initiated by Maximilien, the Duke of Sully, a minister for King Henry IV, during the siege of Amiens in 1597. The Duke established a mobile hospital that could move with the fighting armies. The head and the chief surgeon of the hospital was Pigray, a pupil of Ambroise Paré[1]. The structure of this hospital was later improved by Cardinal Richelieu during the siege of La Rochelle (1627). During the reign of Louis XIV, stationary hospitals were built in garrison towns and in support of the field hospitals.

The first organized military hospitals in Germany were those authorized by the Elector Maximilian I, the Duke of Bavaria, in 1620, for the Catholic League. These hospitals were not mobile, but they were located close to the battlefield and thus named "field hospitals." One of them represented a new concept: it was designed to give the necessary medical treatment to battle casualties at the field and to enable them to be evacuated to a permanent military hospital. Thus, it was one of the first military hospitals to function as a clearing hospital[7].

In the Spanish Army of Flanders during the late sixteenth century, there was no medical service in the field. To the commanders and doctors of that army, it seemed a big hospital at Mechelen, Belgium, may solve the health problems of the troops. It became an issue only when, in the seventeenth century, the army command realized that sickness and injuries among the troops, when not attended properly, may encourage desertion and discourage civilians from joining the services[8]. It brought about the establishment of field hospitals, which had very limited professional abilities: they were expected to give the wounded and sick soldiers only initial treatment and then to transfer them to a fixed rear hospital.

The rise of military medicine in England began with the establishment of the standing army. The army was organized into regiments, and every regiment had a surgeon and an assistant surgeon. The task of these professionals, augmented by soldiers from the regiment itself, was to treat 40 patients at the battlefield and then to evacuate them to base hospitals in the rear.

Field hospitals – the missing link in efficient medical evacuation from the battlefield to rear hospitals – did not appear in England until 1690, during King William III's campaign in Ireland. These hospitals were designed to accompany the armies and thus were called "marching hospitals" or "flying hospitals"[7].

The main task of the marching hospital was to be ready to treat battle casualties evacuated from the regiments, as close to the front line as possible. Later, they were meant to either further evacuate the patients to hospitals in the rear or keep them until they recovered. The marching hospital unit was independent logistically: the hospital consisted of 12 horse-drawn carts, which carried 25 tents. After the hospital had been erected, the carts evacuated casualties to the fixed hospitals. Overall, when assembled, the hospital could accommodate up to 200 patients and it carried all necessary surgical and medical equipment. It was expected that, during active fighting, the marching hospital would be located beyond the range of cannons: less than 2 km from the firing line[9]. The hospital had 17 staff officers: one physician, one master surgeon, eight surgeon's mates (assistants), one master apothecary, three apothecary's mates for dispensing duties and care of medical stores, and three purveyors for commissariat duties[7].

The flying hospital had proved successful in the War of the Austrian Succession when it acted as expected: an essential link between the regimental medical teams and the general hospitals.

The Duke of Marlborough, one of the most distinguished British military commanders in history, was exceptional in his attitude toward the health of his troops: during his march to the Danube (1704), he was involved in the details of the medical plan. The duke insisted on having at least one medical officer in every regiment, foot or horse. Most regiments also had a surgeon's mate. The duke's force was followed by at least one field hospital[10].

The Eighteenth Century

Several military developments may be noted at the battlefields of the eighteenth century: improvements in firearms and in military tactics created new battlefields where, at every engagement, large numbers of casualties were expected. However, advances in military surgery improved the soldier's chances of overcoming injuries when treated properly close to the front line. The increasing size of the armies forced the various state governments to recognize their responsibility in giving proper medical care to their troops. Thus, in most armies, permanent medical services were established. The medical services included regimental hospitals: those small medical units attached to combat units, which gave immediate medical treatment to battle casualties. In some military organizations were also the flying hospitals: marching hospitals whose personnel were better qualified than the personnel of the regimental hospitals. During sieges, the French army utilized special field hospitals, naming them "hospital ambulant." Casualties evacuated from the regimental hospitals were treated at these hospitals. They were further evacuated to fixed hospitals located in towns and cities[1]. This concept was adopted by the Russian army during the reign of King Peter the Great[1]. Though casualties were given best-

available treatment at various hospitals, one of the sustained problems was lack of organization of the evacuation of casualties from the battlefield.

There were exceptions: during the War of the Austrian Succession, the British medical service treated the wounded on the front line and collected them at ambulance stations. Surgeons performed surgical procedures at the forward medical stations situated behind the front line and then evacuated the more seriously wounded to hospitals in nearby towns[7].

In the newly established USA, the standard of medicine generally was low, and the War of the Rebellion began without any permanent structure for medical care. Only during the war itself, and due to congress delegates' requirements, was the European structure of military medical service approved. It included regimental hospitals, flying hospitals, and fixed hospitals[11].

The Napoleonic Wars (1792–1815)

During the Napoleonic Wars, huge armies were exploited in the field. Due to new tactics and the massive use of artillery, the number of battle casualties became huge. Wounded soldiers could remain unattended for long hours on the battlefield and, when they were at last evacuated to base hospitals, transportation in specially designed wagons took more than 24 hours. The lag period until evacuation from the battlefield, combined with the long and tedious evacuation process itself, were among the factors that contributed to a high mortality rate among battle casualties.

Baron Pierre-François Percy (1754–1825) introduced to the French Army of the North a corps of trained stretcher bearers; their task was to pick up wounded soldiers and carry them to the nearest aid post. He also introduced horse-drawn wagons to the army, designed for the treatment and evacuation of battle casualties. Every wagon was staffed by surgeons and surgical teams with adequate surgical equipment, who were able to give medical treatment to casualties at the field and during the evacuation to the rear[12].

Baron Dominique Jean Larrey (1766–1842), the chief surgeon of the Grande Armée, and who participated in most of the Napoleonic campaigns, went even further. He introduced to the medical service in the field the ambulance volante: the "flying ambulance"[1]. This was not a new version of the old flying hospital – the field hospital that served as a midlink between the regimental hospital and the fixed hospital – Larrey actually introduced a new concept to military medicine, and to medicine in general: the importance of time. Until

Larrey's innovation, throughout the history of military medicine, battle casualties had been evacuated from the front line only after the battle was over. Larrey, a military surgeon with vast experience at many battles, realized that the earlier a wounded soldier was treated, the better the prognosis. It meant that the modus operandi of the ambulance volante was to treat casualties at the battlefield itself and even under fire. Thus, Larrey, by bringing the hospital to the soldiers, recognized time as an important independent prognostic factor and became the father of future emergency medicine.

The flying ambulance consisted of 340 men, organized into 3 divisions of around 113 each. It included a chief surgeon, 15 other surgeons, and 5 members of the quartermaster corps. It also included a trumpeter, whose task was to carry the surgical instruments, and a drummer boy in charge of the surgical dressings. Each division also had 12 light and 4 heavy carriages[1].

The parallel figure in the British army to Larrey in that same period was James McGrigor, who served as the principal medical officer of the Duke of Wellington during the Peninsular War. McGrigor believed the process of evacuation of sick and wounded soldiers was tedious and that, in many cases, they were treated too late. He suggested to Wellington the establishment of field hospitals as backup medical units to the regimental hospitals. However, Wellington rejected this idea because he considered any slow-moving transport as compromising his tactical freedom. The outcome was that McGrigor established a chain of general hospitals in various places in the Peninsula[1].

The Crimean War (1854–1856)

The Battle of Waterloo in 1815 was not only the end of the Napoleonic era but it also marked the beginning of an epoch of decay of military medicine. Even the discovery and introduction into surgery of anesthetic materials – ether and chloroform – had but minor influence on military medicine at the battlefield.

At the start of the Crimean War, most of the military medical services of the armies involved were unprepared for the mission. The medical service of the British expeditionary force for the Crimea consisted only of regimental hospitals and general hospitals. A regimental hospital consisted of 1 regimental surgeon and 3 assistant surgeons, 32 stretcher bearers, 16 stretchers, 1 ambulance wagon, and hospital equipment for 12 beds and bedding. Such a hospital was expected to treat and care for 60 casualties[13].

Most sick and wounded soldiers were treated at regimental hospitals and were then evacuated to general hospitals. However, these general hospitals were in Turkey, several hundred kilometers from the Crimean battlefields: a journey of three to four days by boat. Thus, the heritage of Florence Nightingale and her devoted nurses, who managed to significantly decrease the death rate at the hospital at Scutari, were concerned only with the situation at a general hospital far away from the battlefields of the Crimea. Treatment at the general hospitals did not affect the treatment of the soldiers at the front. There were several attempts to open hospitals at the Crimea itself, but again they concerned general hospitals and did not serve as a link between regimental hospitals and general hospitals[13].

The main medical lesson of the Crimean War in the field of military surgery was the need for a field hospital, a medical echelon which could clear the cases from the regimental hospital, treat them and further evacuate them to a general hospital[14].

The Russian hospitals at the Crimea were still as they were when they had been established at the turn of the eighteenth century. However, due to the vision of the chief Russian surgeon, Nikolay Pirogov, nurses served in these hospitals, contributing significantly to the quality of treatment.

The American Civil War (1861–1865)

Military medicine in the USA was influenced to a large extent by the British system. As the lessons of the Crimean War had not yet been studied, American military medicine during the 1860s remained at the same level as at the turn of the century. This meant American military medicine had not kept in pace with the various advancements in military technologies of the time including mines, barbed wire, grenades, mortars, and automatic weapons. The American Civil War was the first war where the railroad was used to transport battle casualties from the battlefield to rear hospitals and one of the first where anesthetics were used extensively. The main cause of injury among the troops was rifles, while the principal causes of mortality among the troops were disease and infection[1].

From the medical point of view, both sides, the Union and the Confederate, were caught unprepared. The number of fixed hospitals located in main towns and cities was small and field hospitals were scarce and their standards quite poor. But worse was the simple fact that there was neither doctrine nor real obligation for treatment and transportation of casualties. Battle casualties were left for days at the field; many of them died from neglect. Furthermore, the level of surgery was not appropriate: most of the operated-on casualties succumbed later to secondary infections.

The man who would transform American military medicine and change forever military medicine in the field was Major Jonathan Letterman, the medical director of the Army of the Potomac of the Union Army. After the failure of medical evacuation the Union Army had experienced at the second battle of Manassas, he was directed by the commander of the army, General McClellan, to improve the function of the medical services of the army in the field.

Major Letterman believed that "... the sick and wounded should be kept with the Army, treated by their own surgeons – life in a general hospital tends to destroy the good qualities of a soldier – so well preserved with their comrades". However, he was aware of the fact that, at the battlefields of the Civil War, the opposing armies inflicted on each other huge numbers of casualties and, at the same time, some of the casualties needed to be treated by skilled surgeons who could not be attached to all medical units.

Taking all these factors into consideration, Letterman conceived a new medical system for the battlefield, which included both the elements of treatment and evacuation: casualties were expected to be evacuated to a field dressing station, which was located next to the battlefield. There, they would get initial treatment including dressing and tourniquets. The second station in the chain of medical evacuation was the field hospital: a mobile hospital carried by 20 wagons. It was located close enough to the first station, but far away from direct fire. It was staffed by several surgeons and equipped to give medical support to a whole division of 7000–8000 men. Most of these hospitals were located at houses or barns, where emergency surgical procedures could be performed. The third station was a large hospital, located away from the battlefield, where different types of operation could be performed[15].

To allow this system to work, Letterman also created an ambulance corps: all ambulances of the army came under the command of the medical department of the army. According to the military orders: "no one was to be removed from the field except by the ambulance corps, who were to wear special insignia." The use of ambulances was restricted to patient evacuation and to carrying medical supplies[15].

Letterman's new medical system was put to work at the Battle of Antietam (17 September 1862). It was a great success: 23 000 casualties were evacuated from the battlefield in one day and treated in the various medical facilities. The system also worked efficiently during the battles of Fredericksburg and Gettysburg. Letterman's system was established officially for all armies in the field when adopted by an act of Congress in March 1864.

Letterman's system was based on the concept that medical evacuation should be controlled by the medical department, intertwined with treatment delivered by medical echelons. In a short time, it became the cornerstone of modern military medicine, and Major Jonathan Letterman thus became the father of modern military medicine on the battlefield.

The Boer War (1899–1902)

The war in South Africa was fought between the British Army and the local Boer population. The most important lesson of that war was in the field of public health. Yet another lesson was in the field of military surgery and medical organization. The Boer War was the first large-scale military conflict in which soldiers who suffered from penetrating abdominal wounds were operated on by military surgeons. It was soon discovered that the prognosis of those who had been operated on was worse than those who had not been operated at all. The conclusion of the South African experience was that penetrating abdominal wounds should not be operated on[16]. It was quite an unusual conclusion, which demanded an explanation. The British used field hospitals in South Africa, but they were located far from the various battlefields. The evacuation from the combat units depended on stretcher bearers of the units, which were not in accord with the field hospitals. Thus, many of the casualties whose wounds were very severe died during the agonizing and tedious evacuation from the battlefield. The survivors had better prognosis when untouched. A second reason for this conclusion was the type of injuries sustained by the British soldiers: the Boers used the Mauser rifle, a small-caliber, high-muzzle velocity weapon, which caused neat wounds, and which did not cause extensive tissue damage. The third reason was the South African soil: it was almost sterile and most battle wounds were not infected.

The main lesson of the Boer War in the field of military surgery was that the evacuation of battle casualties should be coordinated with their treatment. The outcome was the new field ambulance: a medical unit which consisted of a bearer division and a tent division. It included 10 officers and 224 other ranks and was the modern form of the former field hospital: close to the front line, ready to evacuate casualties at all times and able to give them the necessary treatment[17].

The First World War (1914–1918)

Not too long after the Boer War, the British, like most nations, found themselves involved in the Great War. During the first phase of the war, the medical services in the field acted according to the lessons of the Boer War. It meant, firstly, a conservative attitude toward abdominal penetrating wounds. However, when the opponent armies became static, entrenched in trenches and bunkers, this attitude had to be changed.

While in South Africa most of the wounds had been inflicted by rifles, the primary cause of injuries at the Western Front was artillery. The penetrating wounds caused by shell fragments caused extensive tissue damage, shock, secondary infection, and high mortality rate. The correct professional way to cope with the problem was to operate on all cases. Laparotomy – the indicated surgical procedure for penetrating abdominal injuries – had to be performed as soon as possible. However, the distance between the medical units at the battlefield and the evacuation hospitals was too far and the process of evacuation had a detrimental effect on injured soldiers' prognosis[18].

The solution was to create an intermediate surgical facility, located close to the combat units, beyond the range of enemy artillery, where abdominal and other cases could be operated on after a short time lag and evacuated as soon as the patient's condition allowed. As the main task of the intermediate surgical facility was to evacuate casualties from the front line after being initially treated and stabilized, it was named the casualty clearing station (CCS).

However, during the years of the war, these CCSs gradually became the primary medical facility at the front: many thousands of wounded soldiers – mainly severe abdominal and thoracic cases – who could not be evacuated to rear hospitals were operated in these installations[12].

The Second World War (1939–1945)

More than twenty years had passed since the end of the First World War. Yet, when the Second World War broke out, the medical services of the various armies of 1939 did not differ from those that had functioned in 1918[19]. Retrospectively, this might seem quite surprising as, in the time between the two wars, there were many important developments in medicine, some relevant to military medicine. Better prevention of diseases, better understanding of the mechanism of shock, the use of whole blood, and the introduction of sulfonamides were some of them. Additionally, the battles looked quite different than before: modern war was no longer static. The typical modern battle has become the arena for swift movement of armored units, covering long distances during a short time, assisted by heavy artillery and airplanes. A new type of fighting unit had been introduced to the various battlefields: airborne regiments, which needed solutions for their specific medical problems.

Also surprising was that during the first phase of the war, the medical lessons of the Civil War in Spain (1936–39) were not studied. The war in Spain served the Germans as a "dress rehearsal" for the Second World War. However, they mainly concentrated on the organizational elements of evacuation and less on the professional elements. Conversely, the experience acquired by the opponent republicans did not receive real attention. The main reason was that, when the battle was lost, the whole republican army disintegrated. The other reason was that the important book *Field Surgery in Total War*, written by a volunteer surgeon, Douglas Jolly, was not published until 1940: too late at least for the initial phase of the war. Yet, the harsh reality, experienced by both battle casualties and the medical teams at the various fronts, eventually imposed on the medical services several changes, which were similar to Jolly's scheme.

For Jolly, time was a key determinant of outcome in the management of war wounds. To cut short the time lag between wounding and operation, he formulated his "three points scheme." Accordingly, a "casualty classification center" with triage teams was placed in advance of the rest of the hospital. The next point was "number one hospital" or "hospital of the first urgency." Casualties who were defined as urgent for surgery at the classification center were operated at this echelon. With his method, Jolly reduced the time lag between wounding and operation to fewer than five hours. The "number two hospital" treated all the remaining casualties. There, their conditions were assessed and they were treated as necessary before being evacuated to a hospital. Jolly did not create a new type of medical unit: he just used the existing field hospital in a much more efficient way[20]. Based on his experience in Spain, Jolly was confident that any CCS, consisting of trained surgical teams, could act according to his scheme.

In the British Army, casualties from the battalions were evacuated to field ambulances, where basic resuscitation and hemodynamic stabilization could be performed. Those casualties who needed further surgical treatment were transported to the CCS. Since the First World War, the CCS was the principal field hospital at the front line where surgery could take place. From the CCS, casualties were further evacuated to general and basic hospitals.

During the battles of the Western Desert, it became apparent that, for this type of warfare, the CCS was not adequate. When it was understood that the goal of the medical system was to operate on casualties in fewer than eight hours from wounding, the CCS was neither mobile nor flexible enough. The answer was the creation of a "surgical team," which was extracted from the CCS It was light and could be placed closer to the front line. It became known as the "advanced operating center"[21].

The "Hartgill Committee" was nominated and directed to recommend changes that would improve resuscitation and surgery at the battlefield[19]. The committee recommended that field ambulances be reconstituted as fully mobile units. Though they could hospitalize 150 patients, their function was strictly defined as: "to resuscitate, stabilize, and evacuate"[22]. Mobile surgical teams were detached from general hospitals and placed in forward areas, one per division. These units included specialists in various fields of military surgery. From 1942 onward, there were two CCSs per army corps[22].

By the last phase of the war in Europe, it became clear to the consultant surgeons of the US Army Medical Corps that there was a need for surgical units that could resuscitate and operate urgent cases at the combat zone, close to the wounding site. This policy was based on the view that "a wounded man is resuscitated not only to save life but to prepare him for necessary surgery"[23]. These units, called auxiliary surgery groups (ASGs), were considered successful as they provided professional resuscitation, surgical management, and postoperative care close to the combat zone. An ASG included a chief surgeon, an assistant surgeon, an anesthesiologist, a surgical nurse, and two enlisted technicians. Four ASGs were established and located several miles from the front[24,25]. During the invasion of Normandy, every army was allocated an ASG unit. After the war, the ASGs were renamed "mobile auxiliary surgical hospitals," and later, at the start of the Korean War, they became known as mobile army surgical hospital (MASH) units.

The Korean War (1950–1953)

The Korean War was the first military conflict in which helicopters were employed for medical evacuation of battle casualties from the front line. This, together with a relative stabilization of the front, brought about a significant reduction in the time lag from wounding to resuscitation and operation. Thus, it created an opportunity for severe battle casualties, who would have died at advanced stations, to reach field hospitals alive. These hospitals were rather compact surgical units, located near the front line.

MASH units were designed as mobile, flexible military field hospitals, whose task was to provide care for battle casualties within the combat zone. They included 60 beds. The location of these units made them vulnerable to enemy attacks and short-range artillery. At first, they were expected to keep pace with combat units, providing immediate care to wounded soldiers. Later, when the units' movements became quite limited, MASH units were located at several crucial areas and were no longer expected to be mobile. They grew to include 24 surgeons and other doctors, 41 nurses, and 200 beds. MASH units were equipped and staffed to perform all types of surgical procedures[26,27]. MASH personnel specialized in triage, resuscitation, and trauma care, especially the management of shock, which included restoration of blood volume and utilization of whole blood. They also acquired a lot of experience considering professional criteria for further evacuation of casualties to hospitals located at the zone of communication and in the rear[28].

The Vietnam War (1965–1970)

In contrast to the Second World War and the Korean War, in the Vietnam War there was no "front" as traditionally defined: fighting took place concomitantly in several areas against regular, semiregular, and guerrilla enemy units. The outcome of this military situation was that field hospitals were neither affiliated to army units, nor did they follow advancing units in direct support. All military field hospitals in Vietnam were fixed installations committed to area support missions[29].

Military medicine in Vietnam was based on several professional developments in resuscitation and surgery of trauma, acquired during the Korean War and civilian trauma care. Without a defined front and with the support of helicopters for medical evacuation always available, Letterman's principles of medical evacuation from combat units were abandoned. Battle casualties were usually lifted from the battalions directly to the closest field hospital. The cardinal principle of military medicine during the Vietnam War was to get the wounded soldier into a hospital as fast as possible. Helicopters made it feasible for most injured soldiers to reach field hospitals in 30–35 minutes. It also meant that severely injured soldiers who, in previous wars, might not have had any chance to survive their wounds because of long and tedious evacuations, now reached surgical facilities with a high chance of overcoming their injuries[30,31].

At the beginning of the war, the standard field hospital was the MASH unit, which proved itself during the Korean War. However, in 1968, the MASH unit was replaced by a new type of field hospital: the medical unit self-contained transportable (MUST). It was an expandable, mobile shelter with inflatable ward sections. Its heart was a preoperative/resuscitation ward, operating theater, and postoperative care units. It also included radiology and laboratory sections, as well as pharmacy, dental, and logistic departments. Each of the MUST elements could be airlifted and dispatched by truck or helicopter. The expandable surgical element was a self-contained, rigid panel shelter with flexible sides. The air-inflatable ward element was a double-wall fabric shelter providing a free-space area for ward facilities[28,29].

After the Vietnam War

A further development of the field hospital occurred in the US Army Medical Corps during 1978: a new type of hospital called combat support hospital (CSH) was introduced. The CSH was not supposed to be located near the front line. Its main task was to stabilize the injured soldiers brought to the hospital by helicopter and to evacuate them for further treatment at rear hospitals. The CSH contained 44–248 beds and all the elements needed for operations and resuscitation. It had a ground ambulance company and about 600 people to staff the hospital while in full capacity of 248 beds[32].

The CSH represents a departure from the concept of immediate support for the combat units, as had been practiced in Vietnam. However, it should be interpreted as an answer to the new threats and challenges of the modern era around the world, and not as a specific answer to the medical problems of the troops fighting at a conventional battlefield.

The Israeli Experience

The Israeli army (Israel Defense Forces: IDF) originated from the British Army, where many of its founding fathers had served during the Second World War. Among these were physicians who became the forerunners of the future IDF medical service. During the War of Independence (1948) and other military conflicts (1956, 1967), the organization and the mode of operation of the medical services were basically a continuation of the British Royal Army Medical Corps.

It was after the 1967 Six-Day War that the Israeli medical corps had to be ready for a future large-scale battle in the Sinai desert. A hospital in the middle of Sinai, sited near an airstrip, beyond enemy artillery range, was the answer. The hospital could sort and treat 500 casualties and perform about 30 major operations in 24 hours. However, its modus operandi was of an evacuation hospital: its goal being to stabilize the respiratory and the hemodynamic state of the casualties to allow them to be evacuated to rear hospitals. Only 3% of all casualties admitted to the hospital were operated on there[33].

The innovation in the work of the evacuation hospital was in postoperative care: instead of holding the surgical cases, especially the postlaparotomy cases, at the field hospital for at least a week, they were evacuated by airplanes to rear hospitals in fewer than 24 hours from surgery. No serious complications were noticed. Early postoperative evacuation allowed the evacuation hospital to be always ready for new casualties and not to be overwhelmed by them[33,34].

The Lebanon War (1982) was different from previous Israeli military conflicts: while most of the former battles had been fought by armored units in the open, the Lebanese arena was characterized by mountainous terrain and built-up areas. The medical services in the field were expected to give battle casualties appropriate medical treatment at the battlefield and evacuate casualties to rear echelons. The IDF Medical Corps provided the divisions at the front with mobile surgical units, capable of performing advanced resuscitation and lifesaving surgical procedures[35].

However, most battle casualties were evacuated by helicopters from their units directly to hospitals in the rear. It was estimated that the civilian hospital of Upper Galilee, the main hospital close to the front, might be overwhelmed by the number and types of casualties expected to be evacuated there from the battlefield. It was decided, for the first time, to augment the hospital with a military field hospital. The integration between these two different medical bodies was successful[36]. Such an organizational option might increase to a large extent the ability of any peripheral hospital to cope with a mass-casualty situation.

Summary

The crucial place of field hospitals as essential components of medical service in the field has been proved over and again. While the name "field hospital" and the concept of saving battle casualties' lives has remained the same, field hospitals have been changed substantially. These changes have been the outcome of scientific discoveries, technological developments, and professional advancements. Many lives have been saved in these field hospitals, despite the growth of the devastating effects of weaponry.

It was only natural to introduce the concept of field hospitals into the civilian scenario, where natural disasters, as well as disasters due to various technologies, are unfortunately quite common. The recent successful experience of field hospitals in the civilian scenario shows quite clearly that they should stay with us for the future.

References

1. Garrison FH. *Notes on the history of military medicine*. Washington DC: Association of Military Surgeons; 1922: 49–52; 69; 95–6; 99; 121; 127; 138–9; 149; 165–6; 173–6.

2. Majno G. *The healing hand*. Cambridge, MA: Harvard University Press; 1975: 383–5; 393.

3. Miller TS. *The birth of the hospital in the Byzantine Empire*. Baltimore: The Johns Hopkins University Press; 1985.

4. Miller TS. The knights of Saint John and the hospitals of the Latin west. *Speculum* 1978: **53**: 709–33.

5. King EG. *The Knights Hospitallers in the Holy Land*. London: Methuen; 1931: 108.

6. Dolev E, Knoller N. Military medicine in the Crusaders' Kingdom of Jerusalem. *Israel Medical Association Journal* 2000: **3**: 389–92.

7. Cantlie N. *A history of the army medical department*. Volume 1. London: Churchill Livingstone; 1974: 22; 45–46; 80–101.

8. Storrs C. *Health, sickness and medical services in Spain's armed forces c. 1665–1700*. Medical History; 2006: 325–50.

9. Gruber von AE. *Hospital care and the British standing army, 1660–1714*. Aldershot: Ashgate Publishing; 2006: 68–79.

10. Gask GE. A contribution to the history of the care of the sick and wounded during Marlborough's march to the Danube in 1704, and at the battle of Blenheim. *Journal of the Royal Army Medical Corps* 1922: **34**: 274–88.

11. Gillett MC. *The army medical department, 1775–1818*. Washington DC: Center of Military History, US Army; 1981: 15–18.

12. Laffin J. *Combat surgeons*. Sutton: Phoenix Mill; 1999: 62–64; 181.

13. Cantlie N. *A history of the army medical department*. Volume 2. London: Churchill Livingstone; 1974: 37–39; 66.

14. Shepherd J. *The Crimean doctors*. Liverpool University Press; 1991: 697–702.

15. Joy RJT. *Jonathan Letterman of Jefferson: Medical director of the Army of the Potomac. Topic: a journal of the liberal arts*. Washington, Pennsylvania: Washington and Jefferson College; 1983: 26–37.

16. MacCormac W. Some remarks, by way of contrast, on war surgery, old and new. *Journal of the Association of the Military Surgeons of the United States* 1901: **10**: 277–90.

17. Dolev E. *Allenby's military medicine*. London: IB Tauris; 2007: 8–15.

18. Harrison M. *The medical war*. Oxford University Press; 2010: 114–22.

19. Bricknell MCM. The evolution of casualty evacuation in the British Army in the 20th century (Part II) – 1918–1945. *Journal of the Royal Army Medical Corps* 2002: **148**: 314–22.

20. Jolly DW, *Field surgery in total war*. New York: Paul B. Hoeber; 1941.

21. Weddel JM. Surgery in Tunisia: November, 1942 to May, 1943. *British Medical Journal* 1944: 459–62.

22. Harrison M. *Medicine & victory*. Oxford University Press; 2004: 285–86.

23. Churchill ED. The American surgeon. *Surgery, Gynecology and Obstetrics* 1947: **84**: 529–39.

24. Brewer LA, III. The contribution of the 2nd Auxiliary Surgical Group to military surgery during World War II with special references to thoracic surgery. *Annals of Surgery* 1983: **197**: 318–26.

25. Churchill ED. The surgical management of the wounded in the Mediterranean theater at the time at the time of the fall of Rome. *Annals of Surgery* 1944; 120: 268–283.

26. Reister FA. *Battle casualties and medical statistics. US Army experience in the Korean War.* Washington DC: The Surgeon General, Department of the Army; 1977: 55–7.

27. Sako Y, Artz CP, Howard JM, et al. A survey of evacuation, resuscitation and mortality in a foreword surgical hospital. *Surgery* 1955: **37**: 602–11.

28. King B, Jatoi I. The mobile army surgical hospital (MASH): a military and surgical legacy. *Journal of the National Medical Association* 2005: **97**: 648–56.

29. Neel S. *Medical support of the US Army in Vietnam.* Washington DC: Department of the Army; 1973: 59; 65.

30. Byerly WG, Pendse PD. War surgery in a forward surgical hospital in Vietnam: a continuing report. *Military Medicine* 1971: **136**: 221–6.

31. Haacker LP. Time and its effects on casualties in World War II and Vietnam. *Archives of Surgery* 1969: **98**: 39–40.

32. Katoch R, Rajagopalan S. Warfare injuries: history, triage, transport and field hospital setup in the armed forces. *Medical Journal Armed Forces India* 2010: **66**: 304–08.

33. Rozin R, Klausner JM, Dolev E. New concepts of forward combat surgery. *Injury* 1988: **19**: 193–7.

34. Dolev E. Early evacuation of patients from the battlefield after laparotomy: Experiences in Vietnam, Israel and the Falklands. *Military Medicine* 1987: **152**: 57–9.

35. Gasko OD. Surgery in the field during the Lebanon War, 1982: doctrine, experience and prospects for future changes. *Israel Journal of Medical Sciences* 1984: **20**: 350–4.

36. Rozin RR. Integration of military unit and civilian hospital during mass casualty situations: experience during the 1982 Lebanon War. *Military Medicine* 1986: **151**: 580–2.

Caring for Weapon Wounded
The Red Cross Experience from Solferino to the International Committee of the Red Cross Hospitals

Åsa Molde

It all started with the battle of Solferino. In the north of Italy, a fierce battle between the Austrian and French armies took place on June 24, 1859. At least 40 000 dead and wounded were lying around by the end of the day. A Swiss merchant, Henry Dunant, passed by and saw all the suffering and tried to help by tending to the victims. Back home in Geneva, he put his impressions and thoughts to paper in a book called *A Memory of Solferino*[1]. He proposed that volunteers should be trained to take care of the wounded in wartime and that they should be recognized and protected through an international agreement.

The Founding of the International Committee of the Red Cross and the Geneva Conventions

In 1863, Henry Dunant, together with a group of Swiss doctors and lawyers, founded the International Committee of the Red Cross (ICRC). They organized an international conference in Geneva, where it was decided that a distinctive emblem – the red cross on a white background – the reverse of the national Swiss flag, was adopted. The following year, another conference was convened, and the result was the first Geneva convention (GC) of 1864. It states that medical services in armed conflict on land should be protected, and the emblem of the Red Cross should be used as a clearly visible sign on hospitals and ambulances. Wounded and sick should be cared for. These ideas were quickly spread and accepted over the world, and national societies of the Red Cross were created in many countries. It was followed by the second GC, which states the same for victims at sea, the third about protection and assistance to prisoners of war, and the fourth about protection of civilians. They were updated in 1949. Today, 196 countries have signed the first GC.

The ICRC is an impartial, neutral, and independent organization, whose exclusively humanitarian mission is to protect the lives and dignity of victims of armed

conflict and other situations of violence, and to provide them with assistance. The ICRC is the guardian of the GCs, which means it has a role in informing about the conventions and promoting respect for them.

Several examples of the work of a medical doctor as a neutral observer for the ICRC are given in the book by Marcel Junod: *Warrior Without Weapons* (*Le Troisième Combattant*)[2]. He went to Abyssinia in the 1930s and tried to document the attacks by the Italian forces on a Swedish ambulance (a field hospital), which was marked with the Red Cross. Medical staff and patients were killed and wounded, a clear violation of the first GC. He also went to Hiroshima after the atomic bomb and described how most of the civilian population had been wiped out and the incredible suffering of the survivors.

Hospitals Under the Red Cross Emblem

If a country does not have the means to cope with a situation itself, it can ask for help from its sister national societies. This was the case during the Korean War, in which the Swedish Red Cross set up a field hospital to treat the wounded and sick. It existed from 1950 to 1957, even after the cease-fire in 1953. During its first three months, the hospital treated more than 3200 patients, of whom 50% were Americans, 36% North Koreans, and 14% from other nations. Over the years, more than 1000 Swedish doctors and nurses worked there under the flag of the Red Cross, respecting the basic principles of humanity and neutrality[3].

Early Assistance of ICRC

In the 1960s, 1970s, and 1980s, the ICRC sent out single doctors or teams to work in areas of armed conflict where the country itself did not have the means to give proper care. They worked in local hospitals and provided necessary basic equipment and drugs. The team members often came from *one* national society and were sent to places such as

Cambodia and Angola. These could be purely surgical teams, but often also included a general practitioner and obstetrician or midwife. Focus was on weapon wounded, but other emergencies such as car accidents, malaria, and pregnant women needing cesarean sections were sometimes treated.

The ICRC Hospitals

Background

The 1970s and 1980s saw an escalation of armed conflicts in many countries, with limited resources to take care of weapon wounded. To provide better care, the idea of independent hospitals led to the creation of the first ICRC hospital in Thailand on the border to Cambodia in 1979. It existed until 1992, by which time it had treated more than 20 000 wounded from over the border.

Similar hospitals were created in the 1980s in Pakistan for wounded from the conflict in Afghanistan, and in north Kenya for wounded from Sudan and later in Ruanda, Democratic Republic of the Congo, Sierra Leone, Chechnya, and other places. More than 100 000 wounded have been treated in ICRC hospitals.

Setup

ICRC hospitals are owned and run by the ICRC. They are most often needed where a conflict is ongoing for years, so it is a long-term commitment and therefore very costly. The longest running ICRC hospital was in the north of Kenya, in a place called Lokichokio, and existed for 19 years.

Before any action is taken, local authorities must be contacted. Acceptance is essential, and security must be guaranteed, meaning that staff and patients must have safe access and not be attacked. In areas where there are no official authorities, contact is taken to those in charge of the fighting groups to inform them about the role of the ICRC. No arms are allowed in the premises and there are no armed guards. The emblem of the Red Cross on buildings and ambulances, and carried by the staff, is the only protection. However, buildings can also be protected by sandbags and plastic sheeting on the windows.

Contrary to the military, the ICRC is not usually in charge of first aid or transport to the hospital and cannot transfer any patient to another, better-equipped facility. The treatment starts with triage in the admission area of the hospital, and continues with necessary surgery, postoperative care, mobilization, and then discharge when patients have healed. Follow-up is rarely possible.

The treatment is always free of charge. Medical need is the only reasons for admission, meaning that both soldiers and fighters from different groups will be treated, without any discrimination.

The ICRC hospitals are not mobile, but are a fixed structure. The operation theater is usually in a building with a concrete floor and proper walls and roof. Wards, including the so-called intensive care unit, can be in tents. The ICRC organizes basic requirements such as water and electricity and supply of drugs and surgical instruments. No sophisticated technology is used. The laboratory will at least be able to check hemoglobin and hematocrit, but also blood groups. Blood donors can be difficult to find, but all donated blood is tested for syphilis, hepatitis B and C, and HIV. Plain X-ray to show lungs and skeleton is available.

To function as a hospital, support services are needed, such as pharmacy and stores, kitchen, laundry, porters, and guards. The staff is a mixture of expatriates and locally hired staff. Depending on the size of the hospital, there will be several positions responsible for the running of the hospital, such as hospital project manager and head nurse. The expatriate staff comes from many countries, often through a national society. They are volunteer civilians, and have short contracts; for example, three months for doctors, and six months to one year for nurses.

The Work

Originally, only weapon wounded were treated. In the ICRC headquarters in Geneva, standard lists of equipment and drugs were established and most important were the guidelines for treatment[4,5].

To achieve good results, adequate surgery, good nursing care, and physiotherapy are needed. Data collection was possible, and the data bank contains more than 40 000 patients. It has been used in many articles and presentations at international conferences. War surgery seminars have been conducted in Geneva since 1990 to prepare doctors and nurses before their first mission. Nowadays, similar seminars are held around the world for medical staff dealing with weapon wounded.

A large number of expatriate medical staff from different countries pass through these hospitals. Most have not been exposed to weapon wounds before and will learn on the spot how to deal with war wounded. However, many repeatedly return for more missions and can build up their knowledge. Often, there are only one or two surgeons, usually general surgeons, and they must deal with all injuries: head, maxillofacial, chest, abdominal, and limb wounds with fractures. After resuscitation and stopping bleeding, the focus should be on the wounds. Following the basic principles of treating war wounds – good debridement and delayed primary closure – most wounded will heal without complications, even with the limited resources of the ICRC hospital, and mortality rate has been low: 2.2–6.4%[6]. The low mortality rate is partly due to the "natural triage" that takes place for the wounded who cannot reach the hospital because there is no transport and no proper first aid, but is also due to the standardized treatment built on many years of experience.

The focus is on treating weapon wounded in the best way. Gradually, teaching programs have been developed. For example, in some places, there is a senior surgeon who can teach and assist surgeons on their first mission. The teaching and training of local staff has become very important to upgrade their skills and make it easier for them to find a job after the ICRC has left. To run a hospital with many hundreds of beds needs good administration and in this area also, the ICRC has gained a lot of experience[7,8].

The Main Hospitals

In 1987, the fighting in Sudan had increased, and wounded came over the border to Lokichokio in the north of Kenya. Kenyan authorities asked the ICRC for help and it was agreed that the hospital should only treat Sudanese citizens, but employ Kenyan staff.

This hospital existed until 2006 and grew from an initial 40 beds to over 700. It had treated more than 37 000 wounded and performed more than 60 000 operations when it closed due to the end of the conflict in South Sudan. It was a place for training of "first-mission" doctors and nurses who later could be sent to other missions.

In Pakistan, two hospitals were set up to treat wounded from Afghanistan: Peshawar in 1981–1993 and Quetta in 1983–1996. They treated more than 40 000 wounded and were closed because the situation in Afghanistan changed. The ICRC continues to support several hospitals in the north and a big hospital in the south: Kandahar.

In Kabul, the ICRC hospital existed from 1989 to 1992, when it had to restrict the expatriate presence

because of deteriorating security. At the time, there were many hospitals in Kabul, but they mainly took care of wounded from their own ethnic group, while the ICRC hospital was neutral and admitted all weapon wounded who needed treatment.

The ICRC hospital in Novi Atagi, Chechnya, and the new ICRC hospital in Peshawar closed after deadly attacks on expatriate staff (1996 and 2012).

Other Actions

Independent ICRC hospitals were also used, for example in Banda Aceh after the tsunami in the Indian Ocean, and after the earthquake in Muzaffarabad in Pakistan in 2005[9,10]. The knowledge gained during previous years in setting up and running a hospital made it possible to be operational quickly. Tents and material donated by the Norwegian and Finnish Red Cross were used.

Today

Today, the ICRC has no independent hospital, but is supporting more than 400 hospitals in more than 25 countries in different ways: with staff, drugs, equipment, and training. In some places, the ICRC is responsible for some wards in a hospital, which are run like an independent hospital.

Setting up an independent ICRC hospital always requires discussion. This ensures guidelines are followed so the quality of care can be upheld. It also allows staff to be trained efficiently. The difficulties are in finding a place where security can be guaranteed and with enough wounded, and then recognize that it needs long-term engagement to be effective, which also means big costs. However, the ICRC is ready to set up hospitals, transfer knowledge, and use the big pool of devoted volunteer staff with experience of previous missions to take care of weapon wounded, following standards and guidelines that have been developed and tested over many years.

References

1. Dunant H. *A memory of Solferino*. Geneva: International Committee of the Red Cross; 1986. Originally in French: *Un souvenir de Solferino*; 1862.

2. Junod M. *Le troisième combattant*. Geneva: International Committee of the Red Cross; 1947. Reprinted 1989. Translated into English: *Warrior without weapons*; 1982.

3. Kultur (2010). Svenska sjukhuset i Korea – humanitär insats i kriget. Online article (in Swedish). http://www.lakartidningen.se/store/articlepdf/1/15308/LKT1044s2737_2740.pdf

4. Giannou C, Baldan M. *War surgery: working with limited resources in armed conflict and other situations of violence.* Volume 1. Geneva: International Committee of the Red Cross; 2009.

5. Giannou C, Baldan M, Molde A. *War surgery: working with limited resources in armed conflict and other situations of violence.* Volume 2. Geneva: International Committee of the Red Cross; 2013.

6. Coupland RM. Epidemiological approach to surgical management of the casualties of war. *British Medical Journal* 1994: **308**: 1693–1716.

7. Hayward-Karlsson J, Jeffery S, Kerr A, Schmidt H. *Hospitals for war-wounded: a practical guide for setting up and running a surgical hospital in an area of armed conflict.* Geneva: International Committee of the Red Cross; 1998.

8. Hayward-Karlsson J. Hospital and System Assessment, in Mahoney PF, Ryan JM, Brooks AJ, Schwab CW (eds.), *Ballistic trauma: a practical guide 2nd ed.* London: Springer-Verlag; 2005: 513–26.

9. International Committee of the Red Cross. Online article. https://www.icrc.org/en/doc/resources/documents/news-release/2009-and-earlier/6cwm95.htm

10. International Committee of the Red Cross. Online article. https://www.icrc.org/en/doc/resources/documents/news-release/2009-and-earlier/pakistan-news-211005.htm

Chapter

3

Definitions, Needs, Scenarios, Functional Concept, and Modes of Deployment

Maximilian P Nerlander and Johan von Schreeb (corresponding author)

Background

Historically, there has been significant variation in the motivation, type, and quality of international medical teams and field hospitals deployed to natural disasters worldwide. A multiplicity of nations and agencies being involved in a disaster response, each with their own mandate, standards, work habits, and modes of operation, invites inefficiencies and wasteful duplication of work effort. Additionally, shortages of competency-based training for responders may lead to underperformance and medical error[1]. Experiences from the earthquakes in Haiti in 2010 and Pakistan in 2005 propelled an effort from the World Health Organization (WHO) and partners to strive for minimum standards for emergency medical teams (EMTs) responding to disasters, applicable to both domestic and foreign governments/militaries, intergovernmental organizations, and nongovernmental organizations (NGOs). Additionally, these standards are a useful reference for the governments of recipient countries, as well as in-country health providers responding domestically [2]. In this effort, a decision was made to consider field hospitals and the medical personnel staffing them according to the services they provide rather than the physical structure. Thus, the term (foreign) field hospital has been dropped in favor of a system that captures different levels of care. Three levels of foreign medical team (FMT) (types 1–3) were defined in 2013, but in 2015 the term "foreign" was replaced by "emergency" (EMT) to allow a classification system that include both national (N-EMT) and international (I-EMT) categories[3]. Below is a more detailed definition of the type of services each level should include. To register and become a WHO-verified EMT, providers are required to go through a verification process. I-EMTs must adhere to certain minimum standards and modes of operation, according to type of EMT, in order to optimize quality of care, streamline interteam cooperation

and ensure accountability[2]. This is an ongoing effort and, following each new disaster, new aspects are added to ensure the standards are updated and fit to context. The reader is encouraged to refer to the WHO website for the latest version of the standards. EMTs are a surge-capacity function, which may be used to manage excess caseloads of injured and other extra medical care needs during a limited time period. In recent conflicts, this system has been useful to set up care and referral systems close to the frontline. Updated guidance notes for EMTs in conflicts are available from the WHO's website.

Types of EMTs

The classifications of EMTs are based on capability, capacity, and types and level of health-care services offered. Groups of providers that wish to respond to a natural disaster must maintain, or preferably exceed, the minimum standards outlined below. Alternatively, if the team is unable to do so, they should merge with a group providing the required standard in order to deploy. In the coming years, it is likely that only teams verified by WHO will be allowed to enter and practice in affected countries. It is the receiver of the EMTs that define whether EMTs are needed and will be accepted, not the sender. This chapter will focus on I-EMTs and their scope in natural disasters. For deployment to man-made disasters, the same type and levels of standards apply while the operating environment and mandates of the agencies remain very different[4].

Type 1 EMTs

These are limited to daytime outpatient services only, with a minimum capacity of 100 patients per day, and are designed to deal with trauma and other significant health needs. Services include assessment, triage, definitive care for minor trauma, stabilization, and referral as appropriate. Typically, these centers are purely temporary tent- or vehicle-based structures, which can be quickly deployed following a disaster event, preferably within 48 hours. However, it is also possible for these

EMTs to utilize existing structures. Preferably, type 1 EMTs should be able to maintain services on the ground for two to three weeks following the disaster event. Experiences from the 2015 Nepal earthquake highlighted that type 1 EMTs should be either fixed or mobile and thus these subcategories have been added to the registration.

Type 2 EMTs

Groups registering as type 2 EMTs are expected to accept referrals from type 1 EMTs, as well as to provide admission to new patients. Required services include triage, advanced life support, and trauma surgery, as well as inpatient care for nontrauma emergencies. The type 2 EMT is expected to be able to provide basic X-ray services and anesthesia. Obstetric services can be provided either in hospital or by cooperation with a local partner or another EMT. These centers must maintain 24-hour services every day of the week and must have a minimum capacity of 20 inpatient beds and one operating theater with one operating table. The minimum operative capacity is 7 major or 15 minor operations per day. Apart from operational services, type 2 EMTs must also have the resources and expertise necessary to appropriately manage nontrauma emergencies such as infectious and chronic diseases. These EMTs can be composed of either deployable structures or may utilize existing ones as appropriate. Type 2 EMTs are slower to deploy than type 1. While, ideally, type 2 services should be available from the first day, deployment may take days due to the greater logistical burden to provide the required services. An exception to this occurred during the 2014–2015 Ebola outbreak in West Africa, during which the type 2 EMTs had different functions and provided different services, but the concept of different levels of care was useful to streamline protocols and coordination.

Type 3 EMTs

Type 3 EMTs represent the highest level of disaster-related care and are expected to manage patients with complex health needs referred from type 1 and 2 EMTs. These referral centers may employ deployable or permanent structures and are required to provide type 2 services, as well as to provide more complex surgical and intensive care. The minimum capacity is one operating theater and at least two operating tables. For each operating room, there must be a minimum of 20 beds, making for an overall capacity of 40 inpatient beds. The minimum operative capacity is 15 major operations

per day or 30 minor ones. Additionally, the EMT must provide a minimum of four intensive care beds with continuous monitoring and ventilator support. Groups deploying as type 3 EMTs may, on their own accord, invite further specialized resources such as maxillofacial surgery. Similar to type 2, type 3 EMTs may take up to a week to deploy due to the complexity of their services, and should ideally deploy for a minimum of two months.

In addition to the above, the term "specialized cells" refers to groups of specialists in a specific discipline, for example burns care, specialized orthopedic care, rehabilitation, or other areas of competence that may be needed. These always operate out of a type 2 or 3 or local hospital.

The different types of EMTs are to function as surge capacity supporting the existing health system, and must adhere to existing protocols and referral pathways. During the 2010 Haiti earthquake response, international field hospitals acted in isolation without contacts and referrals, which led to suboptimal care. This must be avoided. To coordinate EMTs, a specific emergency medical team coordination cell (EMTCC) is to be set up in the affected country supported by WHO and other EMT partners.

Modes of Deployment

The mode of deployment of I-EMTs is dependent on a wide variety of factors. Comparative studies between disaster areas, as well as analysis of the logistical performance in varying disaster environments, demonstrate that a combination of the predisaster state and vulnerability of the affected area, and the nature of the hazard will heavily influence its postdisaster operations[5–7]. A country with a robust health system and developed infrastructure is likely, due to its inherent lower vulnerability, to be less severely affected, as well as to be in a better position to effectively utilize and integrate international assistance if needed. The challenges faced in the deployment of I-EMTs can be divided into administrative, logistical, and operational. Administrative challenges relate to the host country's ability to effectively receive I-EMTs; this includes issues such as licensing, visas, and permits. Logistical challenges include delivery of deployable structures, medicines, and healthcare materials, which is dependent on functional runways and ports, which may be disrupted due to the disaster. Additionally, different agencies may compete with each other for access to these, as was the case during the 2010 Haiti earthquake[8]. In terms of EMT type and location, the choice of whether to rely on existing structures or deploy temporary ones is affected by quality, location, and integrity of buildings; for example, following an earthquake, structures may remain hazardous[9]. Choices of location are primarily directed by local authorities, but are influenced by the context, accessibility, and security, as well as the nature of the disaster. During the 2015 flood in Freetown, Sierra Leone, which occurred during the Ebola outbreak, a population of 4800 internally displaced persons were housed in camp areas set up in two soccer stadiums. The I-EMTs were located within stadium grounds, which enabled effective Ebola screening practices and the possibility to immediately isolate suspected cases, in addition to providing care to the displaced population[10].

Needs Assessment

For a successful response, it is vital for the I-EMT to understand the needs of the population affected. Is a deployment necessary? What capacities are available? What health-care needs can be expected based on the type of event? What other conditions can be expected that are context-specific and not necessarily a result of the disaster? An effective needs assessment can mitigate discrepancies between needs on the ground and availability of equipment and medicines brought by the I-EMT unit, and is characterized by intense intelligence gathering within the first hours or days post-event. These so-called "remote magnitude assumptions" can, within a few hours, provide sufficient information to guide deployment. Vulnerability of the affected, in combination with the type and severity of the hazard, will provide information about the type and magnitude of assistance that may be needed (see below). However, it should be emphasized that an I-EMT cannot deploy only based on needs. Any I-EMT must ensure that their service is wanted and requested by the affected country. Permission by the host country is needed before deployment. Ideally, this is done by rapidly communicating type, size, and length of deployment of the I-EMT through WHO's EMTCC or other channels such as the virtual onsite operations coordination center (OSOCC).

Once on ground, more detailed information is needed to target and tailor the assistance, and ensure that it is integrated into the existing health system. There is no fixed formula by which to perform a needs assessment, and the method will vary with context. The chief objectives are to determine whether international assistance is required, provide information to direct donor priorities, and to determine a baseline understanding of the disaster by which to compare subsequent outcomes[11]. A variety of methods and sources can be utilized, including local media, liaising with local rescue services who are often first on scene, interviews with key individuals such as community leaders, structured interviews with groups, needs surveys, and structured observation of events[11].

Needs assessments can be challenging in the very early stages of disasters, especially so when communications are affected and local media outlets compromised. Lessons learned from the performance of the Israel Defense Forces (IDF) forward disaster scout teams during 15 overseas responses reveal that the deployment of small teams of highly experienced individuals within a few hours of the disaster has a significant impact on the performance of the subsequent medical response[9]. These teams consist of a logistician, a medical officer[12], communications officer, and an information specialist, and they are tasked with rapid, focused intelligence gathering. In cases of the disaster-affected area being under the authority of a functional government, the team will liaise with local authorities. When this is not the case, such as during the 2010 Haiti earthquake, the team will gather information en route, from other agencies, NGOs, WHO, and local media outlets[9]. Once on ground, they will liaise with national authorities and the UN system. Thanks to the EMT process, a significant number of governments in disaster-prone areas now have the capacity to assess the need for an I-EMT and, if needed, request and coordinate incoming EMTs. The era of self-deploying teams should be over.

Health Needs in Disasters

The well-established epidemiological model of morbidity and mortality being determined by the agent, host, and environment is applicable to disasters as well. Thus, the health needs that I-EMTs are likely to encounter vary with type of disaster, the socioeconomic and material vulnerability of the affected area, and geographical region[13].

Understanding the likely epidemiology of the days, weeks, and months following different types of disasters is key to planning for appropriate health-care provision. For example, during the IDF I-EMTs' response to the Nepal earthquake, where the country's infrastructure had largely been spared, there was a fairly high burden of nontrauma cases early in the aftermath, which went on to outnumber trauma cases during weeks 4–11 post-event.

The type of disaster has a substantial effect both on mortality and on the medical needs that a deploying I-EMT needs to prepare for. Adverse health events can be divided into those that occur as a direct consequence of the disaster, and those occurring indirectly. Direct consequences occur as a result of environmental forces – such as tremors, wind, or rain – or as a result of the consequences of these forces, such as structural collapse and flying debris[14]. By contrast, indirect consequences can occur as a result of the disaster, leading to disruption of usual societal functions, such as transportation, environmental protection, medical care, health programs, and police, fire, and rescue services. Furthermore, indirect consequences also include displacement, damage to property, and personal loss[14]. The epidemiological community makes a chief distinction between earthquakes and nonearthquakes, such as floods, droughts, and storms[15]. In the case of earthquakes, trauma cases predominate in the immediate aftermath and may then be replaced by nontrauma orthopedic and medical needs[13,16,17]. Data from the Brussels-based Center for Research on the Epidemiology of Disasters suggest that the ratio of injured to dead in an earthquake is about 4:1, while in tsunamis the corresponding figure is 1:9. Thus, the need for trauma surgeons after a tsunami is very limited[18]. In the event of nonearthquake disasters, I-EMTs can expect to manage more medical cases. For example, while the direct consequences of a flood potentially cause significant loss of life, flooding events rarely account for a substantial burden of nonlethal injury. However, the indirect consequences that occur as a result of disrupted infrastructure and displacement may result in substantial increases in medical needs [15]. Droughts by nature are not disasters that disrupt infrastructure through environmental kinetic force and thus do not produce trauma casualties. Instead, direct consequences of drought events account for an increased burden of malnutrition and dehydration. Additionally, the indirect effects of droughts may in the longer term produce increases in infectious disease outbreaks, and outbreaks of sexually transmitted diseases, as well as interpersonal violence as large populations are forced to migrate and live in camps[19,20]. Some disasters are in themselves unique and can have knock-on effects on the health system of the affected region. An example is the 2014–2015 Ebola epidemic in West Africa. While constituting an infectious disease outbreak, the magnitude of this event in terms of mortality, morbidity, geographical expanse, and societal consequences certainly mirrors the consequences of more common disasters, with a presence of I-EMTs assisting in managing cases and performing contact tracing and isolation of suspected cases. The three countries chiefly affected by the Ebola outbreak – Guinea, Sierra Leone, and Liberia – had fragile health systems pre-event with substantial unmet health needs. The resource demands posed by the Ebola outbreak thus created substantial strain on staff, hospital beds, lab capacity, ambulance services, and pharmaceuticals. As a consequence, the provision of preventive measures and health care for non-Ebola conditions was negatively affected, such as a significant drop in provision of surgery and maternal health services, as well as other essential health services[21,22]. The 2014–2015 and 2018 Ebola outbreaks in Africa have also been unique in terms of the demands they placed on length of engagement. The international response to the crisis needed to last years rather than the weeks-to-months commitment that is commonplace for more conventional disasters. The temporal scale of the outbreak created its own unique health phenomena; as schools were closed to contain the outbreak, more young people came to stay at home in their villages, which led to increases in children born. Additionally, due to reports of doctors, nurses, and patients being infected with Ebola, individuals refrained from seeking health care in hospitals out of concern of being infected.

Apart from managing the new health needs of the population post-event, I-EMTs must also be prepared to manage baseline conditions prevalent in the affected area pre-event. The level of economic development plays a substantial role in determining these health needs as this affects the overall health status of the predisaster population[23]. The far-reaching consequences of disasters – including disruption of health systems, infrastructure, loss of livelihood, homelessness, disruption to ecosystems, social dislocation, and economic consequences – disproportionally affect developing nations[15]. Thus, in contexts such as low-income countries with rudimentary health systems being affected by a disaster, apart from the burden of trauma patients seen initially, I-EMTs will also need to prepare for managing infectious diseases as there will be a high baseline prevalence of these affecting the population. In addition, the burden of noncommunicable diseases (NCDs) must be addressed. As the world moves toward greater economic development, baseline rates of NCDs such as diabetes and heart failure increase, chiefly so in middle-income countries[24,25]. Following a disaster and subsequent disruption of the health infrastructure, these chronic health needs may be unmet and thus need to be anticipated by a deploying I-EMT.

Role of I-EMTs in the Health System

I-EMTs deploying to a disaster-affected area rarely, if ever, function in isolation, and the quality of inter-action between the I-EMT and the health system of the host country, as well as with other EMTs, can have a substantial impact on the success or failure of the effort. The 2013 WHO EMT standards are part of an effort to streamline this cooperation, and this work is continuously developing, with more infor-mation and tools available for I-EMTs that have ambitions and capacities to deploy. They are expected to formalize their activities by registering with the EMT secretariat at WHO and follow an online-based system to demonstrate capacities and report activities.

IDF experiences from the Philippines during the response to Typhoon Haiyan (locally known as Yolanda) in 2013 found that integrating a military I-EMT with local civilian health-care resources was highly beneficial to a variety of outcomes. While accustomed to operating autonomously in areas with no health system in place, the IDF I-EMT adapted a modified approach and opted for a model of "fully integrative collaboration[26]". This ensured that deployable structures were set up in conjunction to the structures of the existing health facility in the area. Furthermore, a protocol was developed, which facili-tated shared use and control of IDF health-care assets, combined team ward rounds, and clarified differences in roles and responsibilities. This enabled the com-bined health-care unit to deliver care to more than 2600 patients over a 10-day period, facilitated capacity building of the local health-care facility, and stream-lined the I-EMT's exit by enabling effective handover of patient care to the local health-care providers and a smaller incoming international medical group[26]. Similar collaboration between EMTs and the local health-care providers during the 2008 Wenchuan earthquake relief found comparable results, where integrating internationally deployed specialists with local medical teams in existing health-care structures served to optimize patient care[27]. In conflicts, it is essential that military-civilian EMT collaboration

does not compromise humanitarian principles among the latter. (www.icrc.org/en/war-and-law)

Quality and Accountability

Historically, there has been no formalized framework addressing the issue of quality control, record keeping, and accountability to which EMTs must adhere; rather, each organization providing EMTs had its own inter-nal mechanisms and policies to do so[11]. A 2015 literature review on medical record keeping by EMTs deploying to disasters revealed there is significant heterogeneity in documentation practices. This in turn has implications for accountability, appropriate follow-up of patients, and interfacility referral[28]. It can be speculated that, as medicolegal requirements evolve in national health-care systems, and these sub-sequently influence medical training and practice, this may also be reflected in the behavior and attitudes, as well as record keeping practices, of physicians and other health-care professionals deploying for I-EMTs.

The WHO minimum standards for I-EMTs pro-vide a standard of accountability, which teams must adhere to in order to register and be a verified I-EMT. These include requirements to provide needs-based, equitable, and patient-centered care. Moreover, I-EMTs are expected to be accountable to the patients they serve, as well as the national host government and international donors[2]. The ethics component of the WHO standards is based on the World Medical Association (WMA) Medical Ethics Manual, and includes special considerations in times of disasters when the resources are limited, as well as aspects such as patient confidentiality and the need for informed consent whenever possible[29].

Many other efforts have been made to provide minimum standards to guide best practice in disaster response. The health-cluster approach was established by the United Nations (UN)-based Inter-Agency Standing Committee (IASC), and aimed to provide a framework for cooperation between national systems providing disaster relief to achieve agreed objectives and minimize service gaps[3,30]. The high cholera-related mortality in the refugee population of Goma in the Democratic Republic of the Congo following the 1994 Rwandan genocide prompted the Sphere project: a response to ascertain minimum standards in a number of key areas of disaster relief. Apart from health care, these include water, sanitation, nutrition, food, aid, and shelter[31]. The Sphere standards also include best practices at policy level: standards stipulate Ministry of Health (MoH) leadership whenever possible, regular coordination meetings within the health sector, documentation of responsibilities, creation of specific working groups on health-care issues, and the production of regular bulletins[31]. A recent systematic review of published material relating to disaster response revealed that, between the cluster approach, the Sphere standards, and a number of other standards, the cluster approach was most commonly employed, and the authors stipulate that, likely, this is due to the higher visibility of the UN[30].

Summary

In summary, following a disaster any I-EMTs should rapidly estimate type and magnitude of needs and based on this offer their services to the affected country. They should not deploy without an invitation from the host country. Deployments to international disaster zones face a range of challenges, some of which are common between different events, and some which are event-specific. An understanding of in-country health profiles, and the likely epidemiology of the event in question is key to successful outcomes. EMTs must be aware of and adhere to the WHO minimum standards through a registration-verification process to facilitate quality patient care, conducted in a clear framework of responsibility, accountability, and effective cooperation with other local and national responders.

References

1. Djalali A, Ingrassia PL, Della Corte F, et al. Identifying deficiencies in national and foreign medical team responses through expert opinion surveys: implications for education and training. *Prehospital and Disaster Medicine* 2014: **29**(4): 364–8.

2. Norton I, von Schreeb J, Aitken P, Herard P, Lajolo C. *Classification and minimum standards for foreign medical teams in sudden onset disasters*. Geneva: World Health Organization; 2013.

3. World Health Organization/Pan American Health Organization. Proceedings of the WHO/PAHO technical consultation on foreign medical teams (FMTs) post sudden onset disasters (SODs). 2010.

4. Michaud J, Moss K, Licina D, et al. Militaries and global health: peace, conflict, and disaster response. *The Lancet* 2019: **393**(10168): 276–86.

5. Chang SE, Nojima N. Measuring post-disaster transportation system performance: the 1995 Kobe earthquake in comparative perspective. *Transportation Research Part A: Policy and Practice* 2001: **35**(6): 475–94.

6. Holguín-Veras J, Jaller M, Van Wassenhove LN, Pérez N, Wachtendorf T. On the unique features of post-disaster humanitarian logistics. *Journal of Operations Management* 2012: **30**(7): 494–506.

7. Achour N, Miyajima M, Kitaura M, Price A. Earthquake-induced structural and nonstructural damage in hospitals. *Earthquake Spectra* 2011: **27**(3): 617–34.

8. Jobe K. Disaster relief in post-earthquake Haiti: unintended consequences of humanitarian volunteerism. *Travel Medicine and Infectious Disease* 2011: **9**(1): 1–5.

9. Tarif B, Merin O, Dagan D, Yitzhak A. Planning the unplanned: the role of a forward scout team in disaster areas. *International Journal of Disaster Risk Reduction* 2016: **19**: 25–8.

10. United Nations Office for the Coordination of Humanitarian Affairs. OCHA flash update no. 2, Sierra Leone, flooding in Freetown. 2015.

11. von Schreeb J. *Needs assessments for international humanitarian health assistance in disasters*. Institutionen för folkhälsovetenskap/Department of Public Health Sciences; 2007.

12. Logue JN, Melick ME, Hansen H. Research issues and directions in the epidemiology of health effects of disasters. *Epidemiologic Reviews* 1981: **3**: 140–62.

13. Ramirez M, Peek-Asa C. Epidemiology of traumatic injuries from earthquakes. *Epidemiologic Reviews* 2005: **27**: 47–55.

14. Combs DL, Quenemoen LE, Parrish RG, Davis JH. Assessing disaster-attributed mortality: development and application of a definition and classification matrix. *International Journal of Epidemiology* 1999: **28**(6): 1124–9.

15. Seaman J. Disaster epidemiology: or why most international disaster relief is ineffective. *Injury* 1990: **21**(1): 5–8.

16. Alexander D. The health effects of earthquakes in the mid-1990s. *Disasters*. 1996: **20**(3): 231–47.

17. Macintyre AG, Barbera JA, Smith ER. Surviving collapsed structure entrapment after earthquakes: a "time-to-rescue" analysis. *Prehospital and Disaster Medicine* 2006: **21**(1): 4–17; discussion 8–9.

18. Bartholdson S, von Schreeb J. Natural disasters and injuries: what does a surgeon need to know? *Current Trauma Reports* 2018: 1–6.

19. Hendrickson D, Armon J, Mearns R. The changing nature of conflict and famine vulnerability: the case of livestock raiding in Turkana District, Kenya. *Disasters* 1998: **22**(3): 185–99.

20. Parenti C. *Tropic of chaos: climate change and the new geography of violence*. New York: Nation Books; 2012.

21. Brolin Ribacke KJ, Saulnier DD, Eriksson A, von Schreeb J. Effects of the West Africa Ebola virus disease on health-care utilization – a systematic review. *Frontiers in Public Health*. 2016: **4**: 222.

22. Bolkan HA, Bash-Taqi DA, Samai M, Gerdin M, von Schreeb J. Ebola and indirect effects on health service function in Sierra Leone. *PLOS Currents*. 2014: **6**.

23. United Nations Development Programme, Bureau for Crisis Prevention and Recovery. *Reducing disaster risk: a challenge for development – a global report*. United Nations; 2004.

24. Frenk J, Bobadilla JL, Sepuúlveda J, Cervantes ML. Health transition in middle-income countries: new challenges for health care. *Health Policy and Planning* 1989: **4**(1): 29–39.

25. Abegunde DO, Mathers CD, Adam T, Ortegon M, Strong K. The burden and costs of chronic diseases in low-income and middle-income countries. *The Lancet* 2007: **370**(9603): 1929–38.

26. Merin O, Kreiss Y, Lin G, Pras E, Dagan D. Collaboration in response to disaster – Typhoon Yolanda and an integrative model. *The New England Journal of Medicine* 2014: **370**(13): 1183.

27. Jiang H, Dai XZ. Analysis of the rescue patterns and procedures of foreign medical teams following the Wenchuan earthquake. *Journal of Evidence-Based Medicine* 2009: **2**(2): 122–7.

28. Jafar AJ, Norton I, Lecky F, Redmond AD. A literature review of medical record keeping by foreign medical teams in sudden onset disasters. *Prehospital and Disaster Medicine* 2015: **30**(2): 216–22.

29. Momoh P. World Medical Association. *Medical ethics manual*. 2006.

30. Lotfi T, Bou-Karroum L, Darzi A, et al. Coordinating the provision of health services in humanitarian crises: a systematic review of suggested models. *PLOS Currents* 2016: **8**.

31. Gostelow L. The Sphere project: the implications of making humanitarian principles and codes work. *Disasters* 1999: **23**(4): 316–25.

Needs Assessment

Forecasting the Needs and Improving the Immediate Medical Response in Complex Emergencies

Olivier Hagon, Lionel Dumont, and Jean-Daniel Junod

Background

In the urgency of a disaster's aftermath, the general tendency is to "reinvent the wheel." As soon as an emergency is declared, health professionals and others, used to working under regular conditions in their home countries, experience the urge to fly over, aiming to provide care to the victims of the disaster. These actors' heightened state of motivation and excitation related to the disaster often overshadows any doubts they may have about their competence for working in such kind of environment. The typical mistake is to perform medicine "as usual" in a totally disrupted setting. As such, there is frequently confusion between practicing emergency medicine and the specific expertise needed during a disaster's aftermath. In other words, the relationship between emergency and disaster medicine is not really taken into consideration.

The foreign medical team/emergency medical team (FMT/EMT) initiative has started to elaborate on the minimum standards and provide a classification system in disaster settings[1]. Starting with surgery, it has now been extended to other medical fields such as noncommunicable diseases (NCDs), communicable diseases (CDs), and rehabilitation.

The purpose of this chapter is to provide an overview of this changing approach to addressing the health needs during the different phases of a complex emergency. Such an understanding is essential to improve the planning of the required human and material resources, and to ensure their delivery at the appropriate time and place.

Complex Emergency

From a medical perspective, there are several definitions and approaches for regular emergencies (e.g., a myocardial infarct), mass-casualty incidents (MCIs) (e.g., a train crash), and wide-scale disasters (e.g.,

a Haiti earthquake)[2–5]. Each of these categories requires a specific health response.

Increasingly, this kind of situation is being categorized as "complex emergencies." The International Federation of Red Cross and Red Crescent Societies (IFRC) has proposed a definition of complex emergencies, which includes not only a medical but also a sociological perspective[6]. Complex emergencies may be associated not only with the loss of lives, but with widespread violence, displacement of populations, large-scale damage to property and infrastructure, disruptions to societies and economies, hindrance or prevention of humanitarian assistance by political and military constraints, and significant security risks for humanitarian relief workers; all these call for large-scale, multifaceted humanitarian assistance. Moreover, complex emergencies may occur in several different geographical entities (national, international, cross border, and natural contexts) and also have obvious medium-term impacts, not only on the health sector but also on water and food supplies, and may result in economic collapse, social and political instability, and a refugee crisis.

Effect of Natural Disasters

Table 4.1 lists the magnitude of effects that natural disasters have on outcomes such as death, injuries, water and food shortages, and major population movements. Earthquakes cause many deaths, but also injuries, whereas tsunamis, flash floods, and landslides predominantly kill.

In addition, the presence of hazardous materials; chemical, biological, radiological and nuclear (CBRN) substances; and biological or chemical weapons (in armed conflict) will jeopardize the situation. For instance, the nuclear accident in Fukushima that followed the tsunami – itself caused by a heavy, but offshore earthquake – presented significant additional challenges to the aid response.

Table 4.1 Magnitude of effects from natural disasters

Effect	Earthquakes	Tropical storms	Tsunamis	Slow-onset floods	Landlines	Volcanoes/ Lahars
Deaths	+++	+	+++	+	+++	+++
Severe injuries	+++	++	+	+	+	+
Risk of communicable diseases	Potential risk following all major disasters (Probably rising with overcrowding and deteriorating sanitation)					
Damage to health facitlites	+++ Structure/ equipment	+++	+++ Localized	+++ Equipment only	+++ Localized	+++ Structure/ equipment
Damage to water systems	+++	+	+++	+	+++ Localized	+++
Food shortage	Rare (Economic and logistic factors)		Common		Rare	
Major population movement	Rare (Heavily damaged urban areas)		Common (Generally limited)			

Adapted from Pan American Health Organization (PAHO), Natural Disaster[7]

From a medical perspective, the damage to local health facilities depends on the area that is affected. With a tsunami, the inundated seaboard is relatively narrow. Therefore, the surface that is devastated may not be immense, even though many may have perished. With landslides, the affected surface is again limited due to the geology of the phenomenon. Obviously, different topographies (flat land, hills, mountains; mud or rock streams) result in different areas being affected. Depending on the characteristics of all these complex emergencies, multiple and different specific responses need to be organized.

The Immediate Medical Response in Complex Emergencies

Several factors influence how the immediate medical response to complex emergencies can be optimized. All these parameters should be known and integrated in the decision-making process of EMT deployment.

Type of Disaster

As mentioned previously, different disasters require different types of health (and other) care. For example, surgical support is more important after an earthquake than in a tsunami setting (e.g., the Haiti earthquake in 2010 versus the Indian Ocean tsunami in 2004). Slow-onset floods require support for health facilities and water supply rather than surgical assistance (for instance, Hurricane Harvey in Houston, USA, in 2017).

Phases of a Disaster

Following an earthquake, the first priority is search and rescue, followed by emergency relief, early recovery, medium- to long-term recovery, and finally, the community development (Figure 4.1)[8]. Similar outlines can be made for other types of disaster, but beyond broad classification, each is a unique event, which requires careful assessment for how, when, and what help is required. In practice, the stages of recovery do not always follow a neatly defined course or timing.

Geographical, Sociological, and Demographic Characteristics

Obviously, the outcomes of similar natural disasters are vastly different when they strike places such as Port-au-Prince (Haiti), Kathmandu (Nepal), or Fukushima (Japan). The geography, building codes and how they are enforced, economic prosperity (and being part of a larger state that provides support), demographics of the affected area, and many other factors are key determinants to anticipate the health needs.

General information, such as a country's health profile[9], can be found on the World Health Organization (WHO) website. These list life expectancy, the under-5 mortality rate, the proportion younger than 15, the maternal mortality rate, and the population over 60, which are all important and extremely relevant indicators.

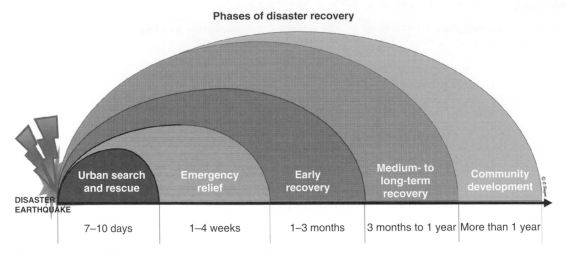

Figure 4.1 Timing of disaster responses following an earthquake

As an example, Table 4.2 lists basic health data for four countries that were hit by a complex emergency: Haiti (earthquake), Liberia (Ebola outbreak), Indonesia (earthquake), and Japan (earthquake, tsunami, and nuclear incident). The case of the Ebola outbreak is unusual. This was a pandemic with a slow onset compared to the others, which were sudden-onset disasters (SODs).

In addition, countries can be classified by their economic development using the World Bank criteria (fiscal year 2018)[10]:

- Low-income country: defined as countries whose gross national income (GNI) per capita is less than USD 1025.
- Lower middle-income economies: countries with a per capita GNI between USD 1026 and USD 3995.
- Upper middle-income economies: countries with a per capita GNI between USD 3996 and USD 12 375.
- High-income economies: countries with a per capita GNI above USD 12 376.

The data thus gathered on the characteristics of the affected population will help the EMT to anticipate the needs (pediatric versus adult or both, surgery versus medical approach, pediatrics and obstetrics needs, and risks for CDs and NCDs).

Again, this needs to be done on a case-by-case basis; for instance, Dumont and colleagues[11] argued that, during the acute phase of the earthquake in Nepal, the need to treat anemia with transfusion was probably overestimated, since the background prevalence of anemia was high[12].

Safety and Security

Even if violence and insecurity worsen in the aftermath of a catastrophe, it remains essential to make a clear distinction between armed conflict and other types of violence that may hamper aid in complex emergencies.

During a complex emergency, desperate victims may resort to violence simply in an effort to survive. Looting of supermarkets or houses is the most commonly encountered situation. Fights and riots are frequent in the case of distribution of food, water, nonfood items, and other support.

During an armed conflict, security becomes a major concern of aid workers. Bombing, shelling, landmines, and terrorist attacks can all present risks for EMT staff members; at the very least, they severely enhance stress levels. Encounters with regular troops, rebels, or child soldiers carrying weapons are all situations that require appropriate behavior from EMT staff members. Support and training from security officers can decrease the risk of major security incidents.

To some extent, armed conflicts *are* complex emergencies, whereas the reverse is usually not the case. In short: *every armed conflict is a complex emergency, but not every complex emergency is an armed conflict!*

Every EMT that is to be deployed in an armed conflict zone must attend to its safety and undergo security training. Importantly, these precautions must be adapted to each specific kind of environment.

Such competences must be acquired and require time to reach adapted standards to ensure the safety and security of the victims, as well as EMT staff

Table 4.2 Baseline comparison between four different countries affected by complex emergencies

Country	Haiti (2010)	Liberia (2014–2015)	Indonesia (2013)	Japan (2013)
General population (thousands)	10 317	4294	249 866	127 144
Population under 15 years (%)	35	43	29	13
Population over 60 years (%)	7	5	8	32
Life expectancy (years)	62 (2012)	62 (2012)	71 (2012)	84 (2012)
Under-5 mortality (per 1000 live births)	73 (2012)	71 (2012)	29 (2012)	3 (2012)
Maternal mortality (per 100 000 live births)	380 (2012)	640 (2012)	190 (2012)	6 (2012)
Total fertility rate (no. of children per woman)	3.1	4.8	2.3	1.4
Five leading causes of death (among the top 10 causes)	1. Stroke (12%) 2. Lower respiratory infections (8.6%) 3. HIV/AIDS (8.3%) 4. Ischemic heart disease (6.3%) 5. Diarrheal diseases (5.1%)	1. Lower respiratory infections (12.2%) 2. Malaria (8.4%) 3. Tuberculosis (5.6%) 4. HIV/AIDS (5.6%) 5. Stroke (5.3%)	1. Stroke (21.2%) 2. Ischemic heart disease (8.9%) 3. Diabetes mellitus (6.5%) 4. Lower respiratory infections (5.2%) 5. Tuberculosis (4.3%)	1. Lower respiratory infections (10.6%) 2. Stroke (10.1%) 3. Ischemic heart disease (8.6%) 4. Trachea, bronchus, and lung cancers (6%) 5. Stomach cancer (4.3%)
World Bank income classification	Low	Low	Low-middle	High

Source: WHO country health profiles [9]

members (whether they operate in a national or international context).

Evolution of Health Needs during a Disaster

"Ideally," a disaster happens in a civilian society with a functioning health system, which will continue to function after the event. The medical need following such a disaster can be divided into several phases, each with distinct specific medical needs (Figure 4.2).

For most SODs, the first wave of victims presents with trauma[13]. Subsequently, nontrauma cases will present themselves at the local hospital or the EMTs for care. An important indicator is the (decreasing) ratio between the number of surgical and nontrauma (medical) cases. Depending on the

type, size, and intensity of the disaster, as well as the local health-care capacity, these two categories usually even out between 7 and 14 days[14,15]. Beyond this broad division, we have observed additional very specific needs during the different phases of a disaster. Consequently, the nature of support (human and material resources) must be continually adapted[16].

For a number of medical interventions, we have tried to trace their needs over time after a disaster, along with the resources that are required to address them (Figure 4.3, Figure 4.4, and Figure 4.5). In the figures, the time points where resources no longer match the needs are indicated, suggesting when action is required to improve the quality of health care for the affected population.

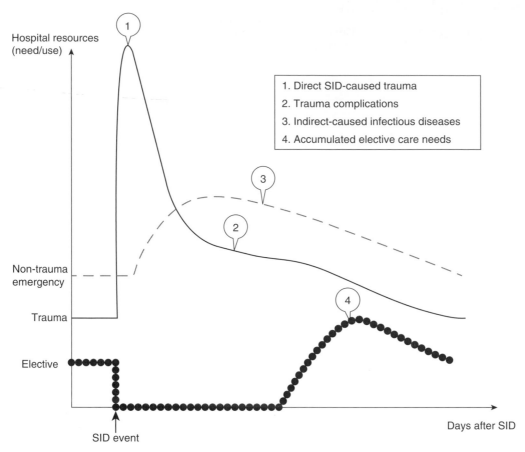

1. Direct SID-caused trauma
2. Trauma complications
3. Indirect-caused infectious diseases
4. Accumulated elective care needs

Figure 4.2 Response magnitude and timing following a generic sudden-impact disaster (SID)[13]

The timescales used in these graphs present a challenge because the same earthquake will differently impact places such as Port-au-Prince (Haiti), Kathmandu (Nepal), or Christchurch (New Zealand), not only qualitatively but also in timing. At least three factors may influence the timeline: the type and scale of disaster, the local capacity for support, and access to the health facilities (being local hospitals or EMT), which may be restricted for various reasons (security, road damage, or remoteness).

In our conceptual scenarios, we decided to take the earthquake as a reference event. As shown in Table 4.2, different types of disaster will have different consequences, which have to be taken into consideration in prospectively constructing a timeline, as well as the anticipated type of pathologies. For instance, during the acute phase of an earthquake, priority is given to emergency surgery, and the resources are adapted according to its needs. Nevertheless, due to the number of patients put on hold due to the disaster, elective surgery would have to restart as soon as possible. This restart is, however, obstructed by the high number of original patients who need complex postoperative care.

In most disaster-prone countries, the fertility rate is more than two children per woman, and as much as one-third of the population is under 15 years old, although there are, obviously, some exceptions[9]. During the disaster aftermath, obstetrical activity remains constant. However, due to the major stress caused by the disaster context, there is an increasing number of premature deliveries in the initial phase[17,18]. Obstetrical personnel (midwives, nurses, and gyneco-obstetricians, if present at all) are usually involved in emergency cases – particularly those requiring surgery – and are thus less available for pregnant women.

Over time, the number of cases with NCDs increases. These include not only adults but also children. From the onset of the acute phase of the disaster, long-term patients suffering with chronic diseases remain in need of care. These include, for instance,

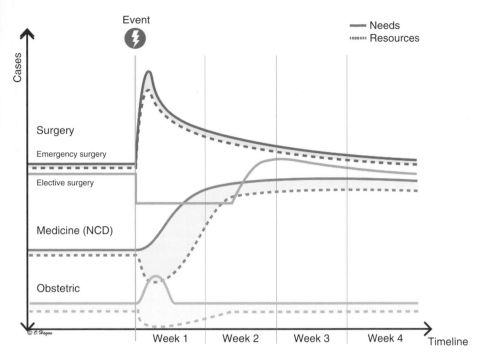

Figure 4.3 Cases that require surgery, obstetric help, or medicines just prior to an earthquake (the event) and thereafter (the needs), and the available health-care capacity (resources)[16]

diabetic patients who need insulin, those with hypertension, and patients with chronic obstructive pulmonary disease. The collapse of the usual facilities (pharmacies, hospitals, and health centers) and the rupture of the cold chain (or the supply chain altogether) will block access to medicines for these patients.

Figure 4.3 shows how emergency surgery decreases following the initial peak of the acute phase, while the need for medicines will progressively increase to reach a steady state at a level much higher than the predisaster baseline. The obstetric needs will acutely increase after the event, but quickly return to normal.

In any circumstances, we may assume that the overall health needs will increase not only due to the increase of new pathologies related to the event but also because of a decrease or even total breakdown of the preexisting capacities of local health structures (including materials, humans, and infrastructure in general).

It is not unusual to see an outbreak of waterborne and other infectious diseases during the acute phase of a disaster. In addition, injuries (wounds and complicated fractures) increase the risk of infection. Their effective treatment is hampered by a lack of antibiotics and other medications, in addition to the rupture of the

cold chain. During the initial phase of the disaster, it is therefore important to immediately update vaccinations for measles, for instance, to avoid a potential outbreak in the near future. And the maintenance of efficient wastewater treatment systems or adequate supplies of drinking water from elsewhere can decrease the risk of outbreak of waterborne diseases.

The deadly consequences of a breakdown of local infrastructure – in this case, sanitation – was dramatically illustrated following the 2010 Haiti earthquake. A UN peacekeeping unit introduced cholera; a disease that was not previously found on the island. By 2015, over 9000 Haitians had died from the disease.

Mental health care mostly involves two indications: one acute (directly related to the disaster) and one chronic (indirectly related to the disaster). Obviously, the victims who were directly affected by the disaster are traumatized and often suffer from acute stress disorder. It is frequently reported that the mental distress persists in the population for a long period: months, and even years[19,20].

The patients who suffer from chronic psychiatric pathologies such as depression and psychosis, as well as patients who are mentally disabled, are in a similar situation to those with NCDs. In addition, the general

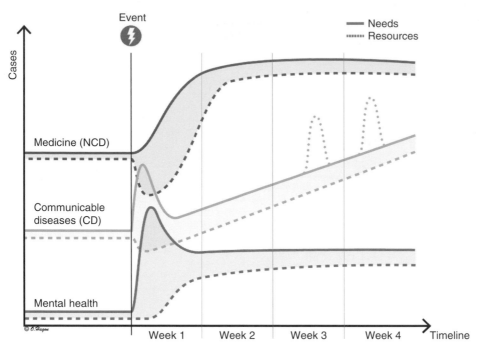

Figure 4.4 Cases that require care for NCD, CD, and mental health just prior to an earthquake (the event) and thereafter (the needs), and the available health-care capacity (resources)[16]

lack of interest of the major part of the EMT or other organizations aggravates the situation.

Figure 4.4 combines cases that require care for NCD, CD, or mental health.

With the large number of patients who have limb injuries, the needs of rehabilitation have to be taken into account from the beginning (and combined with other types of cases in Figure 4.5). Currently, there is only one EMT specialized in this discipline. The minimum standards were published in 2016 and can provide good support[21,22].

During the acute phase, as mentioned previously, the priority is on procuring lifesaving treatments and emergency surgery. At a subsequent stage, the patients who were operated on will require postoperative care, but also various types of rehabilitation support. This will include orthosis, prosthesis fitting, and physiotherapy. The required resources (personnel and material) are very often unavailable or, if present, are "cannibalized" by the emergencies. The challenge is to initiate rehabilitation as soon as possible, using all the different methods. Starting their mobilization during the early period will increase the probability of a successful outcome[23–26].

In summary, the dynamics of the type of changing medical need following a disaster can be described by an initial wave of emergency surgery, which is immediately followed by sustained rehabilitation. After the initial crisis, the backlog of elective surgery is also dealt with. Obstetrics requires immediate attention, but will then return to base levels. Care for CDs and mental-health disorders requires, after an immediate surge, steadily increasing (especially in case of outbreaks) and sustained support, respectively. NCDs (ensuring medicinal supplies) require enhanced attention after the surges in surgery and obstetric care have waned.

Competencies of the EMT

National Versus International Teams
Generally speaking, national capabilities have significantly expanded in a large number of disaster-prone countries. The shift in the name from "foreign" to "emergency" medical team was made to include national as well as international teams. Beyond a simple name shift, this strongly highlights the importance of the local capabilities. The shared culture, language, and customs are

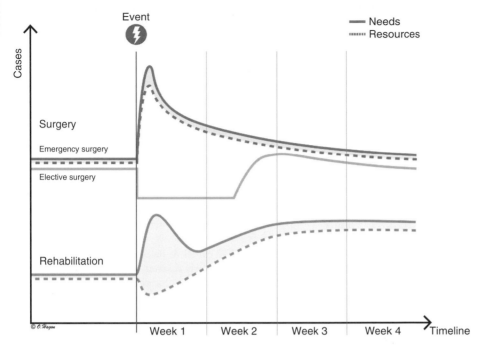

Figure 4.5 Cases that require the combined treatment (surgery and rehabilitation) just prior to an earthquake (the event) and thereafter (the needs), and the available health-care capacity (resources)[16]

all factors that can make a huge difference. Moreover, the national teams usually apply the country's internal minimum standards.

At the next level, regional solidarity – often with common references – facilitates the provision of support from neighboring countries. Their geographic proximity will also decrease the delay of deployment and increase the capacity for lifesaving operations.

Skills

Within the EMT classification process, the core standard WHO "training and skill mix" takes the following points into account[27–29]:

- All staff are specialists in their field.
- Clinical personnel is appropriately trained and experienced in disaster health-care management and in providing care in austere environments.
- Members acknowledge the need to train and provide experience to new staff; scope for junior and inexperienced staff working under direct supervision of experienced colleagues (in the later phase of a disaster response).

- The profile and job descriptions must be defined with minimum skill requirements.
- The composition of the team must have suitable skill mix ratios.
- A training curriculum and continuum is implemented with identified learning objectives, outcomes, and evaluation.

In addition, all staff must be physically and psychologically fit to be deployed, and special attention must be given to the gender balance.

Legitimacy and Regulation

Even though deployment takes place after a disaster, every EMT member must follow the national regulations. It is important to emphasize that the team's ultimate legitimacy is under the national authorities of the affected country. Part of the mandatory conditions that must be fulfilled by each EMT refers to the national regulations.

It is mandatory that EMTs adhere to professional guidelines; for instance, their staff must be registered to practice in their home country and have the license to practice for the work they are assigned to by the agency.

Based on the official documents provided by the EMT, the MoH, supported by the emergency medical team coordination cell (EMTCC), will facilitate the delivery of a temporary license to practice.

Summary

Complex emergencies raise several challenges for the EMT, such as safety and security, as well as the ability to adapt their capabilities to the type of disaster and to the geographical and socioeconomic profile of the affected area. In addition, continuous adaptation to the needs throughout the different phases of a disaster's aftermath is a key condition for an adequate and reliable response from the EMT. Finally, we insist on the fact that strict adherence to the national regulations of the affected country is essential.

References

1. Norton I, von Schreeb J, Aitken P, Herard P, Lajolo C. *Classification and minimum standards for foreign medical teams in sudden onset disasters.* Geneva: World Health Organization; 2013.

2. Schneider SM, Hamilton GC, Moyer P, et al. Definition of emergency medicine. *Academic Emergency Medicine* 1998: **5**(4): 348–51.

3. Below R, Wirtz A, Guha-Sapir D. Disaster category classification and peril terminology for operational purposes.; 2009.

4. Lerner EB, McKee CH, Cady CE, et al. A consensus-based gold standard for the evaluation of mass casualty triage systems. *Prehospital Emergency Care* 2014: **19**(2): 267–71.

5. The International Federation of Red Cross and Red Crescent Societies. What is a disaster? Online article. http://www.ifrc.org/en/what-we-do/disaster-management/about-disasters/what-is-a-disaster

6. The International Federation of Red Cross and Red Crescent Societies. Complex/manmade hazards: complex emergencies. Online article. http://www.ifrc.org/en/what-we-do/disaster-management/about-disasters/definition-of-hazard/complex-emergencies

7. Pan American Health Organization. Natural disasters: protecting the public's health. World Health Organization; 2000.

8. Crutchfield M. Phases of disaster recovery: emergency response for the long term. United Methodist Committee on Relief; 2013.

9. World Health Organization. Country health profiles. Online article. http://www.who.int/countries/en

10. The World Bank (2017). World Bank country and lending groups. Online article. https://datahelpdesk.worldbank.org/knowledgebase/articles/906519-world-bank-country-and-lending-groups

11. Dumont L, Khanal S, Thuring D, et al. Anaesthesia in the wake of the Nepal earthquake: experience and immediate lessons learnt. *European Journal of Anaesthesiology* 2016: **33**(5): 309–11.

12. Khatiwada S, Gelal B, Gautam S, et al. Anemia among school children in eastern Nepal. *Journal of Tropical Pediatrics* 2015: **61**(3): 231–3.

13. von Schreeb J, Riddez L, Samnegård H, et al. Foreign field hospitals in the recent sudden-onset disasters in Iran, Haiti, Indonesia, and Pakistan. *Prehospital and Disaster Medicine* 2008: **23**(2): 144–51; discussion 52–3.

14. Bar-On E, Abargel A, Peleg K, et al. Coping with the challenges of early disaster response: 24 years of field hospital experience after earthquakes. *Disaster Medicine and Public Health Preparedness* 2013: **7**(5): 491–8.

15. Kreiss Y, Merin O, Peleg K, et al. Early disaster response in Haiti: the Israeli field hospital experience. *Annals of Internal Medicine* 2010: **153**(1): 45–8.

16. Hagon O. World Health Organization. Baseline surgical, medical and obstetric needs versus resources both before and after a sudden onset disaster. Minimum technical standards and recommendations for reproductive, maternal, newborn, and child health care. 2019.

17. Torche F, Kleinhaus K. Prenatal stress, gestational age and secondary sex ratio: the sex-specific effects of exposure to a natural disaster in early pregnancy. *Human Reproduction* 2012: **27**(2): 558–67.

18. Ushizawa H, Foxwell AR, Bice S, et al. Needs for disaster medicine: lessons from the field of the Great East Japan Earthquake. *Western Pacific Surveillance and Response* 2013: **4**(1): 51–5.

19. North CS. Current research and recent breakthroughs on the mental health effects of disasters. *Current Psychiatry Reports* 2014: **16**(10): 481.

20. Warsini S, West C, Ed Tt GD, et al. The psychosocial impact of natural disasters among adult survivors: an integrative review. *Issues in Mental Health Nursing* 2014: **35**(6): 420–36.

21. World Health Organization (2016). Minimum technical standards and recommendations for rehabilitation – emergency medical teams. Online article. https://extranet.who.int/emt/sites/default/files/MINIMUM%20TECHNICAL%20STANDARDS.pdf

22. Norton I, Van Schcreeb J, Aiken P, et al. Emergency medical teams: minimum technical standards and recommendations for rehabilitation. 2013.

23. Iezzoni LI, Ronan LJ. Disability legacy of the Haitian earthquake. *Annals of Internal Medicine* 2010: **152**(12): 812–4.

24. Li Y, Reinhardt JD, Gosney JE, et al. Evaluation of functional outcomes of physical rehabilitation and medical complications in spinal cord injury victims of the Sichuan earthquake. *Journal of Rehabilitation Medicine* 2012: **44**(7): 534–40.

25. Rathore FA, Farooq F, Muzammil S, et al. Spinal cord injury management and rehabilitation: highlights and shortcomings from the 2005 earthquake in Pakistan. *Archives of Physical Medicine and Rehabilitation* 2008: **89**(3): 579–85.

26. Rathore FA, Gosney JE, Reinhardt JD, et al. Medical rehabilitation after natural disasters: why, when, and how? *Archives of Physical Medicine and Rehabilitation* 2012: **93**(10): 1875–81.

27. World Health Organization (2013). Global classification process. Online article. https://extranet.who.int/emt/content/global-classification-process

28. World Health Organization (2013). *Classification and minimum standards for foreign medical teams in sudden onset disasters.* http://www.who.int/hac/global_health_cluster/fmt_guidelines_september2013.pdf.

29. World Health Organization (2013). Understanding EMT classification process. https://extranet.who.int/emt/page/understanding-emt-classification-process

Predeployment Operational Planning and Preparations

Arjun Katoch and Elon Glassberg

In this chapter, we offer medical leaders and planners in charge of launching field hospitals guidelines and lessons learned from previous missions regarding mission initiation and international coordination:

Mission Initiation

The initiating body may be a local government requesting medical assistance following a disaster, a government offering assistance, a nongovernmental organization (NGO) that decides to send a field hospital, or even a group of individuals. A call on behalf of a local government requesting aid (whether specific to a country or organization, or a general call for help following a disaster) would assist in smoothing the approval process and in assuring access to the affected area.

Under international law, the national government is responsible for disaster response in its own territory[1]. Diplomacy plays a significant role in the preparation phase of a mission and should never be underestimated. Regardless of whether this is the initiative of the local government or of the organization offering help, establishing contact at the international (diplomatic) level is essential. Diplomatic involvement will help to not only approve the delegations' entry but also establish government to government (or NGO to government) contacts: crucial for the next step in approving and planning the mission. Obviously, the lack of an official approval by the accepting country will technically preclude launching the mission. Furthermore, until such approval is granted, most dispatching organizations will halt preparations, thus emphasizing the importance of swift and assertive diplomatic actions.

Procedural considerations should also be addressed. In tandem with the diplomatic activity, professional contacts (both official and informal) with colleagues in the destination country should be established. These would not only assist in estimating the local needs and ease the work of the recce team but also could assist with establishing contact with health-care professionals and officials, as well as with legal issues like approvals to practice medicine in the foreign country. This important issue is best addressed by a collaborative effort on behalf of the launching organization team, as well as with officials from the deploying country's Ministry of Health (MoH) and diplomats. Practicing medicine requires a license, even during a disaster, and, when involving a foreign country, the requirements vary. A waiver by the local government should be issued (or an official recognition in the one issued in the home country) to allow those doctors, nurses, pharmacists, and so on to practice while deployed. Discussions should also cover areas such as medications (as there could be differences between the countries), as well as establishing a policy regarding nonurgent and chronic cases who may come to the field hospital for help, and more. On the receiving country's side, the official approval given at the government level should be "translated" into a working order for the health officials in the field to try to lower resistance for foreign involvement, should it exist. A mechanism for ongoing collaborations and consultations between the local and the deployed medical professionals should be established, allowing for most of these issues to be addressed as they present. As said, the approval and the licensing issues should be addressed. Detailed guidelines on these issues have been issued by the World Health Organization (WHO) in their emergency medical teams (EMTs) initiative and should be read by the recce team. WHO classified the Israel Defense Forces' (IDF) field hospital in November 2016 as a type 3 team[2].

International Coordination

Normally, if a disaster situation is of such magnitude that foreign field hospitals have to be deployed, there will invariably be many more responders on site. These responders would be international governmental, NGO, and private responders. Conditions that the recce team is likely to find on the ground at the disaster site have been clearly described[3]. On ground, wherever there is a functioning government, there will normally be some sort of coordination center established on site to coordinate both local and international resources. "The quality of disaster response and its coordination is dependent on the experience and administrative and organizational ability of the government of the affected country[3]."

In major disasters, the UN will assist the local government in coordinating international assistance by deploying a UN disaster assessment and coordination (UNDAC) team[4]. The UNDAC team supports the government's on-site coordination by establishing an onsite operations coordination center (OSOCC) to assist in coordination of international assistance[5]. It is mandatory this is established in the event of a major earthquake as specified in the International Search and Rescue Group (INSARAG) Guidelines[6]. The recce team should look out for the OSOCC and obtain a briefing from them. If no OSOCC has been established, it should contact the government coordination center and be briefed by them. There are likely to be many other governmental or NGOs on the ground quite early into the disaster. Most are quite willing to share knowledge and contacts with new arrivals. The recce team should contact such entities. (On-the-ground collaboration will be discussed elsewhere.)

By nature, mobilizing and deploying a field hospital is an organizational and logistical challenge. Whether to another country or within one's own borders, if involving a full-scale field hospital or a smaller medical component, government, or NGO-operated treatment facilities, efforts to match the means to the end are imperative, as the capability is, by definition, deployed at times of various needs (and uncertainty). Predeployment planning is crucial to allow taking advantage of these facilities' most prominent feature of being flexible and adjustable, and to allow for tailoring the capabilities, structure, and staffing to better meet the expected needs, as well as to shorten the time before opening the gates of the hospital and actually receiving patients. It is important to realize that an "ideal" configuration of the about-to-be-launched hospital may not exist under these conditions, and protracted attempts to "improve" the capability before launching a deployment should be generally avoided, as this may cause delays and cost lives at the destination. Nevertheless, thoughtful but practical professional planning and predeployment preparations could prove vital in assuring the mission's success and avoiding many of the obstacles ahead.

One of the most useful instruments in ensuring a smooth deployment is the rapid dispatch of a small advance, reconnaissance team (called recce mission or team) prior to the deployment of the main field hospital.

The Recce or Assessment Mission

Rationale

A field hospital is a large entity with a significant amount of staff and equipment, making it a major effort to move it. It should also be operational at the disaster site as soon as possible without wasting time finding out the situation and needs. Therefore, it is advantageous that a small recce team be deployed in advance to, firstly, confirm the necessity to deploy the field hospital, and, secondly, carry out all the preparatory work necessary on the ground to ensure the field hospital, when deployed, goes smoothly and rapidly to its designated site and is functional without wasting time. The situation in the early hours of a major disaster is quite chaotic and fluid. It is therefore one of the more necessary functions of a recce team to keep the home base informed in real time of the conditions on the ground so adjustments can be made to the staffing and equipment of the hospital prior to deployment to make it more capable of dealing with the requirements at the site.

Purpose of the Recce Team

There may be a need to send a recce or assessment mission to the affected country prior to deployment decisions being taken, or while the main delegation is preparing to deploy. While the purpose of the recce team could somewhat vary depending on the scenario and timing (*should* a mission be launched versus *which* team or *what* capabilities), the principles are the same, as well as the urgency involved. The team should conduct a rapid initial assessment comprising situation analysis, resource, and needs assessment, and would be intended to determine the type of immediate relief response needed. The mission should be clear on what questions need to be answered for decisions to be taken and what type and size the team should be. Coordination with the destination government and/or officials is crucial to assure access for the team and hopefully contribute to the team's safety and success.

The recce team should gather information about:

- the needs, possible intervention strategies, and resource requirements

- local resources, the level of response by the affected country, its internal capacity to cope with the situation, and the level of response from the international community
- the most vulnerable segments of the population that need to be targeted for assistance, particularly pediatric and/or geriatric patients
- professional challenges expected: common mechanisms of injuries (e.g., burns, crush), endemic diseases, congenital defects, the need for obstetric capabilities, and so on
- existing coordination mechanisms in the country
- significant political, cultural, and logistical constraints
- weather, climatic conditions, and season
- in-country logistics; for example, functioning airports or seaports, means of transport, and communication
- mission support: food, medical, and so on
- the presence of any other international relief teams
- any prevailing endemic medical situations (e.g., prevalence of HIV/AIDS, rabies, and so on)
- the need for country-specific prophylaxis (e.g., malaria)
- unusual or site-specific medical conditions and appropriate precautions (e.g., vectors)
- local health and medical infrastructure (including veterinary facilities)

Preparations for the Recce Team Mission

Team Buildup

- Select the team leader of the RECCEE team.
- Team composition: the team should be as small as possible to reduce the logistical burden and allow for maximal maneuverability. As well as the team leader, other members should include at least one medical planner/leader (preferably experienced with similar missions and familiar with the field hospital's capabilities and also charged with providing medical aid to the team members), a logistician (to assist with site selection, transportation, and logistical preparations for the arrival of the main team), and a liaison to the local authorities. Other members may include a communication expert, a representative of an international aid organization, a translator, and more.

- Gather as much information regarding the area to be visited as possible before departure: both background information (including on the medical infrastructure that was there before the event) and up-to-date information regarding the current situation. Consider assigning specific team members to search available data sources, establish communication with relevant experts and locals, as well as with other relevant foreign and international organizations.
- Distribute the tasks, including sector-specific tasks (including route planning and maps).
- Establish a time frame (it is imperative the team be aware of its window of opportunity to affect the capabilities carried by the main delegation).
- Determine the form of the required output.
- The team will take on other responsibilities such as logistics, communications, reporting, media, and so on.
- Logistics and organization: arrange for local currency or US dollars in cash. Organize a transport and movement plan, and prepare accommodation, communication (including satellite phones), supplies, equipment, and translators.

Contractual Arrangements

The following contractual arrangements should be made:

- insurance
- liability for medical malpractice issues
- state of readiness to be maintained for deployment (hours/days)
- daily subsistence allowance arrangements
- documents and official approval to travel to the affected region (where applicable)
- arrangements for evacuation in the event of serious injury/illness
- arrangements/preparations for the possibility of death

Personal Items

The following personal items are required:

- a passport valid for more than six months, preferably machine-readable, and extra passport photos (six), with copies of the passport
- personal medications
- inoculation record, registered in an international certificate of vaccination (WHO recommended)

- documentation to support right to clinical practice
- contact list (team members) and a list of family contacts (leave a copy with the dispatching office)
- local currency or US dollars/Euros in cash, and credit cards
- clipboard, paper, pens, and pencils
- electronics; for example, laptop, tablet, GPS, phones (and chargers)

Predeployment Briefing

The predeployment briefing should include:

- mission objectives
- terms of reference of the mission
- mission tasks, expectations, and methods of operation
- initial plan of action on arrival
- cultural conditions existing in the country/region
- climatic conditions in the country
- security situation, policy, and awareness
- logistics of traveling to the country
- media (including policy regarding interviews, and so on)

Cultural Sensitivity

When preparing for a mission, all members should be aware of the cultural specifics that may exist in the country and how they may affect the mission. The country's cultural, political, and/or religious conditions may influence how the team as a whole approaches its mission and must also be taken into consideration by each individual team member. Where possible, a briefing on the customs and traditions of the country in question should be given by the team leader before deployment.

Arrival in Country

Immediate Action on Arrival

On arrival in the country, there are several actions that should be taken immediately:

- establish contact with the embassy
- assess the situation, including security assessment
- complete entry formalities (forms, telecommunications, medical equipment, and weapons, if any)
- select appropriate team profile level/visibility on entry
- establish team base (base of operations)

- establish capacity to communicate with the dispatching organization and locally (radio, phones, and the Internet)
- logistical practicalities (e.g., bills, transport, money, and food)
- obtain maps, translators, and interpreters
- identify media and agree on media message

Arrange Meetings

Meetings should be arranged with the following:

- local government coordination authority
- line ministries
- local Red Cross or Red Crescent societies or International Federation of Red Cross and Red Crescent Societies (IFRC)
- other international teams in the area

Enquiries to Make

The team needs to ask the local authority the following about the medical situation:

- local medical command structure
- availability of local medical resources
- availability of international and medical resources (e.g., hospitals and field hospitals)
- patient/casualty handover procedure
- fatality management procedures, including disaster victim identification (DVI) as determined by the local government authority

Orientation Phase

- Dispel preconceived ideas and readjust objectives on facing reality.
- Begin the information gathering and management process that continues throughout the deployment.
- Identify the key issues: establish a clear aim/ objectives and then stay focused.
- Ascertain key players' (government, agencies) expectations and gain their confidence. Initiate collaboration with local and international medical and health partners.
- Formalize the objectives and expectations by creating a plan of action.

Plan of Action for the Recce Team

The plan of action should be kept short, simple, and to the point. The following points should be addressed:

- situation: known information on the situation that resulted in the team's deployment, national response, international response, and projected developments
- mission objectives: the specific objectives of the mission, including an estimation of the duration of the mission
- in-country counterparts: the national and local medical management authorities, facilities, and colleagues with whom the team plans to establish contact
- team organization: the organization of the team into subcomponents, depending on the mission objectives
- program of work: a description of the planned activities to achieve the mission objectives
- logistics and resources: information on logistical arrangements in place for, or required by, the team, including available financial resources
- mission support: information on the measures in place to backstop the mission from the home country/organization
- communications: reporting instructions between the team and the home country, and between team members, including between field teams and the team base; if the team is using radio communications equipment (VHF or HF), include frequencies to be used, individual call signs, times for contacts between the base and field teams, and, when appropriate, communication restrictions due to security concerns
- safety and security: information on relevant concerns in the affected country
- international/local media: in the current environment of instant communication/TV coverage, the team must decide on their message and communication strategy for international and national media

Preparation for the Main Team Delegation's Arrival

The recce team needs to prepare for the arrival of the main body of the field hospital to ensure that its entry into the country and move to the disaster site is smooth and quick. To do so it should undertake the following actions[7].

- Identify a suitable location for the field hospital in coordination with the local authorities, both medical and administrative. Keep the OSOCC (if established) informed.

- Liaise with the airport and customs and immigration authorities to ensure smooth entry of personnel and equipment, including medical supplies, into the country. This may include ensuring availability of cargo-handling equipment at the airport to unload the aircraft.
- Establish close contact with the relevant embassy in the country and seek their assistance in dealing with the local authorities if necessary.
- Ensure adequate transportation to meet the needs of the team by locating local relevant resources; for example, local officials (government), NGOs, volunteers, or by rented vehicles. The capabilities should allow transport of both team members and equipment.
- Be ready to brief the incoming main body on issues related to security and cultural sensitivities in the country.
- Arrange for maps, interpreters, and guides if necessary.

Site Selection

- Area requirements for the medical team vary between teams, missions, and over time. As said, at least one of the recce team members should be familiar with the specific capabilities at hand and the technical requirements.
- Ensure the provision of adequate working spaces and accommodation for the team.
- Security: the area should be easily secured to keep out unwanted visitors. Look for secondary hazards, such as overhead power lines, gas pipelines, large trees, or unstable buildings.
- Traffic flow: consider how vehicles will enter and exit the compound.
- People flow: try to design the layout to allow visitors access to the office and work area of the compound without them having to go through the accommodation area.
- Identify a flat grassy area or gravel, which would be suitable for tents for hospital-staff accommodation, kitchen and dining, showers, and ablutions.
- Drainage: allow for the site to be well drained. Provision for drainage of showers and water points should also be considered.
- Hard standing: the team will arrive with several vehicles. A hard standing for vehicles should be provided within the compound. Visitors' vehicles should not be allowed in the compound.

- Generators: one or two large generators will be brought to the site by the main team (to provide electricity, lighting, and so on). Position these as far away as possible from the sleeping and working areas, but allow for easy refueling.
- Toilets: either black bag (single use, take-it-away) or chemical toilets may be used. Disposal of waste should be considered. Handwashing facilities will be required next to the toilets.
- Water supply: a small water treatment facility is required with the unit water supply if no other source is available.
- Vehicles: establish a tracking system of all vehicles and a service and maintenance schedule.
- Helipad: if possible, provide space for a helipad with clear access and egress, both on the ground and for takeoff and landing. A helipad should be as far from tents as possible: at least 150–200 m away. Where possible, flight paths should avoid passing over the camp.

Transfer Responsibility to the Main Delegation

Once the main body of the field hospital arrives, the recce team should brief the commander on the prevailing situation, including safety and security, and cultural issues. They should explain the coordination arrangements being followed by the local authorities and international coordination arrangements, for example OSOCC. The communication links established with the local authorities and embassy should be handed over. Administrative arrangements for local sourcing of water, food, and petroleum supplies should be briefed. It is also extremely important for the recce team to introduce key staff members to their counterparts in the local administration, health, and medical structures.

Take-Home Messages

- It is essential to deploy a recce team to a disaster site prior to deploying a field hospital to get real-time information of the situation.
- The local government is responsible for organizing the response to the disaster. All incoming international assistance supports it.
- The recce team acts as the forward scouts and ensures updated information on the situation on the ground is passed to home base to allow for

informed decision-making for the deployment of the field hospital.

- One of the most important functions of the recce team is to liaise with local authorities to ensure smooth entry of the main body into the country and movement of the field hospital to the disaster site when it arrives, both in terms of logistics and procedures.
- The recce team must ensure the main body is fully briefed on arrival and is integrated into the coordination structures established by the local authorities on site, along with any supporting international coordination structures.

The WHO publication, *Classification and Minimum Standards for Foreign Medical Teams in Sudden Onset Disasters*, is good reference material for the recce team, as well as the field hospital[2].

References

1. Katoch, A. *International natural disaster response and the United Nations; the international disaster response laws, principles and practice: reflections, prospects and challenges.* Geneva: International Federation of Red Cross and Red Crescent Societies; 2003: 50.

2. Norton I, von Schreeb J, Aitken P, Herard P, Lajolo C. *Classification and minimum standards for foreign medical teams in sudden onset disasters.* Geneva: World Health Organization; 2013.

3. Katoch, A. The responders' cauldron: the uniqueness of international disaster response. *Journal of International Affairs: The Globalization of Disaster.* Columbia University, USA 2006: 153–8; 156.

4. United Nations Office for the Coordination of Humanitarian Affairs. UN Disaster Assessment and Coordination(UNDAC). Online article. https://www.unocha.org/our-work/coordination/un-disaster-assessment-and-coordination-undac

5. United Nations Office for the Coordination of Humanitarian Affairs (2018). On-site operations coordination centre (OSOCC) guidelines, field coordination support section. Online article. https://www.unocha.org/sites/unocha/files/2018%20OSOCC%20Guidelines.pdf

6. International Search and Rescue Advisory Group (2015). INSARAG guidelines. Online article. https://www.insarag.org/methodology/guidelines

7. International Search and Rescue Advisory Group (2015). INSARAG guidelines, volume II preparedness and response: manual B. Online article. https://www.insarag.org/methodology/guidelines

Chapter

Training and Accreditation

Anthony D Redmond

Training

It should not need emphasizing, but unfortunately repeated reviews of the response by "foreign" medical teams to sudden onset disasters reinforce that it does [1,2]: those who respond to Sudden Onset Disasters (SOD) must understand and accept that work in a field hospital, like any other specialized branch of medicine, requires adequate training. Those preparing to deploy to a field hospital should also now be familiar with World Health Organization (WHO) emergency medical team (EMT) classification system, and train to match the standards detailed in WHO's *Classification and Minimum Standards for Foreign Medical Teams in Sudden Onset Disasters*: the "blue book"[3].

When considering the training approach, there is a growing consensus that a three-stage process provides the best preparation for deployment[4]. The first step is at a national/local level, where professional competence in the relevant specialty/profession is signed off/accredited, and a current license to practice, or its professional equivalent, is confirmed. The second step is to support adaptation of these technical and nontechnical professional and clinical skills for a low- or limited-resource environment and SOD. The final step addresses nonclinical behavior and skills. Team members must know how to work together effectively in the field, with special emphasis on learning and practicing leadership skills, problem solving, addressing ethical dilemmas, and resolving conflicts within a group. A combination of training methods is likely to get the best results, including individual theory-based education, immersive simulations, and team exercises.

There is, as yet, no internationally agreed curriculum, but work is underway toward gathering open-access training materials and establishing an agreed core curriculum for EMTs. This requires continuing collaboration between WHO, operational EMT organizations (governmental and nongovernmental), universities, professional bodies, and established training agencies. This chapter will describe the key elements to be included in training for a field-hospital deployment, drawing on the author's own experience, and the broader work to date in the establishment of a core curriculum.

Step 1

The safe practice and delivery of health care in a humanitarian emergency is complex and difficult. Even when the procedures and treatments in themselves appear to be relatively simple, they can be far from straightforward in practice in the aftermath of a disaster. Balancing the level of intervention against the need to maintain safe practice requires experience. These events are not for those in need of training to gain experience from those in need of care, but for those in need of care to gain from the experience of those already trained. To this end, it is essential that the first step to safe, effective care during deployment is completion of specialist training (whatever specialty or profession that may be). The question of how new experience in the field is to be gained is of course an important one and requires planning and good governance. It is inappropriate, in the author's view, for trainees, even very experienced trainees, to deploy in the first wave. If they are to be deployed later, they must have a named supervisor/mentor and comply with the level of supervision required at their stage in training at home when deployed to the field.

Training Prior to Selection for Deployment

Some organizations, including the author's[5], have a training and orientation program prior to going forward to the adaptation training in step 2. This can provide participants with sufficient, reliable information to enable them to make an informed decision about whether they are ready for this work, and for the selection committee to consider if they are likely to be able to deploy to a field hospital EMT, and if so, in what capacity.

The essential elements include imparting an understanding of the background to humanitarian responses, the UN system, the cluster system, the major international nongovernmental organizations (NGOs), international organizations such as the International Committee of the Red Cross (ICRC) and the International Federation of Red Cross and Red Crescent Societies (IFRC), government organizations, and major donors.

Understanding the context in which they will work, with a realistic appreciation of the risks and benefits of deploying to a SOD, is an important outcome of this predeployment training. This should include an introduction to working practices and cultures that will be different to their own. It is important, both to those who may deploy and those who are responsible for those who do deploy, to ensure the level of risk involved has been properly and fairly communicated, alongside how those risks may be mitigated. Included in this analysis of risk should be the risk to one's mental and physical health. If there are any conditions that automatically preclude deployment, then they should be flagged up at this stage.

Step 2

Adaptation Training

Before giving care to others, team members need to understand the risks to their own health and how to mitigate them. If they are sick or injured, then they are adding to the disease burden while reducing the strength of the team. The risk of illness and injury cannot be fully mitigated, even in the best prepared and run teams, but it can be reduced. A good understanding of disease profiles of commonly affected countries and the common risks to aid workers is essential for safe deployment. Malaria prophylaxis, compulsory seat belt use, no night driving, and adherence to safety and security standard operating procedures (SOPs) must be high on the list.

Clinicians must understand what is required to deliver and maintain background *essential emergency health care*, both during and after a SOD. This is in addition to recognizing the patterns of illness and injury after different types of SOD. For, while each type of SOD brings its own direct medical and surgical issues, the "everyday" emergencies continue and must be managed. Therefore, in addition to training in the approach to injury management and acute emergencies

directly consequent on the disaster, training must also include the approach to nondisaster-related emergencies, which will inevitably continue to present to the same facility. In what may be the only functioning health-care facility, at least in the region and perhaps for a while, team members must also understand the approach to the management of nonurgent, chronic diseases, which will almost inevitably find their way into a field-hospital setting.

The adaptation of clinical practice to the limitations of a field hospital and a large number of casualties will inevitably raise ethical dilemmas, and training is required in how to predict and deal with these, for both individuals and the team. A particular issue is the appropriateness and scope of resuscitation – if/when to start; if/when to stop – when the prolonged ventilation of the one patient will limit, or maybe even prevent, the mechanical ventilation of many more patients during surgery.

When the next SOD may strike cannot be known for sure, but we know *where* they are most common. Therefore, we can prepare for working in these countries, learn more about their demographics and topography, and identify where certain conditions/ diseases are more prevalent than in other countries and that are essential for incoming teams to know how to manage. Foremost in this list of diseases is malaria. Not only must teams know how to recognize and manage an acute presentation but they must also understand and be aware of how it presents alongside other acute and chronic conditions.

The impact of HIV/AIDS is similarly important to appreciate, and, of course, surgical and maternity teams especially must be made aware of its significance and how to mitigate its risk to other patients and health-care workers.

Tuberculosis, dengue fever, and now Zika virus must be included in training on infectious diseases. The management of diarrheal disease, particularly typhoid and cholera, is an important element in the preparation for deployment, but must include also specific training in safe working practices and the isolation of infectious patients. This will then lead into the recognition and management of suspected viral hemorrhagic fevers, the use of personal protective equipment, and liaison in country with the ministry of health (MoH) and WHO when there is a potential danger of outbreak.

Included in this broader health-care training program should be the management of stings and envenomation. The risk of animal bites must be emphasized, their management explained, and the rabies protocol for the team expanded on and understood; and similarly, the tetanus prevention, management, and treatment protocols.

The special needs of women and children must be addressed, emphasizing the risks of measles outbreak in camps and overcrowded environments, and the recognition and management of malnutrition in children.

How to recognize gender-based violence, including female genital mutilation, must be taught, and the protocol for its onward management explained to the team.

Finally, when discussing the provision of essential emergency health care in a humanitarian context, the team must understand and be able to safely transfer and/or discharge patients within the systems established/supported by the national MoH and WHO.

Specialist Training for the Austere Environment

It is important that those with technical skills are trained prior to deployment in how to adapt those skills to a field-hospital environment. This involves an understanding and mastery of those surgical techniques that are quick, safe, and effective when dealing with large numbers of casualties presenting within a short space of time. The course must also teach consistency of technique and practice to ensure a safe, continuous treatment pathway between surgeons in the same team as they change shifts, and between teams as they rotate through the periods of deployment. Included in this training program must be the techniques of essential emergency surgery to ensure the surgical team can enter all body cavities and carry out damage control/limitation and/or lifesaving surgery. The highly specialized nature of modern surgical training means that most surgeons' day-to-day practice will involve a fairly narrow spread of case presentation and surgical techniques, usually confined to one part of the body or system. It is essential that surgeons in a field hospital can deal with all, or as many as possible, of the cases that may present. These will range from trauma – usually blunt in nature – post-earthquake and SOD, to penetrating in these circumstances. They will also need to deal with the consequences of violence, including gunshot wounds, blast injury, and stabbings. These will continue to occur, even in the aftermath of a SOD; those countries vulnerable enough to need and request outside help may also

be fragile more generally and therefore suffer a higher incidence of background violence. Obviously, if the deployment is to a conflict or a peri-conflict area, a firm understanding of the principles of war surgery is required. Finally, irrespective of the background to the deployment, surgical emergencies will continue to occur. Incarcerated hernias, perforated ulcers, and so on; and importantly, pregnant women will continue to present to health facilities. The team must have the knowledge and equipment to deal with obstetric emergencies, including emergency caesarian section.

The training process must be based on, and use, the equipment that will be available in the field hospital itself. Individual surgeons often have their own preferred instrumentation, but it is impractical to cater for a wide variety of options in a field hospital. Surgeons must accept, and be trained in using, a defined set of instruments and equipment which will be available to them in the field, and become expert in their use prior to deployment.

There are two options to secure a spread of surgical expertise. One is for each individual surgeon to be trained and become competent in all aspects of emergency and trauma surgery; including thoracic, abdominal, vascular, and general surgery, as well as the management of limb injuries, including fractures, and the management of head injuries. Included in this skill set must also be the management of obstetric emergencies. Modern surgical training makes the accumulation of such a broad range of skills difficult to secure, although there are countries that train surgeons more broadly as "trauma" surgeons, and military surgeons may have acquired these skills. However, this may not be the case for many surgeons in civilian practice unless working for a large humanitarian organization such as Médecins Sans Frontières (MSF) or the ICRC. The team may therefore look to broaden the training for its individual surgeons to ensure that each individual has this broader skill set. Alternatively, they may choose to include in the team a broader range of individual specialist surgeons, including obstetricians, each of whom has also had extra training in the management of a wider range of conditions. Another option is simply to run the field hospital with the range of specialist surgeons we would find in everyday practice. This may, however, limit the capacity of the field hospital, as specific surgical expertise is "parceled up" in an individual surgeon and patients queue to be allotted to one, rather than across several, potential clinicians. If the surgeons have been more broadly trained and extended their skills, there will be more surgeons available to work simultaneously across numerous patients. Whatever approach is taken, it is imperative to accept and understand that surgeons, like all other medical practitioners who respond to these emergencies, must only practice within their usual competencies, which can, however, be legitimately extended by appropriate training by an accredited body (such as the Royal College of Surgeons in the UK, for example). However, as stated at the outset, these emergencies are not simply opportunities for surgeons to gain new surgical skills or experience, but rather an opportunity to bring the skills and experience they have already gained to the benefit of those in need.

There are a few courses that address these issues, but the most comprehensive in the author's experience is that run by the Royal College of Surgeons in the UK under the directorship of Dr. David Nott and in collaboration with the ICRC, MSF, and the military[6]. An important feature of this course is that the training is carried out on unembalmed cadavers, allowing for the most realistic skills-based training.

Anesthetists also need to adapt their skills to the *austere environment*. Oxygen supplies, whether piped or in cylinders, will be restricted, if indeed available at all; so, supplemental oxygen will usually be from oxygen concentrators. The supply of oxygen will be a determinant of the depth and duration of general anesthesia and thereby potentially the type and duration of surgery. Anesthetic gases may also be limited, so alternative methods need to be understood and employed (although much can be achieved with continuous intravenous anesthesia; for example, ketamine +/− propofol).

Training should emphasize that "what can be done under local anesthesia, is done under local anesthesia," with local, regional, and spinal blocks demonstrated and candidates' competencies tested and confirmed.

As gas-powered ventilation may be at a premium, the principles and practice of "draw-over" anesthesia may be required to be taught and mastered.

Prehospital Care for the Austere Environment

If providing an outreach service from the field hospital in the form of mobile clinics or other interventions, then teams must receive additional training in the appropriate level of intervention to be attempted, the kit to be carried, and the need to link in with in-country health systems. The safe transfer of patients in an austere environment can be included in this training.

Within this context, specific training can be given on conducting a needs assessment and the health resources availability mapping system[7].

Step 3

Operational Deployment Training

This is not about gaining further clinical skills and/or the clinical management of patients. This has been covered in the previous steps. It is about working safely and effectively within a team, in difficult circumstances, and in an organized and coordinated manner. It is also the final opportunity prior to deployment to identify those who are still not ready for deployment.

It needs to be immersive, using simulation techniques and a simulation exercise (SimEx), and can follow the pattern of a real-life deployment. It should include strengthening team building, team working, and leadership capacities.

Predeployment

The team members must be made familiar with the contents of their personal kit bag, which must be readily available to them at all times during deployment, and fully stocked and accessible when on call. They can be advised on what additional "luxury" items they may consider bringing, while emphasizing it is they, and they alone, that will have to carry it.

It is essential that team members are completely familiar with the on-call mechanism, call-out procedure, and command and control structure they are signing up to; and the type and duration of potential deployments. Now is the time to step back if there are any uncertainties about the deployment that cannot be satisfactorily resolved.

Moving on from personal kit, team members need to be familiarized with the layout of the field hospital in which they will work, their living accommodation, and the feeding, water, and sanitation arrangements. They will have been familiarized with the equipment they will use in the step-2 training, but any lingering uncertainties can be ironed out now.

An essential part of the immediate predeployment preparation is a predeparture briefing by the team leader who will give the background to the deployment, an up-to-date status report including known risks and hazards, and any identified immediate needs. The point of departure and arrival will be clarified, and team members formally introduced to each other and their roles clarified. If not already familiar with the virtual on-site operations coordination center (VOSOCC)[7], team members will be made familiar with how EMTs are now asked to register with the VOSOCC, where requests for assistance can be made by the affected country and WHO, and registered teams can make a matching offer.

Arrival in Country

The processes to be expected and followed on arrival in country can be the subject of a simulation exercise, where team members must negotiate immigration and border control. "Injects" may include queries about the validity of the visa that has been issued and attempts at bribery by corrupt officials. After clearing immigration, reporting to in-country officials and the WHO coordination cell are part of this process.

Arrival at the Scene of the Disaster

The simulated scenario can continue with simulated casualties presenting to the team as they are trying to unload their supplies and beginning the erection of the field hospital. The team should have a plan in place to manage this and know where to access the emergency medical supplies and consumables to deal with these patients at the same time as they are preparing the field hospital. The security issues around this should also be tested.

Setting up the Field Hospital

The drill of setting up the field hospital should be made familiar to the team, and each member should show they understand and can demonstrate the role that they will play during this process.

Running the Field Hospital

A full simulation exercise can demonstrate and test the flow of (simulated) patients through the field hospital, and test team members' ability to triage and retriage casualties as they arrive and proceed through the hospital. In this way, the team practice working together, taking and giving appropriate direction, and familiarizing themselves with the layout and function of the facility.

Full simulations, however, can be financially expensive, so events within the exercise can be run as a "table-top" exercise, where team members are given cards with a patient and their condition marked on it and asked to triage/prioritize the treatment of these patients and distribute them across the floor space of the field hospital.

Within the team's SOPs will be the management of ethical dilemmas and conflicts within the team. These can be tested by appropriate "injects" during the SimEx.

Preparation for Exit

The SimEx is completed with the team demonstrating the preparations they will make for their safe and ethical departure from the field.

Arrival Home and Debrief

Before departing, the team will meet for a debrief on the exercise and discuss as a group where improvements need to be made and the processes that went well. They will comment on their colleagues' performance in confidential written feedback, and the SimEx leads may also wish to interview participants individually to get further feedback, and share with them their assessment of their performance.

During the group feedback discussion, the team can be familiarized with the arrangements for their arrival home, which are likely to include a factual debrief, psychological support where necessary, and health checks/clearance.

Throughout the SimEx, the following issues must be addressed, both during breaks for more "classroom" instruction and by simulation.

- Medical record keeping, daily reporting to the MoH and WHO in the field, and adherence to collating the WHO minimum dataset.
- Communications in the field, including radio communications protocols and the use of satellite communications.
- Media protocol: the safest and most effective policy is to have an identified spokesperson for the team, who will hold discussions and speak on behalf of the team. The media will therefore have a known focal point for the team, so that they can be spared what can be the intrusive presence of the press when they are trying to get on with treating patients. Using professional journalists as part of the SimEx can be a very effective way of training for exposure to the media in these circumstances and testing whether the teams understand and will adhere to media SOPs. A media "inject" into the SimEx, where team members are interrupted by the press and pressurized to give an ad hoc interview, can be a very effective lesson for

members when these interviews are edited (not necessarily benignly) and played back to the team during the debrief session. Included in the media feedback can be a reminder of the use of imagery and the team's policy. Patient confidentiality is paramount, and any images can only be taken with their informed consent and must not be shared with any form of media, including social media, unless and until there is additional informed consent.

- Technical issues: for example, setting up and running a walking blood bank; and water and sanitation.

There will be additional training to these core elements. Leadership training particularly for those identified as potential team leaders will feature in most teams' training programs.

Safety and security will be tested throughout the SimEx, but for those teams who choose to respond specifically into conflict, or peri-conflict, areas, a type of hostile environment awareness training course will be required. This is beyond the scope of this chapter. However, all deployments carry safety and security risks, and these may be tested in simulated "incidents." Many training exercises include a "carjacking" or attempted "robbery" to emphasize the risks and to test the team's and individuals' responses. Some go further and simulate kidnap with "hostages" being hooded and verbally abused. Placing participants under this level of stress is not without its own risks: care must be taken in selection and close scrutiny of candidates maintained throughout to facilitate stopping the exercise as soon as it proves too much. This more intense simulation is usually reserved for those who have been preselected for deployment to a hostile environment.

Just-in-Time Training

The above courses can be run repeatedly, updating when necessary, but providing training and preparation for a generic response. There will, however, be special or unusual events, the most recent being the outbreak of Ebola in West Africa, where, in addition to the training described above, a bespoke training course, specific to that event, is required immediately prior to a team's deployment.

Accreditation

At present, there is no international body that will accredit, or take a degree of responsibility for, the overall training and skills for EMTs/field hospitals. Step-1 training, however, does include accreditation by those professional bodies that grant the relevant professional qualifications. In step-2 training, where technical skills are taught by a recognized professional body, a degree of accreditation in that aspect of training may be granted. For most step-2 training, however, it will be the training organization itself that will accredit them as having satisfactorily completed the course of training, according to their published criteria. It is important that those going through training understand beforehand the learning objectives of the course and the criteria against which they will be assessed (accredited) at the end. This is particularly important in step-3 training when the final selection is being made. The usual criteria are around being a team player, exercising leadership skills when necessary, supporting colleagues, and demonstrating safe practice and conduct.

Although not providing accreditation as such, the WHO EMT verification process does provide external peer review and quality assurance as measured against published core standards. This is the accreditation that EMTs/field hospitals should be looking to achieve.

In summary, therefore, the training process should ensure that all team members have:

- a broader understanding of the WHO EMT initiative, team classification, minimum standards, and core principles
- an understanding of the rationale for and process for mentorship, verification, and registration of EMTs
- a recognition of the need and importance of effective EMT coordination during a deployment through the emergency medical team coordination cell (EMTCC) and the affected country's government
- sustainability during an EMT deployment
- a strengthened team-based approach to decision-making and operational activities
- a broader knowledge and skill of clinical adaptations required for low-resource and austere contexts
- an understanding of the role of the team leader in EMT deployments
- an awareness of the challenges of media engagement during humanitarian emergencies
- recognition of the importance of knowledge exchange and shared learning across all EMTs

The approach to this training should be "blended learning," inclusive of lecture-based sessions, small-group workshops, team sessions, and immersive simulation exercises.

References

1. Redmond A et al. A qualitative and quantitative study of the surgical and rehabilitation response to the earthquake in Haiti. *Prehospital and Disaster Medicine* 2010: **26**(6): 449–56.

2. Peranteau WH et al. Re-establishing surgical care at Port-au-Prince general hospital. *Haiti Journal of the American College of Surgeons* 2010: **211**: 126–30.

3. Norton I, von Schreeb J, Aitken P, Herard P, Lajolo C. *Classification and minimum standards for foreign medical teams in sudden onset disasters*. Geneva: World Health Organization; 2013.

4. Camacho NA, Hughes A, Burkle Jr FM, et al. Education and training of emergency medical teams: recommendations for a global operational learning framework. 2016. Online article. http://currents.plos.org/disasters/article/education-and-training-of-emergency-medical-teams-recommendations-for-a-global-operational-learning-framework

5. UK-MED. Website. www.uk-med.org

6. https://www.rcseng.ac.uk/education-and-exams/courses/search/surgical-training-for-austere-environments-stae/

7. World Health Organization. Health resources availability monitoring system (HeRAMS). Online article. http://www.who.int/hac/herams/en

8. Global Disaster Alert and Coordination System. GDACS – virtual OSOCC – real-time disaster coordination. Website. https://vosocc.unocha.org

Personnel

Pietro D Marghella and Kelly Suter

Introduction

In the early 1990s, a US Navy admiral named Paul David Miller shook up the American defense establishment by introducing a concept that was initially dubbed "tailor force packaging." Miller had become increasingly concerned with what he perceived as the US Department of Defense's (DoD) overly rigid doctrine and policy that underpinned the tactics, techniques, and procedures governing the use of operational forces. Speaking to the demise of the former Soviet Union – our former malefactor partner in the concept of mutually assured destruction – Miller noted that:

> A national security policy that proved successful for forty years is not easily discarded. A military organization that successfully deterred global war, contained a militarily powerful adversary, and projected presence for stability in regional hot spots is not easily reoriented[1].

In Miller's view, US military forces had become stuck in a cold war state of mind. During that period of time, the US DoD had architected its forces around a doctrine focused on force-on-force engagement operations against a sole, state-level peer vying for regional/hemispheric – if not global – hegemony, even though the USA had engaged in numerous regional conflicts and operations other than war in the same extended time frame. Although radical – and, at first, widely rejected – Miller's concept of tailor-force packaging led to what came to be known in the US DoD doctrine as "adaptive force packaging": "A new concept ... which envisions using geographically and mission tailored joint forces to conduct forward presence operations[2]."

Miller's initiative was merely the opening gambit to a more tectonic shift in the USA's approach to force planning: the move away from *requirements-based* (or threat-based) *planning* (RBP) to *capabilities-based planning* (CBP); the former having dominated our approach to the development of operational force structures since the US Defense Reorganization Act

of 1947. The antiquated requirements-based planning approach was largely focused on point (or individual) scenarios. The major shortcoming in this earlier analytical method was that it was more focused on the point scenarios rather than types of threats, limiting the ability to plan for the larger range of threats forces may encounter in the operational environment. CBP, on the other hand, is planning that is conducted (albeit under uncertainty) to accommodate for providing capabilities suitable for a wide range of modern-day challenges and circumstances, while still working within an economic framework that necessitates choice.

The primary distinctions between these types of analyses, then, are in how planners deal with uncertainty, in the reckoning of risk, and in the way of making choices. The core idea central to the CBP approach is to confront – rather than discount – uncertainty, to express risk in meaningful terms, and to weigh costs and benefits simultaneously. The objective of CBP is to put a premium value on portfolios of assets (including organizations and skill sets) which best satisfy operational needs while offering flexibility, adaptability, and robustness to hedge risk across a wide range of possible futures[3]. In many ways, Miller's paradigm-shifting initiative on the employment of military operational assets is now recognized as prescient not only to the transition from RBP to CBP but also to the requirements associated with the "transformation" efforts (led by former defense secretary Donald Rumsfeld) that have dominated the global security environment of the post 9/11 era for the USA and its allies. Also known as the "Rumsfeld doctrine", US DoD initiatives underpinning the transformation included the enhanced use of high-technology combat systems, the reliance on air power, and the use of small, nimble ground forces capable of responding to rapidly developing situations in any combatant command theater[4]. This initiative was and remains so far-reaching that it has fundamentally changed the theoretical and philosophical approach to the process of planning that is conducted in the USA military, leading to changes in the time-proven practices of *deliberate planning* to the more modern and refined approach of *adaptive planning*[5].

So, what is the relevance of all of this to a chapter devoted to a discussion on personnel for field hospitals? First off, it is important for planners involved with the development and deployment of field medical assets – whether in the military or in nongovernmental organizations (NGOs)/private volunteer organizations (PVOs) – to understand how changes in planning doctrine and theory can and should lead to improvements in implementing successful end states for deployable assets (i.e., the ability of those assets to meet operational mission requirements). Secondly, and by extension, to borrow from the concept of operations on adaptive force packaging and the tenets of CBP, any personnel package developed for field medical platforms should mirror the goals already enumerated for both: a priori to satisfy operational requirements while simultaneously offering flexibility, environmental and situational adaptability, and robustness to hedge against risks encountered in the operational environment.

This chapter will examine required operational capabilities and projected operational environments for field-hospital platforms; discuss potential personnel packages for use in these platforms; and offer some considerations derived from lessons learned from recent military, disaster response, and humanitarian engagements, which can assist planners with developing the most capable resources for operational environments.

Discussion

Personnel Planning

Field hospitals and their accompanying personnel packages can be employed for a wide variety of operations. Examples include:

- military operations, with subsets including:
  - combat operations
  - low-intensity conflict operations
  - peacekeeping/peace-enforcement operations
  - security operations
  - humanitarian assistance and disaster relief operations
  - noncombatant evacuation operations (hostile and nonhostile)
  - military operations other than war
  - defense support to civil authorities

- nonmilitary operations, normally supported by civilian NGOs/PVOs, including:
  - humanitarian assistance
  - disaster relief
  - complex emergencies
  - disease outbreaks
  - resiliency building through education and training and community assistance

Historically, planning for the employment of field medical assets was largely the province of military medical planners, since the military was the first formal organization to utilize field medical platforms to support their operations. Over the years, medical planners have developed fairly comprehensive processes associated with deliberate/adaptive planning to determine the required capabilities and the associated staffing and equipment requirements necessary to support the platform's mission. All these processes are now applicable to planning for both military and nonmilitary operations, and include the following:

1. Describing a comprehensive mission statement for the purpose and use of the field hospital platform.

2. Determining the size, constitution, and location of the population at risk (PAR) they would be supporting. As expected, this could vary widely based on the type of operational environment the field hospital would be operating in.

3. Conducting a medical intelligence assessment of the projected operational environment. Planning for operational use of field hospital platforms must include an assessment of geography and topography; dangerous flora and fauna; disease vector risks; availability of water, sanitation, and hygiene assets (or lack thereof); and, in the case of purely military operations, the enemy order of battle, including weapons systems and the availability of asymmetrical or novel weapons.

4. It follows that the medical intelligence (MEDINT) assessment leads to the development of a "force health protection" (FHP) plan for the personnel assets deployed to the field platform.[1] This is meant to ensure that there are no degradations in the capabilities of the deploying forces once they are on mission point.

5. Determining historical casualty rates associated with location and type of deployment to be applied against the PAR (to include both combat casualty rates and those associated with disease and

nonbattle injuries). These should ideally lead to the development of predictive requirements for associated morbidity and mortality.

6. Projecting the period of operational employment (i.e., length of time in the deployed environment).

7. Determining deployment and redeployment requirements.

While it may seem these steps are only applicable to the overall development of a field-hospital employment plan, it is important to note that all these requirements are directly applicable to the process of determining the constitution of the personnel packages that support them. For example, the mission, size of the PAR, the MEDINT "snapshot," application of historical casualty rates, length of operational employment, and deployment and redeployment requirements are all directly relevant to the process of determining the size and makeup by specialty of the field hospital's personnel complement. In other words, planning for the personnel portion of the field hospital is inextricably linked to the basic planning associated with utilization of the platform in the first place.

In the USA, the DoD is the only organization within the family of federal partner agencies that trains full-time professional medical planners for career roles in the mission of determining health-service support requirements against the spectrum of operations they may be involved with in both traditional and nontraditional military operations (i.e., war fighting, peacekeeping and security operations, foreign humanitarian assistance and disaster relief, and now, in the post-9/11 era, domestic support to disaster relief operations).

To facilitate the assurance of comprehensive medical planning, US DoD planners use a sophisticated information management/information technology (IM/IT) tool known as the Joint Medical Analysis Tool (JMAT). The JMAT works by front-loading the PAR, casualty rates to be assigned against the PAR, and the period of operational employment, and then "running" them through a series of algorithms known as the "time-task-treater" files to determine the health-service support requirements (i.e., output) associated with the operation. These requirements include, but are not limited to, identifying providers by individual specialty and number required, type of beds (e.g., medical, surgical, and intensive care) needed to support the PAR, medical logistical requirements, blood, patient movement requirements for theater evacuation, and rations for hospitalized patients – all computed to address the requirements in aggregate on a day-to-day basis for

their projected length of the operational employment. While planners utilizing this chapter for assistance in determining personnel and other operational requirements may not have access to the JMAT or any other mechanism for automating the planning process, knowing the functional areas needing to be addressed can still assist them with their efforts to ensure maximized capabilities and operational readiness.

Sourcing of Personnel

Once planning has been initiated, the sourcing of personnel to staff the field hospitals must be addressed. Military organizations that staff fixed brick-and-mortar medical treatment facilities (MTFs) will find they are the most convenient sourcing organizations for deployable facilities. Medical staff members across the spectrum of professional specialties will already be familiar with the delivery of care within a hospital environment. That said, the field environment can be radically different from that of a fixed facility. Field conditions can run the spectrum from remote and austere to hostile and dangerous. Sourcing MTFs within military organizations should ensure staff members assigned to deployable medical platforms receive adequate training prior to a field assignment. This can be accomplished in any one of several ways:

1. Having a formal field medical service school or training center where personnel who are projected to receive assignments to deployable platforms can receive training in an environment that replicates expected field conditions.

2. Conducting partial- or full-scale live exercises, which involve projected deployment staff setting up and either utilizing portions or complete packages of the field hospital platform.

3. Conducting routine professional military education classes, which cover topics on operational field medicine.

In the late 1990s, the US Navy developed an interesting model for sourcing medical personnel to operational platforms, whether they were for field hospitals, deployable surgical and specialized medical teams, or the hospital ships. Known as the "total health care support for readiness requirements" model, the construct matched personnel one-for-one from fixed brick-and-mortar MTFs to deployable platform billets, which would operate in field environments. The main benefit to this model is that it allowed planners to determine not only exactly where personnel were coming from by sourcing agency and specialty but to likewise determine exactly what backfill requirements would be needed (largely from the military's reserve force) to ensure services would remain at those sourcing facilities since, more often than not, the fixed MTFs would have to play a role in the continuum of care if casualties were returned for definitive treatment and rehabilitation.

For NGO/PVO organizations, the recruitment and sourcing of personnel can be a much more complex matter, since few – if any – maintain a standing cadre of health-care professionals who can be employed in field deployable platforms on a moment's notice. In the USA, NGO/PVO organizations (such as the International Medical Corps, Project HOPE, and Americares) that are medical-centric and public-health-centric, and can deploy personnel to field platforms in response to complex emergency and disaster scenarios, maintain extensive relationships – usually through expressly written memorandums of understanding – with academic-affiliated teaching hospitals, which can source personnel in times of a crisis requiring deployable assets. Teaching hospitals usually have much larger numbers of professional staff (i.e., physicians, nurses) to draw from when events require them, and many believe that the field experience can be value-added to their overall training of junior health-care professionals, at a minimum because they tend to see patients and conditions that are outside of the norm of their usually stable hospital environments.

Other sources of personnel for field hospital platforms include organizations such as national disaster medical systems, which maintain active rosters of volunteers that can be activated (and in some cases, federalized) in times of crisis or disaster (including the Medical Reserve Corps, a USA initiative, which leverages retired health-care professionals for mobilization in times of disaster), dedicated national and state-based organizations such as Voluntary Organizations Active in Disasters, and faith-based organizations.

Beyond issues related to the sourcing of personnel for field hospital employment are those associated with legal, administrative, and medical preparedness for deployers.

Credentialed health-care personnel (i.e., those who require a license to practice such as physicians and nurses) generally have no problem with the portability of their licensure in international disaster response environments. Military and NGO/PVO organizations, which are deployed to provide foreign humanitarian assistance and disaster relief, are generally vetted and accepted by foreign governments when they either request or agree to have foreign response assets support them in times of crisis. In these cases, validation of an individual's licensure or accreditation occurs when the individual has their credentials and licensure vetted to participate with the organization's mission in the first place.

Domestically, licensure review and credentialing may be another case entirely. In the USA, for example, physicians usually maintain licensure in only one state at a time. If a disaster occurs in another state, physicians (other than those in the military) who attempt to deploy without obtaining licensure in the state of the disaster face stiff penalties, including heavy fines and possible permanent loss of license in their home state. This is less of an issue for nurses in the USA as the American Nursing Association has lobbied for and received agreements of licensure portability in some 85% of USA states and territories.

One way to get around the licensure issue in times of disaster is for either the senior national or state public health official, or their emergency management counterparts, to have a standing waiver agreement available for signature approval by an appropriate level of authority (e.g., president or state governor). This would not only grant blanket access to credentialed health-care providers who could deploy to provide assistance but would also eliminate the risk of medical tort liability against these practitioners, eliminating the need for them to maintain medical malpractice insurance outside their home of origin.

The issue of FHP was previously mentioned in the context of needing an adequate MEDINT assessment for deploying forces, but the implications of FHP go beyond simple awareness of what deployers may face in the field. Firstly, it is well known that disaster zones are dangerous environments. Personnel deploying to field environments should be generally healthy and physically capable of operating in what may be a dangerous, stressful, and environmentally challenging arena (e.g., consider the Ebola treatment units [ETUs], which deployed to West Africa during the 2014–2015 Ebola virus disease outbreaks). They should expect to have to work – often well beyond simple eight-hour shifts – for potentially significant periods of time. They will also be required to work in environments that may have suffered significant disruption or complete collapse of critical infrastructure and key resource sectors, placing them at greater risk of injury and illness while in a deployed status. While it seems a common-sense assumption, deploying personnel should recognize they largely assume the same amount of risk of illness and injury as the PAR they have been deployed to support; it is a bad assumption to believe they will somehow remain immune to risk simply because they are providing the medical and public-health support the PAR may need.

The FHP program, which was adopted by the USA military in the wake of the US DoD's experience with the first Persian Gulf War and the subsequent Gulf War illness experience, represents an excellent model to be emulated by any organization – military or civilian – sourcing personnel for field-hospital deployments.

The program consists of three active phases: (1) predeployment phase, (2) deployment phase, and (3) postdeployment phase. In the first phase, deployers receive a baseline health assessment to: (1) check they are qualified to deploy, (2) identify and document any ongoing physical ailments or conditions that may change during their deployment experience, and (3) provide any vaccines, prophylaxis, or medicines they may require based on their current medical conditions or the known threats they may face in the specific geographic location of the deployment (which should, again, be derived from the MEDINT assessment, which goes with the deployment).

The second phase involves active health, injury, and disease surveillance in the deployed location. In the same fashion that deployed health-care personnel track morbidity and mortality data for the PAR they support, an active surveillance program for the deployers themselves should be initiated as soon as they arrive in the geographic theater of operations. The third phase is a follow-up phase. Deployed personnel should be tracked for any changes in their health status that may have occurred because of their deployment. While many international military organizations have some variant of the "Feres Doctrine", which prevents the USA military from being sued because of the adverse health effects associated with their service, this is not the case for civilian volunteer organizations. Tracking the postdeployment health status of participating personnel ensures that any organization – military or civilian – is protecting the health interests of its staff. Tracking also helps civilian organizations to stay ahead of any claims that may arise after the fact, potentially limiting excessive tort liability (an additional way to avoid this, which is widely employed by NGOs/PVOs, is to

have deployers voluntarily sign waivers, which releases the parent organization from any liability associated with their service).

As it relates to planning, recruitment, and sourcing of personnel for field-hospital deployments, it should be noted that there are numerous commercial, off-the-shelf emergency management software programs, which can aid organizations deploying personnel with tracking information related to the personnel they employ. IM/IT professionals associated with the human-resource departments of deploying organizations should look for software programs that, at a minimum, facilitate the creation of recruitment databases, which provide comprehensive individual contact information, help to automate the licensing and credentialing process, and track requirements for updating required training and certification programs such as Basic and Advanced Cardiac Life Support for deploying personnel. Many of these software programs double as emergency management tools, which can be used in the operation centers of the parent organizations and linked to IM/IT platforms in the deployed environment to facilitate the exchange of real-time data.

Personnel Packages

The following provides an example of an organizational makeup of a deployed hospital. It contains three essential levels of staff: (1) hospital executive staff (i.e., C-suite functions), (2) hospital administrative staff (i.e., administrative department heads), and (3) clinical staff (i.e., department heads and additional providers)[6].

This staffing package is based on requirements for a 44-bed hospital supporting a PAR with significant chronic medical needs following a major meteorological disaster in the twenty-first century. Other configurations of deployed Emergency Medical Teams should adhere to the World Health Organization (WHO) minimal staffing requirements. This notional package would require the following number of personnel: (1) 4 executive-level staff (i.e., C-suite), administrative staff, and 10 department-head-level administrative staff (14 health-care administrators and allied health scientists, in total), (2) 30 physician clinical staff (2 executive-level [i.e., C-suite] administrative staff, 16 medical and surgical specialty department heads, and 12 additional clinical providers), and (3) 55 nurses (1 executive-level [C-suite] and 54 clinical nurses). The nursing package is based on the following

Table 7.1 Notional hospital staffing package

Executive staff (C-suite)	Administrative staff (department heads)	Physician clinical staff (executive staff plus additional providers)
Chief executive officer	Patient administration	Emergency medicine (4)
Chief operating officer	Medical records	Cardiology (2)
Chief financial officer	Information management	Ear, nose, throat (1)
Director for administration	Operating management	Geriatrics (2)
Chief of medical services	Fiscal and supply	General surgery (1)
Chief of surgical services	Human resources	Gastroenterology (1)
Director of nursing services	Quality assurance	Obstetrics/gynecology (ob/gyn) (3)
	Staff education & training	Pediatrics (3)
	Laboratory	Neurology (1)
	Pharmacy	Oncology (1)
		Ophthalmology (1)
		Orthopedics (1)
		Urology (1)
		Psychiatry (1)
		Internal medicine (4)
		Pulmonary medicine (1)

formula: 5:1 patient-to-nurse ratio/45 beds (rounded-up) = 9 nurses × 3 shifts per 24 hours = 27 nurses × 2 to accommodate weekends and sick days = 54 nurses). The total staff required would be 99 personnel. This does not include personnel requirements for clinical technical support (e.g., X-ray, lab, pharmacy technicians, phlebotomy, and so on), as well as physical plant support, maintenance, food services, and so on.

Planning Pearls

The following "planning pearls" are not presented in any particular order. They are gleaned from lessons learned from at least the last three decades of experience with operational medicine and the field medical platforms that have supported deployed forces.

- We cannot overestimate the importance of pre-event deliberate/adaptive planning. Most organizations that provide routine responses to military operations, complex emergencies, and disasters routinely engage in deliberate planning ahead of events that have a reasonable chance of occurrence. That said, by failing to engage in deliberate planning ahead of a crisis, the chances of mounting an adequate response decrease in equal – but inverse – proportion to the scope and scale of the event demanding a response.

Considerations on the personnel makeup and constitution of field-deployable medical assets must be made well in advance of an actual response if they have any hope of being effective. In addition, engaging in frequent and realistic exercises gives personnel who will deploy with these platforms a greater familiarity with their roles and expectations in actual execution.[2]

- Speed makes a difference when responding to crises and disasters that necessitate the use of field-medical assets. Military and NGOs/PVOs should recognize that we are at constant battle with the "twin tyrannies" of time and distance when it comes to supporting a PAR. Any delays in response can lead to substantial portions of a PAR being dead, dispersed, or recovered by the time field assets arrive (i.e., the assets will have little to no bearing on the outcome of the mission if significant delays in the response preclude a timely response to their needs). It is therefore imperative that planners associated with fielding deployable medical assets have their personnel packages set and ready for deployment at a moment's notice. Any attempts to configure these packages at the eleventh hour could result in delays that will negatively affect the supported PAR and lead to increases in morbidity and mortality.

- Most nations capable of fielding deployable medical assets are presently not prepared for what could be referred to as "mega-disasters," yet any number of scenarios that may fall into this category loom on our collective horizon. Examples include a pandemic that exceeds the impact of the 1918–1919 "Spanish flu," earthquakes, tsunamis, and nuclear accidents or acts of terrorism. Ultimately, we will always adjudicate our incident-management efforts by lives saved and suffering reduced. We must recognize this places a heavy burden on how our medical and public-health infrastructure responds to these events. Beyond tactical and even operational level deployments of field platforms, planners should carefully consider how medical personnel from available and existent infrastructure can play into deployable platforms, which serve to meet surge capacity demands during periods of severe environmental duress. Beyond field platforms, we must think strategically when considering some of the scenarios that now represent disruptors to the homeostasis of our communities and nations.

- One of the most important lessons to be gleaned from the experiences of international medical- and public-health-centric NGOs/PVOs is how to operate in an austere environment. As a former commandant of the US Marine Corps noted after the 1991 Persian Gulf War: "Don't expect to have the National Naval Medical Center in the desert" (General Charles C Krulak, US Marine Corps, speech presented at the Annual Navy Surgeon General's Conference, April 17, 1992, unreferenced). Personnel deploying to field medical platforms should not expect to have access to as many, or as sophisticated, technological resources as they have available in modern brick-and-mortar facilities under noncrisis conditions. Modern clinical practices in developed nations, which are capable of deploying field medical platforms, are highly technology-dependent. That will prove to be problematic when personnel are operating on what are tantamount to surge-capacity locations of opportunity outside of those established brick-and-mortar facilities. Further, they should expect – and plan for – significant degradations in the standard of care in field environments (and the truism that follows that the bigger the disaster, the greater that degradation will be).

- Planners should consider adding nontraditional personnel components to field-hospital staffing packages based on the scenario prompting the deployment in the first place. For example, a cultural anthropologist could have played an enormously important role in helping to slow or even stop the 2014–2015 Ebola outbreak in West Africa, since most of the practices contributing to the spread of that deadly disease were rooted in the familial and community-based practices associated with caring for the sick and conducting their funerary rituals.

- Another word on the issue of *culture*. In many cases, personnel who deploy to field hospitals and other deployable medial platforms (e.g., clinics and mobile medical and surgical teams) will often find themselves in locations where cultural and religious practices will differ markedly from those in their own countries of origin. That being the frequent case, care must be exercised to be especially knowledgeable and sensitive to these differences to avoid offense or even, in some cases, inciting violence. We have had recent experience with deployed medical personnel being attacked and killed because locals believed they were there to harm them rather than heal them. Leaders in deployed medical units must consider the importance of integrating with local leadership in country to ensure their mission is understood and accepted. They must further maintain constant reinforcement among their staff that they remain respectful of local cultural and religious practices as this will contribute markedly to their safety and the overall success of their mission.

- The founder of the International Medical Corps once noted that one of our biggest failings in deployed environments is our inability to adequately capture (primarily) epidemiological data. The perennial excuse that is cited is, "We're too busy saving lives to bother with data collection" (personal interview with Dr. Robert Simon, October 22, 2014, unreferenced). Continuing with this thinking is a big mistake. Capturing and analyzing the empirical data available from the field experience helps to contribute to the mounting body of evidence-based practices we continue to build in the emerging disciplines of disaster medicine and public-health preparedness. Not bothering with data collection simply leaves too much room for repeating the mistakes we really should have learned from during previous field and operational experiences. Planners responsible for building tables of organization (i.e., staffing packages) for deploying platforms should consider including dedicated personnel who remain solely responsible for data collection and analysis (e.g., a staff epidemiologist, two to four personnel dedicated to data capture and analysis, and one to two dedicated IM/IT professionals charged with data management).

- Planners should carefully consider the state of local health care and public-health infrastructure when architecting personnel packages for field deployable platforms. In third world and failing states, care must be exercised not to over-exceed local capabilities by such a significant measure that on redeployment populations returning to a status quo ante state find themselves in an even worse state as a result of being unable to meet the same standard of care delivered by deployers. Nevertheless, planners should avoid sourcing very highly specialized personnel who would not be otherwise available to the PAR in the first place.

Some Thoughts on Ad Hoc Team Building

Unless personnel are deployed to field hospital units from existing organizations such as military units, often field hospital staff who are put together for the purpose of supporting an operational deployment will never have worked together before. While many newly formed organizations for these types of missions may seize the prospect of initiating impromptu exercises, games, and staff retreats, experience with field operational deployments demonstrates that they are largely unnecessary and a waste of time.

Firstly, it should be assumed that operational deployers are largely mature and experienced health-care and public-health professionals. They are completely capable of – and used to – getting to know new colleagues and working effectively with fellow team members without having to waste valuable (and often unavailable) time with team-building games and activities. Secondly, as experienced health-care and public-health professionals, they are well aware of the value and importance of team work in meeting organizational mission requirements. They already know how to work as part of a team because they do it daily in

their nonoperational work environments. In fact, most have spent their entire professional careers working in teams with people they have frequently never met before. Above all, health care requires this skill, as well as the ability to rapidly adapt to the environments and situations they have cause to confront.

Nevertheless, the real focus is not how to help health-care workers carry on superficial conversations and get to like one another but to create an environment where their natural team tendencies, their intuition, their skills, and their talents can flourish. This should be the goal of building a strong health-care team within an emerging field environment: giving them fertile ground to do, and do well with, what they have been trained to accomplish, and the results will almost invariably follow.

The following are offered as a series of suggestions to create an environment that supports the natural ability of health-care and public-health professionals to form teams and work effectively within them:

1. Communicate prior to deployment. While this is not always possible, it is definitely advantageous. If the team can meet once or twice before deployment – in person, by phone, or by Skype – it will start the team-building process. If they cannot meet in person, pass around the contact information for those who will be working in the field hospital and encourage communication. They will do the rest. Experience shows that emerging staff will begin contacting each other to coordinate ahead of the deployment because they understand the value of this early contact. Experience also demonstrates that they will begin discussing the equipment that should be brought and who will bring it, begin sharing knowledge about the location and the crisis, and they will even discuss what kind of personal items they are packing. As the team members begin to organize themselves, they will get to know each other and they will breed professional and personal familiarity without even realizing it.

2. Communicate during the deployment. It is unnecessary to have constant, formal administrative "round-table" discussions during deployments to build the team and debrief, especially after particularly bad days. Most people tend to believe that these constant meetings distract them from the core mission of providing the medical and public-health support the affected

populations they are there to support need the most. Instead, invite the team members who are not working to dinner after work. Give them a safe, comfortable, and relaxed space to converse and, again, they will do the rest of the work. They will get to know each other. They will become invested in the lives and experiences of each other. They will provide emotional and psychological support to fellow team members (most of the time, that is all they need as health-care workers: the chance to share a difficult experience and to hear encouraging words from someone who is in a similar situation and understands). These informal moments can result in amazing team-building.

3. Ask and listen. Health-care workers have an abundance of experience in knowing what to do best in a team. One only has to look to the different roles and functions that each member of a code-blue team has to assume in order for that team to function effectively and achieve their goals of bringing back a heart-attack victim from the brink of death. They know the best place for their experience and expertise to function at its maximally well-suited capacity. Ask health-care workers what they excel at and where they feel most comfortable in team. Almost invariably, they will give you the truth (for the most part, there will be only a few who either under- or overestimate their strengths and weaknesses, since they recognize above all else that lives hang in the balance of the honesty of their personal assessments). Deployment team leaders should carefully listen to their answers and use that information to build the structure of the team. Be aware that it will take some rearranging until the team becomes efficient, but continue to ask and remain fluid in rearranging team organizations based on that feedback. Leadership will soon find their staff know where they belong and will eventually fall into their most functional roles. When a health-care member is "in their element," they are especially efficient, effective, and helpful. Leadership should simply become facilitators to helping these professionals fall into their "rightful" place, and eventually will find that they have gelled into a highly functional and capable team.

4. Finally, and almost above all else, limit micromanagement. There is almost nothing more damaging to a competent team of health-care professionals. It throws off their flow. It causes division among the team members. It facilitates an environment where team members do not feel valued, heard, or appreciated. In medicine and public health, each team is connected by a common thread, and if one team member goes down, the rest of the team feels the effects. Field-hospital leaders should focus on helping their staff gain their operational footing by facilitating their staff's ability to find their professional niches, and then letting them do what they do best.

Summary

At the dawn of the twenty-first century, one could argue that we are seeing an increase in the frequency – and scope and scale of impact – of disasters worldwide. The confluence of such factors as a significant increase in the global population (300% since 1918–1919, thereby creating a larger PAR), 70% of the world's population living within 100 km of the littorals (placing them at greater risk of seismic, meteorological, and hydrological disasters), the rise of the "megacity" globally (leading to the phenomenon of "clustering," where the PAR already places an enormous burden on available critical infrastructure, which tends to immediately collapse when disasters occur), and climate crisis (which may be contributing to a variety of the complex emergencies and disasters we are experiencing in the first place) only points to the fact that we will be seeing a concurrent increase in the number of times we will have to deploy field medical assets in the first place. Ultimately, it is the personnel who support these important resources that will make the most significant difference in lives saved and reduced suffering. That said, no two disasters are ever the same. Planners who are responsible for sourcing personnel to deployable platforms are cautioned to remain deliberate, adaptive, and flexible to ensure that the right people and skill sets are in place to help ensure a positive outcome to their incident management efforts.

Notes to the Text

1. This particular initiative is often overlooked, especially when organizations deploying field personnel do not have doctrine and policy associated with protecting their deployers. Many times, we make the wrongful assumption that deployers do not become part of the PAR when they enter the field environment, but the

fact is that, in the environment they are operating in, they are facing many, if not all, of the same risks as the PAR they are there to support.

2. Engaging personnel who are to scheduled to be sourced to deployable field hospitals in exercises is a relatively simple matter for military personnel. However, this is not the case for many medical- and public-health-centric NGOs/PVOs, who rely on volunteers who frequently deploy from brick-and-mortar health-care facilities, which are not directly affiliated with the organizations that deploy them to field units.

References

1. Miller PD. *Both swords and plowshares: military roles in the 1990s*. Cambridge: Institute for Foreign Policy; 1992.

2. Powell CL. *Chairman of the joint chiefs of staff report on the roles, missions, and functions of the armed forces of the United States*. Washington DC: Government Printing Office; 1993.

3. National Research Council (2005). Naval analytical capabilities: improving capabilities-based planning. https://books.google.com/books?id=KuJVAg AAQBAJ&q=

4. Rumsfeld DH (2002). Transforming the military. https://www.foreignaffairs.com/articles/2002-05-01/transform ing-military

5. Office of the Chairman of the Joint Chiefs of Staff. *Joint Planning. Joint Publication 5.0*. Washington DC: Government Printing Office; 2017.

6. White KB, Griffith JB. *The well-managed healthcare organization*, 8th edn. Chicago: Health Administration Press; 2016.

8

Leading the Mission
Organizational Structure and Operations

Yitshak Kreiss and Yoel Har-Even

Introduction

Due to the complexity and uncertainty of health care in an emergency-setting environment, effective field-hospital leadership is essential. This type of leadership demands a structured management and task-orientated chain of command. This chapter will describe a comprehensive conceptual model for effective field hospital leadership and the organizational structure and operational system supporting the hospital leadership, and will propose a basic framework for field hospital leadership development.

Command and Control

The lines of command and control in the field hospital include the hospital leadership group (HLG), the hospital operation and organizational structure, and the leadership functions and processes. These are described in more detail below.

The Hospital Leadership Group (HLG)

The HLG is the operational staff of the mission leader. The HLG comprises several professionals and its main role is to enhance the leadership capabilities and functions, and to augment the medical outcome and team performance.

The main objectives of the HLG are to:

- guarantee mission accomplishment
- integrate the work of the different hospital units
- enable maximal security for the staff and patients
- analyze the internal and external environment and adjust accordingly
- be responsible for the needs of the staff and patients
- implement logistic support
- execute strategic and tactical planning
- allocate resources in a sapient manner
- establish local and international collaboration

Figure 8.1 shows a generic structure of the leadership group for a complex mission. However, it is important to remember that this is a basic structure, which can be adjusted to specific types of missions by adding or removing staff members.

Designated Roles and Responsibilities

The following describes the various roles, along with their responsibilities, of each member of the HLG:

Deputy/Chief of Staff

- acts as a stand-in and replacement for the hospital leader, in his or her absence
- is responsible for the output of the HLG and for synchronizing the various elements within the medical mission's management
- coordinates and synchronizes all elements of the mission, including logistics and auxiliary services
- ensures the daily routines are carried out and maintains them
- communicates with rescue mission, in the event there is one
- sets up the hospital and ensures it is dismantled at the end of the mission
- responsible for the process of "lessons learned" and "conclusions reached" during and following a mission, regarding his or her area of responsibility

Chief Medical Officer

- reports directly to the hospital leader on all medical issues within the hospital compound
- serves as the most senior medical authority and, as such, is the primary authority in the medical decision-making process and in determining treatment policies
- ensures the medical personnel have certifications and ensures their professional

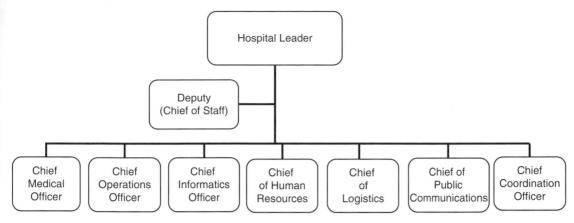

Figure 8.1 Example structure of the HLG

fitness to accomplish the medical tasks, prior to deployment

- coordinates all the activities of the hospital's ethics committee
- organizes knowledge management and on-the-job learning
- holds medical staff meetings to discuss medical issues, dilemmas, and treatment policies
- records and organizes lessons learned from investigations and meetings

Chief Operations Officer

- coordinates patient flow to and from the hospital, as well as the patient evacuation process
- ensures operational continuity
- manages and organizes the activity of the hospital headquarters
- responsible for the security of hospital personnel and equipment
- organizes and prioritizes planned and unplanned activities
- coordinates the various teams' activities outside of the hospital
- gathers and records all operational data pertaining to the hospital
- reports to the hospital leader on all ongoing operational aspects

Chief Informatics Officer

- distributes informatics infrastructure and communications equipment

- responsible for all medical data collected and accumulated throughout the mission, including data recording and storage
- formats medical data for reporting to local authorities and the dispatching organization
- manages informatics personnel
- responsible for operating and maintaining all equipment pertaining to informatics infrastructure and communications
- reports to the hospital leader

Chief of Human Resources

- responsible for utilization of personnel
- distributes personnel between the various hospital departments, including task shifting as needed
- manages personnel shortages and replenishments
- manages the logistical care of personnel casualties
- looks after the personal needs and welfare of personnel
- ensures personnel rest and recreation
- reports to the hospital leader on all functions and processes related to the human resource component of the mission

Chief of Logistics

- responsible for all logistical issues pertaining to managing and running the hospital, from preparations and deployment through debriefing on return home
- manages the logistics department

- ensures ongoing medical and logistic supplies and conducts all purchasing and equipping as they arise

Chief of Public Communications

- answers directly to the hospital leader on all issues and tasks pertaining to outreach and communications to the local public population
- acts as a spokesperson to, and coordinates communications with, the mass media and social media.
- coordinates all activity connected with communications and the local population pertaining to their medical treatment

Chief of Coordination

- maximizes capabilities by collaboration
- responsible for all contact and coordination with the authorities in the host country
- responsible for all contact and coordination with international governmental and nongovernmental organizations (NGOs)
- briefs local health authorities, the Emergency Medical Team Coordination Cell (EMTCC), and the health cluster

- establishes contact and coordination with adjacent local and international medical teams and search-and-rescue teams

Organizational Structure

Hospital Structure

To allow the hospital to operate effectively and independently, it is necessary to define, alongside the HLG, the organizational structure that enables effective operation of the hospital. The organizational structure illustrated in Figure 8.2 is a model tested over three decades by the Israel Defense Forces (IDF) Medical Corps field hospital in numerous missions. This structure is generally similar to the basic structure of a small- to medium-scale hospital during routine times. At the same time, it allows for the more focused and simple management processes that are required in nonroutine scenarios, such as emergencies or disasters.

We have chosen to place the mental health-care professionals under auxiliary services due to the basic intention that their main task is to treat the medical team. Having said that, and as mentioned, this is a basic workforce configuration, which can be adjusted and, of course, the mental health-care professionals can be called on to treat those patients or the affected population in need of help and assistance.

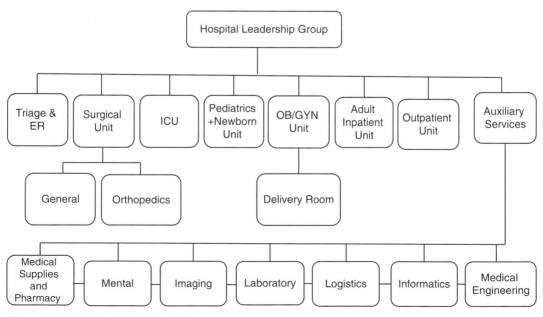

Figure 8.2 Organizational structure model

Leadership Functions and Processes

The operation of a field hospital requires a wide range of functions and processes. This section focuses on the central functions and processes, which are key for the effective leadership of a field hospital in any scenario, and methods for adapting them for extreme situations.

Setting and Operating with Clear Vision and Organizational Values

This is important for every leader in any situation, and requires modifying the mindset to strategic thinking, consolidating organizational thought, developing a vision, aligning viewpoints, and setting goals. The importance of these skills greatly increases during emergency field-hospital scenarios when uncertainty and time pressure emphasize the need for an almost automatic response.

Hospital leaders are expected to keep mission and organizational values in mind in the decision-making process and stay true to their values, even when it may be tempting to back out[1]. A clear vision based on well-established values guides leaders and individuals to act properly, sometimes against instincts or even under life-threatening situations, as in extreme disasters such as the earthquake in Haiti[2], the 9/11 attack in New York City[3], or the genocide in Rwanda[4,5]. This is essential not only for the leaders but also for medical professionals who should be educated to understand they have a responsibility to contribute to the effective operation of the hospital in which they work and to its direction and objectives.

Clear vision is also the major driving force to move individuals and teams in light of the "drop-in-the-sea" phenomenon. In an environment of a massive number of victims in which there are only limited resources by definition, leaders may face frustration, which may have a negative impact on hospital function. In such cases, the clearer the vision is, the stronger the values are, and the more they are shared, the more it will be understood that numbers are not the only thing that counts, but rather the value of saving lives and the role of bringing hope.

Planning: Strategic and Tactical

Field-hospital emergency missions are usually characterized by a highly demanding environment with multiple constraints mandating continuous environment analysis, effective resource allocation, and rapid operation, especially in the early-response phase. Therefore, planning is crucial as a key factor for preparedness, readiness, rapid response, and, subsequently, effective decision-making[2,6]. This process is composed of planning at both the strategic level and the tactical level.

The strategic level is concerned with defining goals and determining the missions and resources to achieve them, such as the type of hospital to deploy, the potential length of deployment, the type of environment at the deployment area, and resource considerations. It should be *continuous*, beginning before the mission, through day-to-day operations, to the planning of an exit strategy, and, just as importantly, with a view beyond the scope of the crisis, on the day after and during the recovery phase. The planning process must be *adaptable* to the rapidly changing environment and *integrative*, combining all the elements essential for effective decision-making, including political, social, demographic, logistic, and medical aspects.

However, strategic-level planning alone is not enough in times of emergency or crisis. The HLG should also be able to create short-term planning at the tactical level, which includes role rotation of medical personnel, flexibility in team structure, and creative solutions. The HLG should design the outcome-oriented planning process framework by choosing a destination, evaluating alternative routes, and deciding the specific course of the plan[7]. Moreover, due to the unpredictability of the situation, hospital leaders should be able to shift from the strategic level of planning to the tactical level and switch between them according to the changing environment, the needs and the required adjustments[2,8]. For example, during the Haiti mission, after the earthquake in 2010, the IDF field-hospital leadership needed to decide on the optimal type of field hospital to erect in response to this earthquake[2]. The options included a "light" hospital, which would provide primary treatment to many patients, or a more sophisticated hospital with advanced capabilities from a wide variety of specialties, which would limit the number of potentially treatable victims. The IDF leadership's choice of the latter option was based on prior experience with disasters in general and earthquakes in particular where local hospital infrastructure is often destroyed and many victims who need hospital-level care require evacuation either to facilities lying outside the affected region or to mobile hospitals deployed locally with capabilities to treat such injuries. We understood that expected delegations would mostly be bringing "light" hospitals and clinical facilities, and so we decided to transport a sophisticated field hospital capable of providing advanced care. This decision proved to be appropriate in Haiti, but we soon faced having to cope with changes in the medical requirements of an earthquake zone over time. In the first few days, we had to concentrate our efforts on treating earthquake-related injuries, and so we transformed one orthopedic treatment station into a surgical unit with full anesthetic and monitoring capabilities, thus doubling our surgical capacity. We also shifted medical staff members, especially nurses, from nonsurgical units to general and orthopedic surgery units. A few days later, when patients presented with less urgent medical needs, we again readjusted staff assignments, organization of the units, and the indications for hospitalization. Such intramission adaptability, as we have learned, is possible when there is maximal versatility in staff training and capabilities, and in utilization of equipment and adjustment of organizational structure. Most importantly, it requires a clear understanding of commitment to the goal at the individual level, as well as continuous, adaptive, and integrative planning processes at the leadership level.

Executing Communication and Negotiation, and Adopting Collaboration as a Strategy

These capabilities may be developed gradually in routine times, but should be practiced intensely and adopted more rapidly in emergency settings, which demand quick teambuilding, managing multidisciplinary staff, resolving conflicts, and building group resilience and endurance. Field-hospital leaders should become the mediators internally and externally to minimize miscommunication and maximize agreement and understanding. They are also required to develop their team members' personal qualities of communication and negotiation to work effectively with each other.

In crisis situations, working alone is simply not an option and collaboration is therefore vital. It may be simple when it concerns coordination of patient transfer or sharing supplies, but when it comes to working together, side by side, treating the same patient or in the same operating room, it becomes much more complex. This task will be even more complicated in an unfamiliar environment with

potential barriers impeding the collaboration such as language, political and legal issues; differing attitudes; variability in accepted working procedures; and a lack of time to create firm interpersonal connections. Therefore, the skills of communication and negotiation should be adapted and developed toward communicating with new partners and building the outer circles of cooperation[9].

The strategy during emergency situations is to encourage operating a wide variety of communication channels and negotiating with local operators, international organizations, the local population, and other medical teams. We recommend educating the hospital leaders to adopt collaboration as a strategy and to understand they are obligated to overcome barriers of language and culture, and to find methods to bridge differences in working procedures and regulations.

Analysis of a Complex Environment

The ability to analyze a complex environment in an orderly manner is an essential element of effective leadership during field-hospital emergency operations. This environment, which is influenced by safety considerations and a high level of uncertainty, requires the leader to process information in an organized manner, and to analyze several operational alternatives in a vastly limited window of response time.

Moreover, in emergency situations, the medical outcome may be influenced by nonmedical parameters. It is therefore essential to educate and train medical leaders to broaden their perspective and to add additional aspects to their emergency analysis. These include the following:

- Political issues: it is important that the leader understands the political environment to operate the hospital effectively. Safety parameters, evacuation destinations, using the environment resources, and coordination with local and international teams differ between field hospitals working in areas with a well-functioning health administration and those in conflict zones, refugee camps, or areas with nonfunctioning governmental systems.
- Legal and ethical considerations: part of the effective medical leadership required in operating field hospitals is to learn the legal and ethical aspects of the deployment area, the guidelines for operating foreign teams in the hospital in regard

to credentials and licensing, and the impact of the local legal system.

- Social and cultural considerations: a major factor influencing the outcome of any health system is the cultural environment and attitudes to health care. This may be even more prominent in times of crisis because societies differ in the way they change their behavior during emergency or crisis, including, for example, health-care consuming habits, level of acceptance of foreign health-care professionals, the basic trust the local society has in its government and health systems, and the basic attitude toward life, death, and care for dead bodies. Effective environmental analysis may direct leaders to adjust modes of operation; for example, in areas where patients are concerned about referral to a foreign hospital, teams can contact them or ask local medical personnel to escort patients to the hospital. Hospital leaders should bear in mind that trust building takes time and requires deep understanding and acceptance of cultural diversities, so they should rapidly address this issue and work inside and outside the hospital to build trust with the local population.

- Medical factors: in the routine operation of a hospital, the medical factors are familiar to the hospital leadership, but during a disaster or in an emergency, the medical factors, by definition, are unfamiliar and uncertain. Therefore, a rapid, holistic, and integrative assessment is essential. Hospital leadership should analyze the number and types of injuries and their flow patterns, the functionality of local medical infrastructure, existing neighboring teams, evacuation routes and facilities, types of local morbidity, and medical hazards. The hospital leaders should be ready to cope with different and unfamiliar types of morbidity in the deployment area and therefore create mechanisms of consultation and knowledge generation in real time.

- Expect the unexpected: in any type of crisis management, the leader should expect unexpected threats to the mission. We do not recommend preparing for all potential threats, but the hospital leadership is encouraged to be aware that immediate and unexpected hazards – such as threats to safety, shortages of personnel or essential supplies, decrease of evacuation facilities, or sudden change in the environment – will always

happen and the hospital leadership must create a mechanism for rapid assessment and response. Hannah and colleagues[10] suggest that the ability to give meaning and to simplify complex situations to formed schemas for individuals constitute critical intervention points for leadership. The leader's judgment and action (or inaction) will determine the potential impact on the outcome.

Rapid Decision-Making Based on Situational Assessment

This capacity is essential for any leader, especially for field-hospital leaders in emergency settings who must make complex decisions under conditions of time pressure, uncertainty, and scarce resources.

Different types of decisions are required during emergency management, both at the leadership level and at the individual level. Many of them – such as hospitalization dynamics, policy of surge capacity, workload of professional personnel, and level of security – change from mission to mission and along the mission phases, and have the potential to threaten the success of the mission. Therefore, field-hospital leaders must design the decision-making process in accordance with the specific type of mission and the different phases of the scenario. We suggest the hospital leadership build a structured command and control process, based on continuous situational assessment as a basic tool for rapid decision-making. One model for such a design may be composed of the following systematic process, which includes setting a daily routine for the hospital with periodic planning sessions and situational assessment, establishing a reporting system with response to immediate crises, and appointment and operation of the designated committees such as infection control, supply, and ethics.

One example for such a decision-making challenge is how to deal with the need for surge capacity during field hospital operation when there is no centralized triage mechanism in the area. When the hospital is at full capacity – usually more quickly than is anticipated – it cannot continue to admit patients after hospitalization capability is fully utilized. During the acute phase of the response in Haiti after the earthquake, to cope with this extremely frustrating situation, new patients were accepted as soon as space became available, and were discharged sooner than was ideal to make room for new arrivals. Due to there being no centralized triage mechanism to direct patients to one facility versus another, we notified each "light" hospital and other health facilities that, for every patient referred to the field hospital for a higher level of care, we would expect the referring facility to be willing to accept one of the field hospital's patients for immediate postoperative management in exchange. This policy enabled the throughput of the operating rooms to be maximized by increasing the number of operations and procedures that the field hospital was in a unique position to perform, while ensuring that patients received appropriate postoperative care.

Probably one of the most complicated examples of the unique decision-making capacity required for the medical leader in an emergency field hospital operation is the challenge of unusual ethical dilemmas, which have immediate impact on life and death. Emergencies and disasters pit personal, professional, and public interests against each other, and create complex ethical dilemmas, which are at the center of emergency management. These dilemmas include treatment priorities, triage considerations, limits of care, withholding treatment, and dealing with surge capacity and resource allocation according to survival chances and not according to the individual needs. Field-hospital leaders must be prepared to confront these complex ethical issues to be able to make decisions and take relevant action[6]. We encourage field-hospital leaders to use generic tools during emergencies, but also to create onsite leadership supporting mechanisms such as ethical committees, adjusted to the specific environment, which will help establish an ethical and practical system of medical priorities in a chaotic setting. Such a structured system of decision-making was described after the earthquake in Haiti[11] and similar processes were reported after Hurricane Katrina struck in 2005 and Hurricane Sandy in 2012[12–14].

Managing People and Building Their Endurance

Probably the most important factor predicting mission success is endurance, both at the hospital level and at the individual level. Therefore, one of the major roles of the field-hospital leadership is to continuously strengthen team endurance before, during, and after the mission. Building this kind of endurance in an unfamiliar environment that precipitates or sustains a crisis or event, such as a natural disaster or conflict, in a disorganized setting, is challenging but crucial. The field-hospital workers may experience specific risks and situations related to the provision of humanitarian care, such as[15]: reduced levels of security and protection; damaged or absent infrastructure, including limits in the availability of food, water,

lodging, transportation, and health services; unstable climate conditions; lack of running water; provisory toilets, and limited sanitation and hygiene conditions.

These external stress factors augment the more prominent hospital internal stress factors, such as the heavy workload with long working hours, the mental and physical stress facing ethical and moral dilemmas related to the event, the close contact with the affected population, and the language and cultural barriers with the patients and their families. This extremely stressful environment must direct hospital leaders to actively develop their people's endurance and to be more directive and transactional[10].

The first step is to acknowledge the need for building endurance, the fact that it takes time, and that it is much harder to build during the mission, so the process is continuous and must begin prior to deployment. Leaders must understand the milieu of their team and their organizational behavior, and work continuously to motivate them to develop and strengthen their commitment to the mission.

At the individual level, especially during the stressful early phases of deployment, hospital leaders should dedicate time to identify and understand their people's needs, possibly even before they are expressed, using informal one-to-one talks to build a bond with them. Leaders should understand and accept their team's quirks and weaknesses, address their desires, ambitions, tensions, and fears to help each person reach his or her potential and to steer their people effectively toward the mission. In the later phases of the mission, leaders should be aware of the cumulative effects of hard work, austere conditions, intense interpersonal interaction, and homesickness; all of which can have a negative effect on individual and team. At this stage, the first signs of burnout appear in the medical staff, which can manifest differently from one person to the next. It is therefore expected of the medical leaders, at all levels, to actively try to identify the first signs of burnout and treat them with the help of all the means at their disposal, including professional involvement of the mental-health team.

At the institutional level, leaders may effectively strengthen endurance by employing the following strategies:

- Teaming: field-hospital leaders should rapidly enhance transformation of the individual professionals into a strongly cohesive team, establish a shared identity, and constantly reinforce the team message. This continuous teaming process includes another component:

subteam building, which is the forming of special teams for tough assignments, balancing talent and expertise in each group, and ensuring the groups are keeping the same pace and helping each other.

- Anti-chaos measures: the best way to manage and motivate medical staff working in a disorganized environment or in chaos is to create order. Leaders can set personal examples, demonstrating memorable behaviors and symbolism, maintain routine, operate under a strict schedule and organizational discipline, and establish order when needed[2,14]. This leadership challenge is more prominent in nonmilitary or newly formed civilian field hospitals. In these facilities, personnel may come from a wide variation of backgrounds with differing ideologies, experience, and levels of commitment. Moreover, these facilities may lack a structured hierarchy or chain of management and pose added leadership challenges. In such situations, field-hospital leadership should focus on trust building, common language, and professional procedures.

- Keep sight of the big picture: an important dilemma in leading people in emergency situations is the question of how much information to share with personnel. Sharing information and exposing medical crew to the big picture may help them cope better with the stress, but it can sometimes increase their mental burden and cause frustration due to fact that the capacity to help a few in a disaster area is only a "drop in the sea." Our experience proves it is better to share the big picture in most cases, but to continuously work to identify those groups and individuals who may need a different or modified approach.

- Insisting on rest and debriefing: when faced with people who are in danger and need of assistance, medical personnel in emergency situations tend to work round the clock and can quickly wear themselves out. This can lead people to work less effectively over time and may endanger their mental health. The leader should sometimes go against this tendency and force his or her staff to rest and recharge. The leader should also establish mechanisms for regular debriefings to provide staff with opportunity to relieve stress. This task should continue even postmission due to the possibility of late-onset reactions to disaster scenarios among medical personnel[16].

Crisis Leadership as a Web Interaction

The influx of knowledge and information during a crisis is so extensive that a single person alone cannot retain it all[17]. Therefore, effective crisis leadership is also the outcome of a web interaction of groups rather than just the direct influence of a leader [19,20]. This dynamic leadership evolves while different proxies interact inside this web and create new types of behaviors and actions, making those organizations more creative, flexible, adaptive, and effective in dealing with the uncertainties. The hospital leadership role is, therefore, to create the opportunities for their crew members to develop their own individual leadership and to encourage them to express it. This type of "shared leadership" may augment effectiveness of the formal hospital leadership and lead to creative, out-of-the-box, original, and innovative solutions, which are essential in crisis scenarios. Shared leadership will increase the commitment of individual leaders to the mission and, through them, the whole staff. When team members feel included in the decision-making process, this increases their faith in the leaders.

Shared leadership has an additional benefit. It allows formal leaders to sometimes find the direction they need not only in their commanding level, which may be far away from the arena, but also in their team members, who are exposed to the same environment. For example, when making life-and-death specific ethical decisions, or deciding on admission policy, hospital leaders may find the guidance they need from team members. The overall responsibility does not change as ultimate responsibility always remains with the leader but sharing leadership can not only contribute to the effectiveness of the decision-making process but also can relieve the mental stress on the formal leaders themselves.

Crisis Leadership Development

While medicine focuses on decision-making at the individual physician–patient level, leadership involves stepping back and examining problems at a higher level, thus requiring the ability to view issues broadly and systemically[21]. As medical education evolves with the passage of time and adapts itself to an ever-increasing knowledge base, the area of leadership remains underdeveloped[22]. Health-care professionals are trained in the diagnostic, therapeutic, and administrative aspects of patient care, but not enough in the theoretical and practical aspects of assuming and delivering leadership. The curricula in many schools fail to incorporate an organized leadership training (designated courses or practice) as part of both graduate and postgraduate studies and this stems from a lack of recognition of the critical role medical professionals must play as leaders. This is even more crucial when it comes to leadership during emergency, crisis, and disasters.

This chapter describes the required leadership skills and capabilities for field hospitals in times of emergency. Assuming that effective leadership requires basic personal capabilities and motivation to lead and influence others, one should bear in mind that effective leadership can be built and developed like any other skill[23]. Moreover, while many leaders possess character traits essential for leadership during routine times, and may have acquired relevant leadership skills in the course of their lives and careers, health-care institutions should incorporate formal crisis leadership training as an essential component of every health-care education and can do so by adopting a comprehensive conceptual model to use as the core for education, training, and preparedness.

Just as pre-mission training is essential for all medical teams intending to deploy to disaster zones and austere environments, preparation of team leaders is just as important to develop the appropriate skills to fulfill their role in leading their teams in these challenging scenarios.

Take-Home Messages

Leadership is one of the most researched social phenomena, with a wide spectrum of definitions, parameters, and theories. Some parameters discussed in this chapter are generic and might apply to leadership in all emergency situations, and not specifically in field hospitals; nevertheless, field-hospital leadership has its own uniqueness and complexity.

Regardless of their background, education, training, environment, and skills, each hospital leader will use a different leadership style by finding a unique element within him- or herself: embracing and utilizing it. Leadership style depends not only on the leader's personality but also on the environment he or she is operating in and on their team members. No matter which leadership style is used, the most important factors for effective leadership are the interface between personality, skills, and capabilities; the interaction with those being led; and influencing the immediate surrounding environment. Effective field-hospital leaders should possess the ability to switch between leadership styles suited to the different situations and adjust them accordingly.

References

1. Fields, SA. Leadership in times of crisis. *Family Medicine* 2009: **41**(2): 86–8.

2. Kreiss Y, Merin O, Peleg K, et al. Early disaster response in Haiti: the Israeli field hospital experience. *Annals of Internal Medicine* 2010: **153**(1): 45–8.

3. Giuliani, R. Life leadership it's about preparation and performance. *Leadership Excellence* 2005: **22**(6): 17.

4. Eriksson, JR. *The international response to conflict and genocide: lessons from the Rwanda experience*. Volume 1. Steering Committee of the Joint Evaluation of Emergency Assistance to Rwanda; 1996.

5. Heyman SN, Eldad A, Wiener M. Airborne field hospital in disaster area: lessons from Armenia (1988) and Rwanda (1994). *Prehospital and Disaster Medicine* 1998: **13**(1): 21–8.

6. Merin O, Miskina IN, Lin G, et al. Triage in mass-casualty events: the Haitian experience. *Prehospital and Disaster Medicine* 2011: **26**(5): 386–90.

7. Montana PJ and Charnov BH. *Barron's management book*. 4th edn (2008).

8. Bar-On E, Abargel A, Peleg K, Kreiss Y. Coping with the challenges of early disaster response: 24 years of field hospital experience after earthquakes. *Disaster Medicine and Public Health Preparedness* 2013: **7**(5): 491–8.

9. Shirley PJ, Mandersloot G. Clinical review: the role of the intensive care physician in mass-casualty incidents: planning, organisation, and leadership. *Critical Care* 2008: **12**(3): 214.

10. Hannah ST, Mary B, Bruce A, Cavarretta FL (2009). A framework for examining leadership in extreme contexts. Management Department Faculty Publications. Online article. http://digitalcommons.unl.edu/managementfacpub/39

11. Merin O, Ash, N Levy G, Schwaber, MJ, Kreiss Y. The Israeli field hospital in Haiti – ethical dilemmas in early disaster response. *The New England Journal of Medicine* 2010: **362**(11): e38.

12. Paschal, D. Launching complex medical workups from an urgent care platform. *Annals of Internal Medicine* 2012: **156**(3): 232–3.

13. Powell T, Hanfling D, Gostin LO. *Emergency preparedness and public health: the lessons of Hurricane Sandy*. JAMA 2012: **308**(24): 2569–70.

14. Hurricane Sandy puts NJ hospital under extreme stress, highlighting vulnerabilities, areas requiring improvement. *ED Management* 2013: **25**(1): 1–5.

15. Gushulak BD. Humanitarian aid workers (2014) Chapter 8, *Yellow Book*. Website. http://wwwnc .cdc.gov/travel/yellowbook/2014/chapter-8

16. Knobler HY, Nachshoni T, Jaffe E, Peretz G, Yehuda YB. Psychological guidelines for a medical team debriefing after a stressful event. *Military Medicine* 2007: **172**(6): 581–5.

17. Uhl-Bien M, Marion R, McKelvey B. Complexity leadership theory: shifting leadership from the industrial age to the knowledge era. *The Leadership Quarterly* 2007: **18**(4): 298–318.

18. Tobi SPC. Military leadership in an era of complex systems (In Hebrew). *Views of Leadership* 2011: **3**: 29–51.

19. Pearce CL. The future of leadership: combining vertical and shared leadership to transform knowledge work. *The Academy of Management Executive* 2004: **18**(1): 47–57.

20. Tobi SC, Zomer GA. *Principles of military leadership development* (In Hebrew). IDF leadership School; 2012.

21. Collins-Nakai R. Leadership in medicine. *McGill Journal of Medicine* 2006: **9**(1): 68–73.

22. Pronovost PJ, Miller MR, Wachter RM. Perspective: Physician leadership in quality. *Academic Medicine* 2009: **84**(12): 1651–6 10.1097/ACM.

23. Gonen I, Zakay E. *Leadership and leadership development: theory to practice* (In Hebrew). Ministry of Defense, Publishing House, the Education and Youth Corps, Leadership Development School, Israel Defense Forces; 1999.

Coordination and Organization of Medical Relief to Affected Areas

Kobi Peleg, Moran Bodas, and Ian Norton

Introduction

Providing humanitarian relief to affected populations is a top priority following a major sudden-onset disaster (SOD). These global-scale disasters can generate huge numbers of casualties and extensive damage to local infrastructure, including medical facilities. In many cases, the need to handle the surge in demand for immediate lifesaving procedures, as well as long-term public health management, surpasses the ability of the local health-care system. This is especially true if medical facilities sustain damages, and/or if health-care personnel are affected. Consequently, and as is often the case, the affected population is in dire need of medical aid to support the overloaded and crumbling local health-care system. The international aid during the initial life-saving phase usually takes the form of urban search and rescue (USAR) teams and emergency medical teams (EMTs) sent by donating countries and nongovernmental organizations (NGOs) not affected by the disaster. This chapter focuses on the latter.

Most destructive natural disasters and associated casualties take place in specific regions and in a small number of countries. Asia sees the most disasters, fatalities, and affected populations. Africa has the highest death rate[1]. According to the UN University's World Risk Report from 2016, the global hotspots for a high disaster risk are in Oceania, Southeast Asia, Central America, and the southern Sahel region in Africa. The countries most gravely affected typically belong to the low-income or developing categories. This means that they already face sanitation problems, limited access to suitable drinking water, and limited public awareness of threat reduction and mitigation measures[2]. Consequently, major disasters striking these regions often result in a high number of casualties and a need for external assistance[1]. Major changes are occurring within regions with a growing number of middle income countries in historically disaster prone regions are becoming more resilient with national response teams and the rise in regional entities such as ASEAN

(Association of Southeast Asian Nations) offering support between countries in their region.

The main form of medical relief to affected areas is the EMTs, formerly known as foreign medical teams (FMTs) (the term was changed to expand the definition so as to include local medical entities in the affected country). These are groups of health professionals and support staff operating locally or outside their country of origin by providing health care to disaster-affected populations. These health professional groups of physicians, nurses, paramedics, and other health professionals comprise a significant element of the global health workforce, and play an important role in saving lives and supporting the health-care provisions to people affected by an emergency or disaster[3].

In most countries, medical professions are highly regulated, and exercising medical practice is subject to vigorous regulation, accreditation, licensing, and quality control. However, up until very recently, regulations concerning the medical practice in disaster-stricken areas were almost never enforced. In the chaos following the crisis, suboptimal medical care was often encountered. Inevitably, this had hindering effects on achievement of the main goal of saving as many lives as possible and reducing the suffering of the affected population.

The need for increased accountability of humanitarian response, specifically the medical one, has been confirmed from evaluations of many disasters in the past, in particular the Indian Ocean tsunami in 2004 and the 2010 earthquake in Haiti. Usually, under the circumstances of these and similar disasters, the ministry of health (MoH) of the affected country faces a no-win situation: they require urgent medical care, which should be not only be speedy but also effective and professional, but end up with many teams pouring in, some without advance notice or proper registration[4,5].

For these and other reasons, there has been a growing debate over the efficacy of the health-care system based on the medical teams arriving in disaster areas to provide medical treatment to the affected population. The main problems have less to do with the professionality of the teams, rather with the lack of organization, coordination, and integration of these teams into a single and effective health-care system. Experience has shown that, in many cases, the deployment of EMTs is not based on assessed needs. In some cases, teams arrive in affected areas on their own merits regardless of actual necessity. Such teams are often unfamiliar with the international emergency response systems and standards, and may not integrate smoothly into the usual coordination mechanisms[6].

The purpose of this chapter is to describe the development process of the international system for EMT organization and coordination, which was set forth by the World Health Organization (WHO) and other global leaders in an effort to generate a better, more reliable, efficient, and standardized coordination system for medical relief to affected areas.

The Medical Requirements in Disaster-stricken Areas

Before we account the drawbacks of the medical relief system until its recent regulation by WHO, we should first describe the medical needs often present in disaster-stricken areas. Providing medical aid to affected areas comprises several efforts. The first is immediate lifesaving procedures performed on casualties resulting directly from the adverse event. These efforts include emergency and disaster medicine

procedures, such as resuscitation, hemodynamic stabilization, lifesaving surgery, amputations, and so on. Providing immediate, lifesaving medical care efficiently and rapidly is of utmost importance to saving as many lives as possible.

It is important to note that in most cases, especially following a devastating natural disaster such as a large earthquake, the local medical system is strongly impacted. Many of its facilities might be deemed inappropriate to provide medical care due to danger from after-shocks or loss of critical infra-structure, power and access to safe water required for medical care. In addition, a substantial number of the workforce is expected to be absent, be it because they were personally harmed or because they choose to firstly attend to their personal and familial needs before reporting for their duties. The weak and unstable local health-care system is in dire need of substitutes, and these are usually provided in the form of EMTs responding from within and outside the affected region.

However, it is important to understand that, even in events with major trauma impact such as earthquakes, the acute phase of medical care is temporary. Even in events with major trauma impact such as earthquakes, the acute phase is relatively short and, 7 to 10 days after the event, there will be a significant decrease in trauma patients and a rise in patients seeking care due to nontrauma-related complaints and routine medical problems. (see Figure 9.1). These include patients in need of treatment for illnesses or other medical conditions that preceded the disaster, for example, diabetes, pregnancy care or communicable disease such as dengue. Consequently, a very

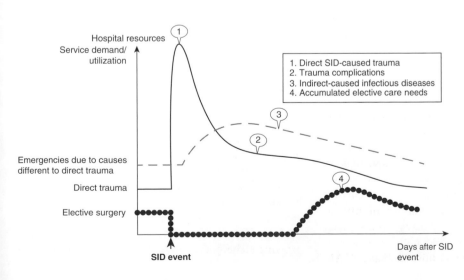

Figure 9.1 Conceptual model for the variation over time of needs/use of hospital resources for nontrauma emergencies, trauma complications and elective surgery before and following a sudden-impact disaster (SID)[8]

different set of medical skills and resources is required to accommodate the shifting needs of the affected population.

Another important aspect of medical relief to affected areas is public health. It is commonly thought that disasters bring about public health emergencies While outbreaks are sometimes seen following a major disaster, it is not the disaster itself that causes them; rather it is the lack of access to suitable drinking water and food supplies, lack of shelter or increase exposure to mosquitoes after floods that give rise to different outbreaks, including diarrhea, respiratory illness or vector borne disease. For example, the contamination of water following the devastating earthquake in Haiti (2010) led to the worst cholera outbreak in the history of the country, affecting ~700 000 and killing about ~9000[7]. However, this need not be the case. If efforts are made (as soon as the response phase is initiated) to secure the affected population with alternative sources of drinkable water and food supply, access to shelter and bed nets outbreaks can be avoided, especially if coupled with public health messages on issues like food hygiene and hand washing. EMT response is now seen as part of a wider public health approach with prevention as important as direct medical care, including public health messaging by the EMTs to the local population.

Other aspects of medical relief in emergencies include restoration of critical services, rehabilitation of the injured, and mental health. [6] and these services are provided both by general EMTs and by "specialist care teams." Historically neglected by

EMTs these aspects are important to consider even in the first days. Providing affected populations with proper health recovery plans and supporting their mental wellbeing are of crucial importance in the stabilization and rehabilitation of the population.

The Medical Relief System in the Mirror of Time

The establishment of the UN in 1945 marked a turning point in the globalization of the humanitarian system. The main beneficiaries of humanitarian aid shifted from Europeans to other populations in need, worldwide. The decolonization process had a profound impact on the emergence of NGOs. In parallel, it also gave rise to a growing number of nonaligned, third-world countries, which continue to express their rights to sovereignty from major power blocs [9,10].

The expanding humanitarian sector entered the 1950s with many elements recognizable in today's system already in place: governance mechanisms, specialized task forces and agencies, and NGOs, all engaged in conflicts, natural disasters, disease outbreaks, and food and nutrition crises, such as the Nigerian Civil War (1967–1970) (see Figure 9.2)[9].

One critical incident took place in the beginning of the 1970s. In November 1970, a severe cyclone and storm surge hit the coastal areas of the Ganges Delta, in what was then East Pakistan, killing an estimated 300 000 people. By the end of 1971, an estimated 10 million refugees sought safety[11]. The East

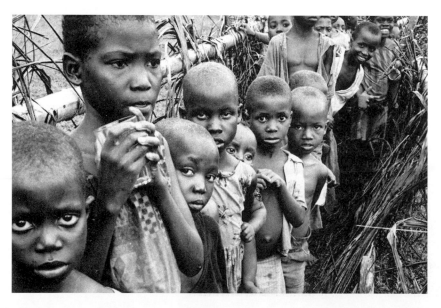

Figure 9.2 Nigerian Civil War, 1967–1970; Umuosu, September to October 1968: food distribution in a feeding center (© ICRC/HD Fink/ng-n-00030–29)

Pakistan crisis, as it was subsequently called, was an extensive refugee crisis that encouraged the UN to take affirmative actions to promote global humanitarian efforts[9]. Arguably, this incident marked the new era of humanitarian and medical relief to affected areas, which led to the current architecture of this system.

The 1970s were a time of rapid evolvement of the humanitarian system. A devastating famine crisis struck countries in the Ethiopia and Sahel region of Africa (Chad, Gambia, Mali, Mauritania, Niger, Senegal, and Upper Volta/Burkina Faso), leading to a global effort to assist the affected population with resource mobilization. However, there is general agreement that these efforts were poorly coordinated within the system and between the system and local governments[9].

Additional crises and disaster situations span across the 1980s and 1990s, including natural disasters (e.g., Ethiopian famine [1984–1985], Armenian earthquake [1988], Somali famine [1991–1992], and Hurricane Mitch [1998]), and armed conflicts (e.g., Bosnia [1991–1995], Somali civil war [1991–1993], First Gulf War [1991], Bosnian War [1992–1995] [see Figure 9.3], Rwandan genocide [1994] [see Figure 9.4], and Kosovo [1999])[9]. These incidents all displayed elements of poor coordination of medical relief operations.

In 1991, the Inter-Agency Standing Committee (IASC) was established by the UN as a platform for coordination between UN agencies on the global level. These efforts were made in light of the understanding that coordination of external relief to affected areas is fundamental for effective humanitarian action[16].

Despite the good intentions, the 6.5-magnitude earthquake that hit Bam, Iran, on December 26, 2003 was another example of the difficulty of medical relief coordination. The devastating earthquake left the local health-care system dramatically impaired and international aid was evidently required. Even though the international community dispatched sufficient quantities of resources, the coordination of these resources was substantially lacking. In fact, Abolghasemi and colleagues[17] claim:

An important lesson learned from the Bam earthquake experience is that the assumption that receiving greater amounts of relief items results in a more effective response, is false. As encountered in the Bam earthquake, extensive international assistance could be burdensome on the management and coordination of the activities, transport, storage, and distribution of relief items.

This incident highlighted the importance of developing a robust mechanism of organization and coordination of medical relief to affected areas[17–19].

The literature provides an elaborate account of other cases demonstrating the multitude of difficulties and deficiencies of the medical relief system up until recently. For example, studies have shown that medical teams focused primarily on trauma care and neglected other aspects of health care such as primary and public health, essential obstetrical care, and pediatrics[20–22]. In addition, medical teams were also criticized for poor medical records keeping[23],

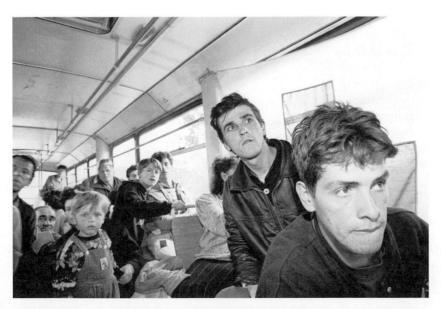

Figure 9.3 Bosnian War, 1992–1995; Počulica, Bosnia, 1993: the ICRC evacuates former detainees, women, and children from Zenica(© ICRC/A Feric/yu-n-00082–05)

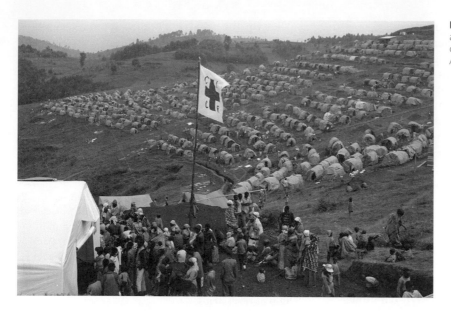

Figure 9.4 Rwandan genocide, 1994; an ICRC medical unit in a camp for displaced people in Cyangugu (© ICRC / P. Fuller / rw-n-00077–02)

administration of technically improper surgical procedures[4], and deficiencies in the fields of training and education, leadership, coordination and management, integration between different teams, organization, and standardization[8,24].

Up until the late 2000s, humanitarian aid missions were often arriving on scenes of affected areas with little to no coordination, as well as insufficient understanding of the situation on the ground, the needs it entails, and inadequate awareness of other teams and delegations operating in the area. As a result, a suboptimal health-care system was operating in the field, one in which the benefit of each medical team was often lost[4,6,8,19,24–28].

The humanitarian reform of 2005, followed by the perceived failure of the humanitarian aid to respond effectively to the Darfur (Sudan) crisis in 2004, introduced new elements to improve capacity, predictability, accountability, leadership, and partnership. The most notable aspect of the reform was the creation of the cluster approach[16]. According to the UN disaster assessment and coordination (UNDAC), which is part of the UN's Office for the Coordination of Humanitarian Affairs (OCHA):

> Clusters are groups of humanitarian organizations (UN and non-UN) working in the main sectors of humanitarian action, e.g. shelter and health. They are created when clear humanitarian needs exist within a sector, when there are numerous actors within sectors and when national authorities need coordination support[29].

The cluster approach was first utilized in the humanitarian response to the 2005 Pakistan earthquake. Arjun Katoch, who was then the deputy head of UNDAC, recalls:

> The UNDAC team led by Gerhard Putman Cramer (of which I was the Deputy Team Leader) used [the cluster approach] as a basis for organizing and writing the Flash Appeal for the Pakistan earthquake. This was approved by Jan Vandermootele, who was the UN Resident Coordinator in Islamabad then (subsequently also the UN Humanitarian Coordinator). There was no conscious decision by either OCHA or the IASC to "deploy" the cluster system. We just decided to use it based on the reform report, as it was a logical continuation of the "sectors" used earlier in natural disaster coordination in the field. These clusters included a health cluster. That was the first use of a health cluster[30].

Additional attempts were made to promote better humanitarian response. For example, efforts were made to share knowledge, experiences, and lessons between members of the humanitarian action community. However, these were often ineffective. Following each disaster incident, practitioners would publish their insights into the humanitarian aid extended, but these were highly specific, cultural-biased, and non-representative. Consequently, generalization of findings was difficult, and there was no practical way to derive overarching conclusions and comprehensive guidelines.

In an effort to achieve better organization and management of medical teams responding to provide humanitarian aid to affected populations, WHO appointed local health officials working on its behalf to assume responsibilities for medical relief coordination during emergencies. Despite good intentions, the expectations for better coordination of medical aid were short lived. The appointed officials, normally tasked with day-to-day health-care issues in the developing countries they were stationed in, were holding insufficient knowledge and expertise in emergency management. Subsequently, coordination of medical aid remained lagging.

An outrage over this suboptimal mechanism was gradually heard, culminating with the 2010 earthquake in Haiti, which is widely agreed as the pivotal point of change in recent years[8,15,18,19,24,28,31]. The 2010 Haiti earthquake was pivotal in the sense that it brought the need of enhancing the EMT system to center stage. Perhaps most prominently, it brought a renewed and strengthened interest toward the accountability of EMTs. Today, it is recognized that there needs to be greater accountability, more stringent oversight, and better coordination of the work of EMTs[3]. It is now widely agreed that standardizing the capabilities of EMTs, their resources, and interoperational guidelines will further improve resource utilization and will facilitate a better mechanism of saving lives[6,8,19,24,25,28]. Yet, to date, there is no single accepted definition of accountability in the humanitarian context[32].

In the aftermath of the Haiti earthquake, WHO recognized the necessity of change in the EMTs system:

> Serious questions have been raised about the clinical competence and practices of some EMTs deployed in recent years. It is now recognized that there needs to be greater accountability, more stringent oversight and better coordination of their work[3].

The remaining question was:– how?

The New EMT System

Following Haiti's earthquake in 2010, the EMT Working Group of the WHO then working under the auspices of the global health cluster (GHC) initiated an effort to standardize the EMT system. The objective was originally to establish a mechanism to assist authorities of affected countries, or in their absence WHO, to formally accept and support only those agencies meeting basic professional and operational requirements[4].

The original conceptualization of the new EMT system drew inspiration from an already well-established mechanism of humanitarian aid to affected areas – the USAR system, which is coordinated by the International Search and Rescue Group (INSARAG). Through a process of lesson learning, common consent, and experience spanning some 25 years, the USAR community has been able to attain a high level of coherence and interoperability, resulting in a highly efficient response to disaster-stricken areas[31].

Of course, no copy–pasting was possible, nor recommended, between the INSARAG and the new EMT system. In fact, several similarities and differences between the two were discussed. Among the similarities are the design to achieve greater clarity and understanding with the aim to improve response coordination, and the clear definition of capabilities by responding entities. Among the differences are (1) the greater mix of actors and complexity of the health-care system compared to the USAR community, (2) the longer periods of deployment needed by EMTs' compared to USAR teams, (3) the number of potential beneficiaries, which is usually greater with the EMTs work, and (4) the differences between the coordinating bodies of the two systems: OCHA for INSARAG and WHO for the EMTs[4,6, 31]. The INSARAG model served as an example for the EMT system on how guidelines can be set up. This was specifically true in terms of classification and technical reference guide[6].

And so, the WHO rethinking process culminated in 2013 with the newly devised *Classification and Minimum Standards for Foreign Medical Teams in Sudden Onset Disasters*. The aim of this document was: *"to develop a simple classification system and registration form to define type, capacities, services, and minimum deployment standards for EMTs that want to respond to the immediate aftermath of a sudden onset disaster"*[6]. To this end, the document lists six guiding principles (see Box 1) and 13 core standards (see Box 2) that are to be observed by all EMTs, as well as the minimum technical standards per type of EMT and for each service. These variables are the reference for a global registration system[6].

The document provides international EMTs with benchmarks to meet when offering their services to affected countries. The standardization of services achieved by the proposed guidelines allows countries offering EMTs to clearly state the services and capacities that they are offering, and countries requiring such support to better communicate their needs[6].

Box 1 The six guiding principles of EMTs' work as set forward by the WHO's GHC[6]

1. The EMT provides safe, timely, effective, efficient, equitable, and patient-centered care.
2. The EMT offers a "needs-based" response according to the context and type of SOD in the affected nation.
3. The EMT adopts a human rights-based approach to their response and ensures they are accessible to all sections of the population affected by the SOD, particularly the vulnerable.
4. The EMT undertakes to treat patients in a medically ethical manner consistent with the World Medical Association Medical Ethics Manual. In particular, the EMT undertakes to respect with confidentiality that patients will have the right to be informed about their medical condition and communication on prognosis and alternative treatments in a language and culturally appropriate fashion, and that all informed consent for medical procedures is obtained in such a manner unless obviously impossible.
5. All EMTs are accountable to the patients and communities they assist, the host government and MoH, their own organization, and donors.
6. EMTs commit to be integrated in a coordinated response under the national health emergency management authorities, and collaborate with the national health system, their fellow EMTs, the cluster, and the international humanitarian response community.

Box 2 The 13 core standards of EMTs' work as set forward by the WHO GHC[6]

1. Agree to register with the relevant national authority or lead international agency on arrival and collaborate with interagency response coordination mechanisms at global, national, and subnational levels, as well as with other EMTs and health systems.
2. Will undertake to report on arrival what type, capacity, and services they can offer based on the international EMT classification system.
3. Will undertake to report at regular intervals during response and prior to departure to the national authorities and the cluster, using national reporting formats or, if not available, the agreed international reporting format.
4. Will undertake to keep confidential records of interventions, clinical monitoring, and possible complications.
5. Will undertake for the individual patient to have records of treatment performed and referral for follow-up planned as needed.
6. Will undertake to be part of the wider health referral system and, depending on type, offer to accept or refer, or both accept and refer patients to other EMTs, the national health system or, if approved, other countries.
7. EMTs will adhere to professional guidelines: all their staff must be registered to practice in their home country and have licenses for the work they are assigned to by the agency.
8. EMTs will ensure that all their staff are specialists in their field, appropriately trained in either war or SOD surgical injury management. The majority should have training and experience in global health, disaster medicine, and providing care in austere environments. Acknowledging the need to train and provide experience to new staff, there may be scope for junior and inexperienced staff in the later phase of a disaster response and working under direct supervision of experienced colleagues.
9. EMTs will ensure that all pharmaceutical products and equipment they bring comply with international quality standards and drug donation guidelines.
10. EMTs are self-sufficient and do not put demand on logistic support from the affected country, unless agreed otherwise before deployment.
11. EMTs comply with minimal hygiene and sanitation standards, including adequate management of medical waste.
12. EMTs must ensure the team and individuals within it are covered by adequate medical malpractice insurance. EMTs must have mechanisms to deal with patient complaints and allegations of malpractice.
13. EMTs must have arrangements in place for the care of their team members' health and safety, including repatriation and exit strategies if required.

The WHO standard divides EMTs into three distinct categories, and EMTs are expected to declare which category they belong to: type 1 (primary health and emergency care), type 2 (basic field hospital), or type 3 (full field hospital). Classification to a given category is made depending on the EMT's capacities and capabilities, as well as any additional specialist services they can provide. Breakdown of EMT type is performed by addressing the following criteria: initial assessment and triage, resuscitation, patient stabilization and referral, wound care, fracture management, anesthesia, surgery, intensive care, communicable disease care, maternal health, child health, chronic disease emergency care, mental health, rehabilitation, laboratory and blood bank, pharmacy and drug supply, radiology, sterilization, and logistical support. The defining scales are described in the WHO's standard to determine EMT required capacities for each criterion. EMTs are expected to confirm that they are able and willing to meet the guiding principles and adhere to the minimum standards. The EMT can then, following consultation with the receiving country, provide services within a functioning national hospital or health center, or offer to bring a field facility with them[6]. Recent changes include the splitting of the Type 1 description into Mobile and Fixed teams given the large numbers deployed to Philippines Typhoon 2013 Nepal Earthquake 2015 with marked differences in capacity and requirements. The Typology of Specialist care teams has also expanded to over 20 with teams now recognized for outbreak response, rehabilitation, specialist surgical care types etc.

The efforts to generate a new EMT system did not conclude with a simple typology and standards. For the new system to work and achieve its objectives, namely to achieve better coordination of EMTs' work in affected regions, there was a need to establish registration, certification, accreditation, and licensure mechanisms. The WHO's is ensuring this through the global classification process (see Figure 9.5). The EMT global classification process allows organizations to declare their compliance with WHO's *Classification and Minimum Standards for Foreign Medical Teams in Sudden Onset Disasters*[6] and begin the steps toward classification. This mentorship and verification method has three main goals. First, to create a fair and transparent mechanism for application, screening for eligibility, validation, and verification of EMTs. Second, to strengthen capacity, optimize cost effectiveness, and maximize probability of success for organizations eligible for the verification process. Third, to provide guidance and support to organizations throughout the classification process toward successful site verification of evident capacity to meet minimum standards.

According to WHO's data, as of September 2019, 27 teams have completed a peer review process and been classified as meeting the minimum standard for international deployment while 70+ teams are in process. Over 130 countries are also in the process of developing their own National EMTs for local response.

The coordination of EMTs presents unique complexities, some arising from the sheer numbers of EMTs responding to an incident. While the new standardization is key in maintaining a robust mechanism for assuring the quality of EMTs, there remains a need for a simple, unidimensional matching mechanism of supply and demands. Managing this task is assigned to the EMTCC usually stationed within the Ministry of Health Emergency Operations Centre (H-EOC). The core purpose of the EMTCC is the overall coordination of the surge of responding EMTs (local and international) to best meet the excess health-care needs following a SOD or other health emergency. The EMTCC overlooks and organizes aspects of leadership, coordination, communication, quality assurance, and supportive services[33]. It is important to note that the overall authority over the medical relief operations remains within the hands of the local government. The EMTCC in some countries will be entirely staffed by local officials, while in others it will be led by local officials with support from international experts drawn from WHO, EMT coordinators from teams and from UNDAC experts.

In conclusion, the new EMTs system has been growing and developing through a maturation process throughout recent years. This new and revised system is expected to lead to better coordination between aid providers and aid recipients. In fact, this system was put to the test several times in recent years. In the reminder of this chapter, we would like to explore the realization of this system from concept to real life in recent SODs and draw the lessons that can be learned from these experiences.

Putting the New EMT System to the Test

Despite its status as a work-in-progress, Typhoon Haiyan, which struck the Philippines on November 8, 2013, forced the developing new EMT system to be tested. Typhoon Haiyan was the strongest to ever make

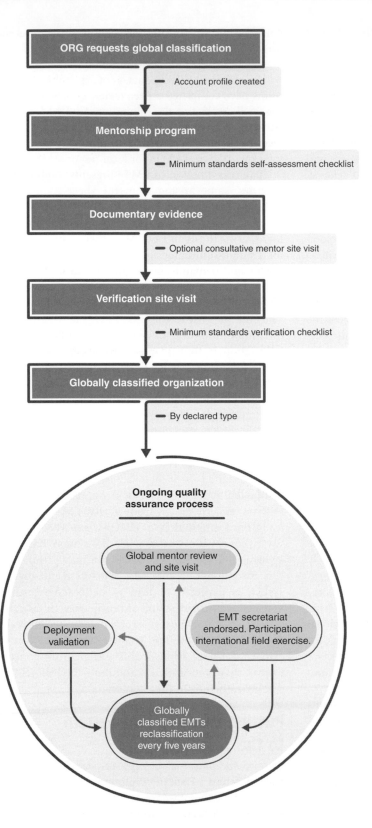

Figure 9.5 Global classification process of EMTs[34]

landfall in the western North Pacific Ocean. It left devastating destruction, affecting the lives of 16 million people. One of its more crucial effects was the devastating blow to the local health-care system[35].

As in many other cases, EMTs from around the world rushed to provide medical relief to the affected population in the Philippines. Albeit, this time, the need for a more coordinated approach was mutually agreed on and the EMT typology and standards were presented to the Minister of the Department of Health of the Philippines as an option to register arriving teams which he immediately agreed to.

The EMT work in the Philippines was far from perfect, with reports of teams arriving without approval, lack of optimal coordination resulting in some areas being underserved, accountability issues, questionable professional standards of care, and absence of clear exit strategies[36,37]. Nevertheless, there is relatively wide agreement that the experience with EMT work in the Philippines was a positive step forward. For the first time, a systematic distribution of EMTs according to Type was done and it proved to be useful[36–39].

A second and more prominent occasion on which the new WHO standardization was tested was the earthquake in Nepal. On April 25, 2015, a 7.9-magnitude earthquake struck Nepal. This was a devastating natural disaster, which some refer to as the worst one Nepal has seen in decades. According to the Nepalese Government, the death toll of this earthquake culminated at 8962 people, and an additional 22 302 were injured. An estimated 3 million became displaced. The earthquake affected 35 of the 75 districts of the country, 14 of those severely[40].

Excluding the Ebola outbreak in West Africa during 2014–2015, which was a very different situation, the 2015 Nepal earthquake was the first incident in which the new EMT system was tested fully. During the response to the Nepal earthquake, considerable efforts were made to coordinate all EMTs, of all three types, register them on their way in, and to allocate resources among them in an orderly and efficient manner. Medical resources introduced by incoming EMTs, combined with the local exiting resources, were compared and matched with the medical needs on the ground. Overlooking these efforts was a special team led by the Ministry of Health official in charge of international medical team coordination and supported by a WHO staff member, ordinarily responsible for EMTs organization and standardization, together with three UNDAC disaster-medicine experts. These were joined by staff from the Ministry and volunteers from various EMTs to staff the first ever example of an EMTCC.

The team's main task was to coordinate EMTs with the local health care system. To this end, the international coordination team joined forces with the local MoH and medical corps, who were tasked with the coordination of foreign medical aid. The local authorities, with the assistance of a WHO/UNDAC representatives, registered incoming EMTs, including their classification type, their equipment and resources, personnel, expected length of stay, and other capabilities. Importantly each team had to present their medical/nursing licenses and received national authority to practice in Nepal for a temporary period without delay. In parallel, the local authorities gathered requirements' reports from the field, as well as situation reports from local health districts and EMTs already working. The information obtained was utilized to coordinate EMTs so that resources were matched with requirements a rising from the field. Much of this information was only available to local authorities in the first days, so having national and international medical coordination in one place allowed unique ability to match needs and offers.

In practice, this coordination effort included a daily meeting attended by a senior representative from the Nepalese MoH, the Nepalese surgeon general (or senior representative), and at least one expert from the EMTs and the WHO and UNDAC joint group. During said meetings, representatives from the Nepalese MoH and medical corps would provide a situation awareness update and inform of needs arising from the ground. An assessment was then made to explore the arrivals of new EMTs, status of the operational EMTs, and possible relocation of EMTs or allocation of resources between EMTs. In extreme cases, in which EMTs were performing in an unsatisfactory manner, the local MoH could consider discontinuing their field operation.

Immediately following this meeting, a more extended coordination meeting took place each day. This multiplayer meeting was attended by representatives of all EMTs, representatives from WHO and the local MoH, and the surgeon general. On most occasions, these meetings included more than a hundred participants. The extended forum would look into the daily geographic information system distribution of the different EMTs using UNDAC's InfoMap (MapEquation) software. The meeting was short, to the point and nationally led with international support.

The process allowed for an efficient day-to-day evaluation and maintenance of the foreign medical assistance and referral system to the Nepalese people to allow the best achievable medical care at each location.

Overall, the new EMT system was proven successful following the Nepal 2015 earthquake. Local and foreign EMTs were managed and coordinated better than during previous events. The improvement was noticed not only at the headquarter level but also on the ground. EMTs were better coordinated among themselves, allowing for a more efficient resource allocation between EMTs, minimizing gaps in medical equipment requirements, coordination of secondary relocation of patients, reduced shortages in oxygen and medication supplies, effective transportation of EMTs from one area to another, and so on. While there is no doubt that, for the first time, the EMT system performed remarkably well, there remains much to be done to perfect the EMT system.

Summary

Through trial and error, leading world experts in the field of disaster medicine and humanitarian aid, in service of the people affected by emergencies and disasters, were able to advance the global EMT system. The processes of standardizing and harmonizing the medical relief efforts of EMTs in times of crisis are of utmost importance for the overarching goal of saving lives. The new EMTs system utilized during the 2015 Nepal earthquake was a step forward in establishing a more robust system of medical aid management to affected regions and worked comparatively better than previous disasters. Teams are increasingly undergoing international classification and working to improve their standards and professionalism in the interest of better patient care. Yet there remains much work to bring the system to perfection, particularly through strengthening national EMTs and preparing each MoH to rapidly set up and manage an EMTCC within its own Health EOC, with support as required form the international community.

References

1. Strömberg D. Natural disasters, economic development, and humanitarian aid. *Journal of Economic Perspectives* 2007: **21**: 199–222.

2. United Nations University – Institute of Environment and Human Security (2016). World risk report. http://weltrisikobericht.de/wp-content/uploads/2016/08/WorldRiskReport2016.pdf

3. World Health Organization (2013). Registration and coordination of foreign medical teams responding to sudden onset disasters: the way forward. http://www.who.int/hac/global_health_cluster/fmt_way_forward_5may13.pdf

4. World Health Organization/Pan American Health Organization (2010). Working groups background paper registration, certification and coordination. Presented at the technical consultation on international medical care assistance in the aftermath of sudden onset disasters, Cuba.

5. Fisher D. Regulating the helping hand: improving legal preparedness for cross border medicine. *Prehospital and Disaster Medicine* 2010: **25**(3): 208–12.

6. Norton I, von Schreeb J, Aitken P, Herard P, Lajolo C. *Classification and minimum standards for foreign medical teams in sudden onset disasters*. Geneva: World Health Organization; 2013.

7. Pan American Health Organization (2013). Epidemiological update – cholera. http://www.paho.org/hq/index.php?option=com_docman&task=doc_view&gid= 23696+&Itemid=999999&lang=en

8. von Schreeb J, Riddez L, Samnegård H, Rosling H. Foreign field hospitals in the recent sudden-onset disasters in Iran, Haiti, Indonesia, and Pakistan. *Prehospital and Disaster Medicine* 2008: **23**(02): 144–51.

9. Davey E, Borton J, Foley M. (2013). A history of the humanitarian system: western origins and foundations. London, UK: Humanitarian Policy Group. https://www.odi.org/sites/odi.org.uk/files/odi-assets/publications-opinion-files/8439.pdf

10. Rysaback-Smith H. History and principles of humanitarian action. *Turkish Journal of Emergency Medicine* 2015: **15**: 5–7.

11. Loescher G. *The UNHCR and world politics: a perilous path*. Oxford, UK: Oxford University Press: 2001: 156.

12. Bar-On E, Abargel A, Peleg K, et al. Coping with the challenges of early disaster response: 24 years of field hospital experience after earthquakes. *Disaster Medicine and Public Health Preparedness* 2013: **7**(5): 491–8.

13. Heyman SN, Eldad A, Wiener M. Airborne field hospital in disaster area: lessons from Armenia (1988) and Rwanda (1994). *Prehospital and Disaster Medicine* 1998: **13**(01): 14–21.

14. Bar-Dayan Y, Mankuta D, Wolf Y, et al. An earthquake disaster in Turkey: an overview of the experience of the Israeli Defense Forces field hospital in Adapazari. *Disasters* 2000: **24**(3): 262–70.

15. Kreiss Y, Merin O, Peleg K, et al. Early disaster response in Haiti: The Israeli field hospital experience. *Annals of Internal Medicine* 2010: **153**(1): 45–8.

16. World Health Organization (2016). Emergency medical team coordination cell (EMTCC).

Coordination handbook – draft version 10. http://www.searo.who.int/about/administration_structure/hse/emt_coord_handbook.pdf?ua=1

17. Abolghasemi H, Radfar MH, Khatami M, et al. International medical response to a natural disaster: lessons learned from the Bam earthquake experience. *Prehospital and Disaster Medicine* 2006: **21**(03): 141–7.

18. Peleg K, Kellermann AL. Medical relief after earthquakes: it's time for a new paradigm. *Annals of Emergency Medicine* 2012: **59**(3): 188–90.

19. Naor M, Bernardes E. Self-sufficient healthcare logistics systems and responsiveness: ten cases of foreign field hospitals deployed to disaster relief supply chains. *Journal of Operations and Supply Chain Management* 2016: **9**(1): 1.

20. Lind K, Gerdin M, Wladis A, Westman L, von Schreeb J. Time for order in chaos! A health system framework for foreign medical teams in earthquakes. *Prehospital and Disaster Medicine* 2012: **27**(01): 90–3.

21. Nickerson JW, Chackungal S, Knowlton L, McQueen K, Burkle FM. Surgical care during humanitarian crises: a systematic review of published surgical caseload data from foreign medical teams. *Prehospital and Disaster Medicine* 2012: **27**(02): 184–9.

22. Gerdin M, Wladis A, von Schreeb J. Foreign field hospitals after the 2010 Haiti earthquake: how good were we? *Emergency Medicine Journal* 2013: **30**(1): e8.

23. Jafar AJ, Norton I, Lecky F, Redmond. AD. A literature review of medical record keeping by foreign medical teams in sudden onset disasters. *Prehospital and Disaster Medicine* 2015: **30**(02): 216–22.

24. Djalali A, Ingrassia PL, Della Corte F, et al. Identifying deficiencies in national and foreign medical team responses through expert opinion surveys: implications for education and training. *Prehospital and Disaster Medicine* 2014: **29**(04): 364–8.

25. Hopmeier MJ, Pape JW, Paulison D. Reflections on the initial multinational response to the earthquake in Haiti. *Population Health Management* 2010; **13**(3): 105–13.

26. Growth of aid and the decline of humanitarianism. *The Lancet* 2010: **375**(9711): 253.

27. Van Hoving D., Haiti disaster tourism – a medical shame. *Prehospital and Disaster Medicine* 2010: **25**(3): 201–02.

28. Peleg K, Kreiss Y, Ash N, Lipsky AM. Optimizing medical response to large-scale disasters: the ad hoc collaborative health care system. *Annals of Surgery* 2011; **253**(2): 421–3.

29. United Nations Office of Coordination of Humanitarian Affairs (2016). Cluster coordination. Website. https://www.unocha.org/our-work/coordination

30. Katoch A. Personal communication (October 30, 2016).

31. Tatham P, Spens K. Cracking the humanitarian logistic coordination challenge: lessons from the urban search and rescue community. *Disasters* 2015: **40**(2): 246–61.

32. Tan YA, von Schreeb J. Humanitarian assistance and accountability: what are we really talking about? *Prehospital and Disaster Medicine* 2015: **30**(03): 264–70.

33. World Health Organization (2016). Emergency medical teams. Website. http://www.who.int/hac/tech guidance/preparedness/emergency_medical_teams/en

34. World Health Organization. The WHO EMT Initiative. Website. https://extranet.who.int/emt/

35. McPherson M, Counahan M, Hall JL. Responding to Typhoon Haiyan in the Philippines. *Western Pacific Surveillance and Response Journal* 2015: **6**(1): 1–4.

36. Brolin K, Hawajri O, von Schreeb J. Foreign medical teams in the Philippines after Typhoon Haiyan 2013 – who were they, when did they arrive and what did they do? *PLOS Currents* 2015: 7.

37. Peiris S, Buenaventura J, Zagaria N. Is registration of foreign medical teams needed for disaster response? findings from the response to Typhoon Haiyan. *Western Pacific Surveillance and Response Journal* 2015: **6**(1): 29–33.

38. Read DJ, Holian A, Moller CC, Poutawera V. Surgical workload of a foreign medical team after Typhoon Haiyan. *ANZ Journal of Surgery* 2016: **86**(5): 361–5.

39. Shrivastava SRBL, Shrivastava PS, Ramasamy J. Deployment of foreign medical teams: an initiative to reduce the aftermaths of public health emergencies. *Biology and Medicine* 2015: **S3**: 006.

40. Government of Nepal. (2019). Disaster Risk Reduction Portal. Website. http://drrportal.gov.np/

Chapter 10

Field Hospital Logistics
The Technical Component

Terry Trewin

Introduction

Building a hospital in a developed and well-resourced country is a difficult task and can take years. Replicating key functions and elements of that same hospital in a disaster area within days is challenging to say the least. Health facilities are an essential pillar of all communities and a building block for disaster recovery, and health professionals are expected to lead by example. Demonstrating this leadership in areas such as hygiene and sanitation by health responders should always be a key consideration of logistics personnel. Deployable self-sustaining field hospitals take meticulous planning, resourcing, education, training, and exercising to get it right.

This chapter will discuss key elements that differentiate a generic humanitarian camp to a field hospital and it is those very key elements, whether you are a leader, clinician, or technical logistics team member, which will illustrate the complexities surrounding the practicalities of preparing and responding with a self-sustaining field hospital to disasters.

Field hospitals have been deploying to disasters for many years and, while it would be arrogant to think there are no more lessons to be learned, we must be mindful that with the experience, information, and technology that are now available there are very few excuses to arrive at a disaster unprepared.

Self-Sustaining Field Hospitals

A self-sustaining field hospital is a facility that can lead, manage, and fundamentally look after itself for predetermined periods without being a burden on affected communities or health systems, and, importantly, without compromising health care or the safety and security of its personnel and patients.

It also should be understood that field hospitals sometimes cannot transport all the necessities to operate a health-care facility, such as water or fuel. In those cases, careful planning needs to be in place

and the communication of those needs to the hosts is essential well prior to any mobilization.

While water and fuel are two obvious elements to consider, the intricacies and contingencies of a functioning field hospital are vast.

- Can you incinerate biological waste?
- Do you have enough laundry detergent for surgical scrubs?
- Do you have a second washing machine for contaminated clothing?
- Do you have enough clinical waste bags and what do you do with them when full?
- Can you repair the autoclave in the field?
- Can you secure your shelters on soft and hard ground?
- Can you transition from trauma to an outbreak emergency?
- Can you manage a fire or hazardous material spill in your facility?

Technical Logistics Personnel

The term "logistics" is broad and generically covers many areas of warehousing, stock movement, and stores management. While the freight movement of a field hospital may be a standard task, it is the complexities of building a field hospital, and then ensuring it continues to function, which demand a more technical role.

Medical on-site ground support demands a specialist skill set supported by a capability and capacity to ensure health professionals can deliver uninterrupted patient care within hours of arriving and for the duration of the deployment. Disaster zones are chaotic and the ability to function without contributing to the chaos is essential.

Personnel with particular skillsets are a necessity and those with multiple skills are highly desirable: cross training where practicable is essential.

Typical base skill sets include:

- electrical
- mechanical
- construction/building trades
- electronics and communications
- emergency management
- safety and security
- environmental health: water, hygiene, sanitation, and vector control
- medical waste management

Specific training for repairs and maintenance is required relative to the equipment being deployed; for example:

- autoclaves
- X-ray
- incinerators
- morgues
- IT and communication systems
- oxygen and associated devices
- monitoring devices
- surgical equipment
- toilets/showers
- isolation wards
- laboratory equipment
- cold chain
- vehicles

Having the skills to build and run a field hospital is only one part: ensuring the technical logistic personnel have the necessary tools and equipment to perform their roles is also important. Spare parts and servicing equipment are a must. A low-cost autoclave part or fan belt for a generator could bring a surgical mission to a standstill.

It is not uncommon for emergency medical teams (EMTs) to surge technical logistics personnel in the build phase and scale back during normal operations and again surge for demobilization.

In the context of logistics, it should not be overlooked that clinical needs planning may sometimes unintentionally overshadow or compromise the welfare of health responders. While appreciating working in disasters is hard, uncomfortable, and testing, occasionally important elements of team welfare can get overlooked. Tunnel vision in emergency management can be a common problem; this can be exacerbated when key logistic personnel are not present during planning and decision-making processes. A proper leadership structure with logistics personnel included can mitigate many issues.

EMT Personnel

EMT personnel are a critical asset to mission objectives: this must be considered and reflected when conducting risk assessments.

Health-care personnel working in disaster areas are expected to perform high-functioning tasks for long periods in extremely testing conditions, which will obviously test their mental and physical fitness. For example, for a nurse, working a 14-hour night shift and then expected to sleep between shifts in a nylon tent on the ground in stifling heat over a 4- to 14-day rotation is undoubtedly problematic to their well-being, which will ultimately impact on team and clinical performance. While acknowledging the practicalities, the positives of looking after your personnel are significant.

Typically, planning for personnel begins with a knife-and-fork approach, which in turn leads to many questions:

- Do they have a knife and fork to eat with (or chopsticks)?
- Do they have a plate?
- What are they going to put on the plate?
- How do they heat their food?
- How do they wash their hands before they eat from the plate?
- Where does the dirty water go?
- Where do they sit?
- Do they have a table?
- Is the table out of the weather?
- Is there a light?
- What do they do with food scraps?
- Who empties the rubbish?
- Where does the rubbish go?
- Where do they wash the knife, fork, and plate?
- How do they dry the knife, fork, and plate?

Health-care personnel should be well presented to patients and the community: EMT personnel should wear an identifiable uniform with the basic principle of one on, one dirty, and one clean. The following questions need to be considered:

Does the uniform protect them from:

- work hazards?
- climate?
- vectors?

How do the team wash and dry their uniforms?

- Do they use handwash?
- Do they machine wash?
- Do you have laundry soap?

- Do you have enough?
- Where does the water go?
- Does the EMT have procedures around contaminated clothing?
- Who supplies footwear?
- Who sets the standard in foot care?

Where does the team sleep?

- Do they have climate appropriate bedding?
- Do they have mosquito netting?
- Do they have a stretcher to get them off the ground?
- Are they in individual tents or dorm living?
- Where do they sleep between night shifts?
- Is the accommodation secure?
- Do you have evacuation plans and key muster points?

Health personnel need to wash/bathe regularly:

- Do they have the facilities to have a regular shower?
- Do they have hot or cold water?
- Do they have soap?
- Do they have shampoo?
- Do they have a towel?
- Do they have privacy?
- Do they have security?

So, from the above examples, it is clear to see how easy it is to overlook necessities and unfortunately increase the likelihood of heading down the "lessons learned" path in regard to caring for EMT personnel.

As discussed previously, the benefit of caring for EMT personnel is a positive for the team and ultimately the patients you are there to assist.

The Facilities

There are a wide variety of shelters for EMTs: a health facility can be compartmentalized, incorporating different shelter types. These types may range from a simple quick erect triage shelter and outpatients through to a complex surgical theater and logistical areas such as:

- mess/kitchen
- medical stores
- food stores
- logistic stores
- shower/washing areas
- toilets
- disabled toilets and showers

- water treatment area
- accommodation

While not exhaustive, the following fundamentals of a shelter system should be considered:

- Climate-specific: a shelter system needs to be climate matched to the region of operation. Shelters designed for the European winter will be challenged in the tropics and vice versa.
- Weight: shelter systems need to be manageable when no heavy lift equipment is available.
- Water rating: shelters must be waterproof to protect the patients, staff, and electrical equipment from inundation.
- Wind and snow rating: from a safety perspective, shelters with high wind and snow ratings should be considered. This should also include fixings for both hard and soft surfaces. The constant noise from wind and rain on lightweight shelters should also be considered.
- Configuration: shelter systems should be configurable to a variety of layouts: areas of allocation may not be symmetrical such as car parks, streets, and hospital grounds.
- Size: shelters need to be fit for purpose and ergonomic for staff and patients. Staff cannot walk around bent over for days, and patient spacing needs to be appropriate.

Layout

Once functionality, safety, and security have been considered, the field hospital should be laid out with patient flow, security, and functionality as key priorities. This typically begins with waiting areas and triage through to outpatients, emergency, wards, and advanced treatment areas such as surgical. Field hospitals that incorporate staff facilities should have clear segregation between the hospital and staff areas.

The layout of a field hospital should consider climate and geography; for example, shelters erected in areas prone to rain should be positioned in such a way that water runoff will not create problems. A shelter with a roof area of 100 m^2 that receives 10 mm of rain may have a runoff of up to 1000 L; erection at right angles to a downward slope will be problematic for other parallel running shelters: if you consider two or more parallel shelters, the issue should be obvious.

With consideration given to patient flow and positioning, ingress and egress for emergency vehicles and freight must also be planned. Trucks delivering water, fuel, and stores, or removing waste, need ample room to access and exit critical areas. Ambulances or patient transport vehicles will require turnaround points.

The placement of critical areas and their compatibility with other functional areas is a crucial consideration; examples include fuel dumps next to wards or incinerators, waste-collection points near kitchens or mess facilities, and waste or incinerators near the accommodation.

Facilities such as toilets and showers should be located within an easy walking distance of accommodation and wards: no further than 50 m in well-lit and secure areas.

Understanding the layout, footprint, and variable configuration is essential to selecting, or more so articulating, your requirements to a host nation, which is critical to getting a suitable and adequate deployment site. Geospatial information systems should be used to view and measure sites before deployment; this will consequently reduce on-site assessment time and mistakes.

Water, Sanitation, and Hygiene

Water

Health facilities are high consumers of clean water; whether it is for human consumption, sterilizing equipment, surgical procedures, or for decontamination during outbreak emergencies, health facilities require a constant supply of potable-grade water, which meets or exceeds the World Health Organizations (WHO) minimum standards. It is impractical to consider transporting all the water required to operate a field hospital in isolated areas. Consequently, one of the first steps to deployment is to assess the available quantities and quality of available water: this should be a priority request to host nations. Typically, the only water transported is emergency drinking water for EMT personnel.

Water Quality

Locally sourced water must still meet the WHO minimum standards of quality[1] and the EMT cannot delegate that responsibility if it serves it to its staff and patients, and uses it in medical procedures. The EMT still has a responsibility to ensure the water it distributes is of high quality.

Table 10.1 Water quality requirements

Requirement	Unit of measure	Minimum
Turbidity	Nephelometric turbidity units (NTU)	Less than 1.0 NTU
Chlorine	Parts per million (ppm) or milligrams per litre (mg/ L)	0.2–0.5 ppm free or residual chlorine
E. coli or thermotolerant coliform bacteria	Colony forming units (CFU)	0 CFU per 100 ml sample (undetectable in 100 ml)
Total dissolved solids (TDS)	TDS (including desalination)	Less than 600 mg/L or ppm
Chlorine waterborne outbreaks	ppm or mg/L	Concentrations of chlorine in outbreak emergencies may need to be increased immediately within the treatment train. Concentrations higher than 0.5 ppm are recommended

WHO recommends a multibarrier approach to water quality, which means multiple layers of protection. This includes, but is not limited to:

- flocculation
- filtration
- reverse osmosis
- ultraviolet radiation
- disinfection

EMTs should always confirm the source and quality of water they receive. Water may be excellent at the source, but delivered in a disused sewage or fuel tanker. If EMTs are pumping water from streams or dams, they should travel upstream to ensure the water is not being contaminated. Consultation with health officials and community leaders is essential.

The WHO EMT Guidance Notes

Water Quantity

Minimum quantities of water in health settings are not solely related to drinking water. Volumes for each specific area can include:

Hygiene and sanitation:

- handwashing
- clothes washing
- showering and bathing, including patients
- general cleaning
- floors and wall cleaning
- equipment cleaning
- flush toilets

Medical requirements:

- surgical equipment cleaning
- sterilization processes
- wound cleaning
- surgical use

The quantities listed below are the recommended minimum guidelines for an EMT. Teams should strive to exceed these minimum quantities as worthy preparedness for surge capacity or contingencies when systems fail. An example is: you may calculate 5 L × 100 outpatients per day, but if 50% of your patients show up with carers, your calculations could be up to 250 L short. While this meets the minimum recommendation, should you consider 10 L per outpatient?

Table 10.2 Water quantity requirements

Need	Volume: liters per day	
Outpatients	5	Consultation
Inpatients	40–60	Patient/day
Surgery	100	Intervention
Maternity	100	
Dry or supplementary feeding centers	0.5–5	Consultation
Wet supplementary feeding centers	15	Consultation
Inpatient therapeutic feeding center	30	Patient/day
Cholera treatment center	60	Patient/day
Severe acute respiratory diseases isolation centers	100	Patient/day
Viral hemorrhagic fever isolation centers	300–400	Patient/day
EMT personnel	100	Per day

Source: WHO EMT Guidance Notes

Contingency planning is essential for field hospitals, and water storage is no exception. Having the ability to store excess water for emergencies is critical: when the supply chain breaks, the hospital stops.

Sanitation

Proper sanitation that meets the WHO or globally accepted standards is essential for health facilities [2,3]. Sanitation typically refers to the management of contaminated waste, such as sewage (human waste) and the byproducts of health facilities and the medical procedures they provide.

The provision of correct sanitation management is the burden of any health facility and carries significant responsibilities. The ability to collect, treat, and dispose of contaminated waste is a minimum standard of any EMT. EMTs must have the capability and capacity to be self-sustainable in the field and must lead by example.

EMTs must understand there are both standards and expectations for all personnel to follow. The ongoing cholera outbreak in Haiti, which started in 2010, is a classic example of poor sanitation compliance.

Careful planning and the technical knowledge and expertise are essential. Standards that need to be explored, but are not limited to, include the following:

- disposal methods
- distance from water sources; both surface and groundwater
- distance from food crops
- distance from accommodation/community
- numbers of toilets
- construction of toilets

Hygiene

Hygiene is a process of maintaining a standard of cleanliness for EMT personnel, patients, visitors, and the facilities. Promoting and using good hygiene practices are commensurate with the expectations of a proper health facility, with the common objective being to reduce or eliminate the spread of disease.

EMT facilities are expected to model good hygiene practices, which not only meet or exceed accepted standards but also demonstrate and promote good practices to communities and other medical teams wherever they deliver health care. The ill and injured require high levels of hygiene from those there to help.

Hygiene broadly ranges from handwash facilities, hygiene promotion and cleaning schedules, who is responsible for what, and the capacity to sustain good practices during a deployment. This should not be neglected in disasters. EMT personnel, patients, and visitors need to wash their hands regularly, and this needs to be facilitated by the EMT. Whether a simple drum-and-tap method with soap or a reticulated and pressure-fed sink, they need to be strategically placed throughout the facility and typically placed where all will unwittingly encounter them. In addition to clinical handwashing stations inside the facilities, handwashing stations need to be put where personnel, patients, and visitors will encounter them on their journey in and around the facilities such as:

- triage
- entry and exit points
- toilets
- kitchens
- mess facilities

It is the responsibility of the EMT to maintain soap supplies and proper drainage for such stations.

Leadership personnel need to maintain hygiene vigilance in their EMT, including personal hygiene and the cleanliness of the facility. Good communication skills, team briefings and schedules, and deciding who is responsible for each task will support this critical initiative.

Waste Management[4]

Proper waste management is another critical element to self-sustainability and an obligation the EMT has to the community they are there to assist, as well as the environment.

Typically, the EMT needs to understand what sort of waste they will generate and make significant efforts to reduce this in the preparedness phase. Secondly, they need to estimate how much they will produce, which can be done during training and exercise sessions, and in consultation with maintenance teams at regular hospitals.

It should be obvious that the amount of waste generated will change significantly from an EMT type 1 mobile team to an EMT type 3, although the management and disposal will remain similar.

Understanding the acceptable methods of waste disposal by the host country, and whether arrangements are in place for hospital waste, will assist with understanding what deployable equipment is required. It should not be taken for granted that a host country meets globally accepted standards on waste disposal, and, if this is the case, it is unacceptable for a visiting EMT to contribute to bad practice. As a result, EMTs should have contingencies to manage waste in a way that is safe and meets international standards and expectations. The waste management practices that are in place in the host country should be a priority question when offering to assist.

Education of EMT personnel on waste reduction and segregation is critical to a successful waste management program. This will need to feature regularly in team briefings as personnel become fatigued during deployments. This should be supported by clearly labeled waste receptacles and color-coded waste bags.

Managing sharps in the field can be complicated when personnel fill sharps containers with nonsharps-designated items, particularly during vaccination programs. Plastics and general rubbish items can quickly fill sharps containers, which can be complicated to manage in isolated environments.

Ideally, waste should be managed and treated as close as possible to where it is generated, this will reduce the likelihood of accidents or spills, and the EMT can ensure its waste is secure and being managed properly.

Waste remains the responsibility of the EMT until it is properly disposed of. Handing medical waste to an opportunistic contractor can lead to disaster for the EMT. If engaging contract assistance, an EMT should always be confident its waste is being disposed of correctly: this may mean traveling with the waste to ensure it is disposed of correctly.

When using contract assistance, the EMT has a responsibility to ensure the waste is packaged correctly and the drivers have sufficient personal protective equipment to protect themselves in the event of an accident.

Secure and correctly engineered landfill sites or functioning medical waste management facilities may be rare to find in disasters. Consequently, for an EMT to be self-sustainable, it must be able to manage its waste until proper and acceptable facilities are functioning. Transporting waste home to a country of origin is not acceptable and is likely to contravene agreed conventions on the transborder movement of hazardous waste.

Medical waste may be of high value to scavengers or counterfeiters, and all efforts should be made to ensure all medical waste is rendered as safe as practicable, inert, and unusable.

Once the waste is segregated into general, medical, recyclable, combustible, and noncombustible, the management process can begin. It is estimated that over 95% of waste from an EMT will be general waste; typically no different to general household waste. A small percentage will be medical waste.

If incineration is to be deployed, it must be of a sufficient temperature to provide complete combustion, and open fires are typically not sufficient. Temperatures exceeding 850°C are recommended, or the use of nearby smelters, brick kilns, or crematoriums.

Where no medical waste management exists for sharps containers, encapsulating them in concrete is an ideal solution. Being approximately only a small percentage of waste from the EMT, sharps containers can be filled with a concrete mixture, secured, and allowed to dry before disposal. Small bags of premixed cement within deployable EMT caches are an ideal contingency for the waste management of sharps containers. Cement slurries mixed with expired pharmaceuticals and allowed to dry is also a contingency to ensure they are rendered safe.

Burying biological waste may be necessary for some situations, but this can only be done with consultation with local authorities. There may also be cultural implications if burying amputated body parts. There are specific rules about what may be buried, and standards must apply. If burying anatomical parts in an emergency situation, this should be no less than 1500 mm above the water table, more than 600 mm from the surface, and greater than 50 m from any surface water. They should be covered with immovable objects to prevent animal scavenging.

Electrical

Self-sustaining EMTs need to consider proper planning around electrical generation, its use, distribution, and safety.

Understanding the need is the first step to effective power management. Whether the team is small and agile, or a fixed type 3 surgical facility, carefully calculating consumption will mitigate unnecessary weight and burden of heavy electrical generators and underestimating the need. Typically, electronic medical monitors are not big consumers of electricity, but on the other end of the scale, autoclaves, X-ray machines, and environmental control units are.

It should go without saying, but educating staff in electrical safety is a necessity, particularly in a field hospital setting or existing structure where additional dangers may be present. The more safety features that are in place when distributing electricity throughout

a facility, the better. This should be done in consultation with appropriately qualified electricians. Devices such as earth stakes and residual current leakage devices (safety breakers) should be mandatory and incorporated in all electrical systems. Waterproof fittings must be considered when inlets or outlets are exposed to the elements.

Calculating the usage of an EMT is very important for understanding what generators are required.

- electrical devices are generally labeled with a current draw, either expressed in watts or amps
- a basic calculation of electrical demand can be determined once all items are added together
- as a rough and conservative estimate, 1000 W = 1 kVA.

So, a typical hot-water urn may consume 2000 W: consequently, a generator greater than 2.0 kVA will be required.

If the consumption is expressed in amps, again a rough estimate can be achieved by multiplying the amps by voltage.

So, if the hot-water urn used 8 A × 220 V = 1760 W, it would require a 2.0 kVA generator or greater.

As an example, a staff mess tent and kitchen may require the following equipment:

So, from the above example, a generator greater than 5.0 kVA needs to be allocated to this area of the EMT facility, and any additional equipment not factored into the equation will create complications. Therefore, careful planning is required, and contingencies need to be in place. This type of planning needs to be conducted for all areas within the facility.

Table 10.3 Electrical power requirements

Equipment	Watts
10 L hot-water urn	2000
Fridge[a]	2000/600
Microwave	600
Lighting	200
Fans	200
Total	5000

[a] Some appliances may require a surge on startup such as fridges and air conditioners. For example, the running draw of a refrigerator may be 600 W, but the startup draw may be significantly higher in the vicinity of 2000 W.

Autoclaves and environmental control units are typically big consumers of electricity and may require higher voltages to run, such as 440 V (3 phase).

Medical facilities using sensitive electronic equipment should consider the more stable source of invertor type generators or surge protection to prevent surges and spikes in supply. Consulting professional electricians to ensure wiring standards are met and the highest possible safety standards apply is a necessity.

Safety and Security

It is not uncommon for the words safety and security to be used concurrently, and consequently sometimes to be processed as the same thing. But in the context of an EMT, they are two completely different areas to consider, although both require risk analysis and management. One of the key steps in understanding the risk to an EMT is identifying what a critical asset is and the impact it will have on mission objectives. Obviously, your personnel are a crucial asset and what might affect them should be a priority of your risk management. The international standard for risk management is "ISO 31000:2018 Risk Management."

Safety-planning measures need to be considered throughout all phases of preparedness and response, and this includes training. It may be unrealistic to use all safety plans from a typical fixed hospital, although many will translate directly to the field. Fire safety, trip hazards, and lifting are typical examples of what can be slightly modified to reflect the field scenario. More specific plans for driving vehicles, buddy systems, and working around aircraft, for example, will be more specific. Plans may need to be finalized in the field, such as muster points and escape routes.

Security planning is a necessity to keep critical assets safe. Understanding security processes, procedures, and actions begins in initial team training and continues throughout the mission until everyone returns home. Security assessments are critical before any deployment and must be ongoing throughout that deployment. Personnel need to understand and be prepared for what to do in an emergency and who and how to call for assistance. While security is everyone's responsibility, key personnel within the EMT need to identify the main point of contact and liaison for security-related issues.

Summary

Topics covered in this chapter only provide a general overview of the some of the key elements to support and run an EMT facility in the field. Effective field hospitals require considerable planning and training and are heavily resource dependent. If you take "lessons learned" seriously, running into a disaster unprepared should be a practice of the past.

Liaising early with the host country and detailing what you can and can't do and what you need to function effectively is important. The WHO EMT initiative promotes documentation for teams offering to assist, which details exactly what services they are offering. This is an ideal time for logistics personnel to detail what they have and what they may need on arrival. Water, fuel, and an appropriate location are key discussion points.

Contingency planning is essential to ensure the self-sustaining uninterrupted provision of medical care can continue to be delivered among the chaos of disaster.

Health professionals should lead by example to both the community and other health-care teams. Professionally presented personnel and facilities, which meet global expectations and minimum standards in sanitation and hygiene, are no longer a "nice to have."

Considerable investment in training and preparation is necessary across the many facets of a successful EMT and its facilities. Studying others and their techniques: what works and what does not, what mistakes they made, and what has been learned is very important.

References

1. *Guidelines for drinking-water quality*. Fourth edn. incorporating the first addendum. Geneva: World Health Organization; 2017. License: CC BY-NC-SA 3.0 IGO.

2. *Water and Sanitation for Health Facility Improvement Tool*. Geneva: World Health Organization; 2017.

3. *Water, Sanitation and Hygiene in Health Care Facilities*. Geneva: World Health Organization/ UNICEF; 2015.

4. Essential Environmental Health Standards in Health Care. Geneva: World Health Organization; 2008.

Auxiliary Medical Services in a Field Hospital

Yoel Har-Even, Guy Lakovski, Melanie Morrow, Michel Somekh, and Tami Halperin

Introduction

Setting up a field hospital with advanced auxiliary medical services (AMS) is a feasible mission. The chosen equipment and workforce enable smooth and professional work, with the ability to diagnose and treat most of the anticipated problems, and to stabilize most others prior to evacuation. Accurate planning of the service to be provided and the equipment is necessary. Training the medical staff regarding the need to use auxiliary services sparingly is an important part of running a field hospital.

The work of all the AMS departments begins well before a disaster occurs and continues well after it ends. Their work is of importance even during routine times, long before the outbreak of a disaster, and involves purchasing and equipping medical devices and instruments suited for work in the field, with an emphasis on the mobility of the equipment and its ability to function without electricity (at least for several hours until the hospital connects to the electricity grid). Given certain disaster scenarios, consideration must be given to the

equipment's ability to operate under extreme weather conditions and, of course, it must correspond to the specifications as defined by the medical professionals of the different disciplines.

Following the occurrence of a disaster/incident, as much information as possible is collected on the given scenario, the size of the disaster, the estimated number of casualties, and the type of injuries, as well as the treatment required on scene.

Based on this information, the goals of the humanitarian mission are determined, with the field hospital a part of the mission. At this point, the departments and medical capabilities the field hospital will have are decided, which are determined by the hospital's commander and senior medical personnel who will head the hospital's planned departments.

At this planning stage, the department of AMS is incorporated into the hospital structure so that a list of equipment and accessories can be made in preparation for establishing the hospital and recruiting professional staff (Figure 11.1).

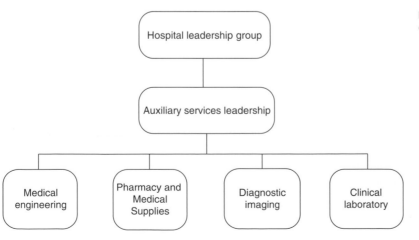

Figure 11.1 The structure and organization of the AMS department

The functions and tasks of the AMS department are to:

- prepare and plan for the mission within the given time constraints
- assist in preparing the required equipment for shipping to the country of destination
- organize and assist in establishing the field hospital as quickly as possible in the country of destination
- ensure regular, continuous activity of all the field hospital's departments by providing maintenance of the equipment, running the obligatory testing of the equipment, and enforcing safety and security requirements
- assist and take part in preparing the equipment for its return journey home at the end of a mission
- ensure the equipment is maintained in good working order in between missions
- take part in the debriefing sessions that are held throughout the mission and at its closing

Medical Engineering

Background

The work of a medical engineering department begins well before a disaster occurs and continues long after it is over. Medical engineering deals with the acquisition of equipment suitable for work in the field, with emphasis on the equipment's mobility and ability to operate without an electricity source (at least for several hours until the hospital connects to the electricity grid), the ability to operate under extreme weather conditions, and of course, it must correspond to the specifications as defined by the medical professionals of the different disciplines.

When the field hospital is at the planning stage, the medical engineering department is incorporated into the hospital structure so that a list of equipment and accessories can be made in preparation for establishing the hospital and recruiting professional staff.

The Role of a Field-Hospital Medical Engineering Department

The department is responsible for providing maintenance services: repairing and ensuring the smooth running of all the field hospital's medical devices, including all the various gas systems. They must be able to guarantee the competency of all devices throughout the hospital's various departments, while maintaining the

safety of both patients and caregivers. Only standard medical devices are allowed, in order to avoid exposing patients and caregivers to any danger. Those operating the equipment must receive appropriate training.

The role of the medical engineering department remains the same no matter what type of disaster the field hospital is attending. The only difference will be the nature of the equipment, the quantities, and the personnel (the qualifications required and the number of people needed for the specific mission: more detail on this is in the section on personnel later in the text).

The Required Core Competencies

- installation of all the field hospital's medical equipment
- provision of the training and technical support for operating the equipment, including the gas systems
- Repair of the medical equipment and medical gas systems

In a field hospital, there is no option to send a piece of equipment for repair off campus (i.e., sending faulty devices, which cannot be repaired in-house, to an external workshop/supplier). Due to the nature of the missions and the distance from home, the department should use all the means at its disposal to maintain the medical equipment to the highest standard. This ensures the hospital has maximum independence as there is no option of receiving a repair service from external suppliers. The medical engineering department is, in fact, called on to use all its professional skills to keep everything in working order.

This is also true in between missions, where the medical engineering department is responsible for storing and preserving the functionality of the equipment. Before embarking on a mission, they must conduct test runs. Charging the batteries of equipment that includes rechargeable batteries is critical and important.

Personnel

- two to three technicians/medical device engineers, of whom one will serve as head of the department
- the number of technicians is recommended to be one medical device technician for every four intensive care unit (ICU)/operating-room beds

Division of Labor

The objective is to maintain the physical strength and availability of technicians throughout all working hours of the field hospital, including nighttime. If necessary, night shifts should be implemented to provide a seamless response to service calls from the operating rooms and to provide technical support for faulty medical devices during these hours. Devices that do not urgently need to be fixed at night can be repaired during normal working hours.

For the morning shift (when the hospital opens for activity and starts receiving patients), there will be at least two technicians present who will conduct a daily round of all the hospital departments; checking in with the head of each department regarding the condition of their medical devices, whether any devices need fixing or changing, the condition of the oxygen system, and whether oxygen cylinders are needed.

For the night shift, there will be one technician on call every night. If the field hospital has three technicians, the night-shift technician will rest during the day, not performing daytime activities to be alert for the night work. If there are only two technicians, the night-shift technician will perform minimum duties throughout the day (depending on the hospital's workload) to better provide optimal response throughout the night.

Essential Equipment

- medical devices, in working order, and replacements
- working tools
- testing equipment
- disposables
- desks and chairs
- cupboards and storage boxes
- storage tent and workshop tent
- spare parts and batteries

Main Functions and Tasks

- provide support in all aspects of deploying medical equipment and gas systems
- maintain all medical devices; both proactive checks and repairs
- repair medical equipment, including the gas systems installed in the hospital
- train and provide technical support to those operating the medical devices
- manage the inventory of spare parts, technical rotation, and testing of the medical devices

Department Action Required Prior to Deployment

- Collaborate with the heads of department to prepare the list of medical equipment needed that is specific to the mission.
- Prepare a second list (based on the above) of all the spare parts, disposables, accessories, tools, and testing equipment needed, as well as professional technical literature, including user and maintenance manuals.
- Raise funds and join forces with other hospitals/nongovernmental organizations (NGOs) to recruit specialist or fragile equipment, or equipment that is not in frequent use (such as that for newborns, infants, and children).
- Test all equipment prior to packing it. Charge all devices with rechargeable batteries and replace all faulty equipment before departure. In between missions, conduct routine maintenance checks to catch any faulty equipment ahead of time. This routine will ensure equipment is kept in good condition and will leave just the batteries to be recharged as a precaution prior to a swift departure.
- Actively participate in packing the equipment, with emphasis on marking the boxes that hold spare parts, disposables, tools, and testing equipment. Boxes should be grouped according to department and clearly labeled.
- Unique and important testing equipment, as well as expensive and important items, should be packed together with the technician's personal luggage.

Action Required at Deployment

- Take part in establishing and organizing the field hospital.
- Distribute the medical equipment among the various departments and connect them to electricity. Ensure the devices are in working order and were not damaged during transport.
- Establish the infrastructure for medical gases and ensure it is working and is up to standard.
- Instruct the medical teams on how to work and operate the equipment.

Routine Action Required in a Functioning Field Hospital

- Accurately list all equipment by department. This register is important for keeping track of the equipment when the field hospital is dismantled and packed for the return journey.

- Maintain a list of all equipment that has been repaired or replaced and ensure the list is always up to date.
- Proactively conduct tours at the various departments, both in the morning and evening, to check the status of all medical devices.
- Repair broken or faulty devices.
- Replenish the disposables.
- An appliance that the department is not able to repair will be replaced or exchanged (depending on availability and inventory). Any device found to be deficient/dangerous, which cannot be repaired, should be removed from circulation. Patient and team-member safety is paramount.
- Instruct users on using all the field hospital's medical equipment and provide technical support.
- Manage the inventory of spare parts, disposables, and technical rotation of medical equipment, and replace medical equipment if necessary.
- Manage purchasing requests and orders for spare parts, disposables, and accessories
- Register and manage the inventory of medical devices by department and note the status of any device being repaired.
- Dispatch a daily report on the competence of all medical devices.

Pharmacy Services

Background

If the pharmacy and the role of the pharmacist in a field hospital is considered prior to deployment, there are many benefits to the field hospital. The pharmacist is involved in many predeployment projects and is an integral part of ensuring medicines and medicine information are handled efficiently in country. At the end of a deployment, the pharmacist will assist in hospital operation during the mission and implementing changes.

Field Hospitals: Rules

The World Health Organization (WHO) lists minimum standards that need to be met with regards to medicine supply within the emergency medical team (EMT) framework according to the type of deployment[1].

The medication requirements as set out by WHO can be seen in Table 11.1. Medicines should align with

Table 11.1 Medication requirements according to EMT type

EMT type	Medication requirements
1	Outpatient drug supply to treat for the EMT's declared capacity for two weeks, the WHO essential medicines list or equivalent, and tetanus prophylaxis
2	Inpatient and outpatient drug supply, including surgical and anesthetic drugs, and enhanced essential drug list
3	Intensive-care-level drug pharmacopeia

the latest version of the WHO essential medicines list (EML), which is updated every two years[2,3]. The EML outlines medicines that should be available to satisfy the priority health needs of a population. This considers the medicines' efficacy, safety, public health relevance, and cost-effectiveness. Most countries use the WHO EML to develop their own local EML. Medicines in field hospitals should, wherever possible, align with the host country's EML. Field hospitals need to be able to manage cold chain safely and carry vaccines including tetanus and pediatric hepatitis B vaccine. The medicine requirements increase as the complexity of the hospital increases.

All medicines that are carried and used within the hospital must be of a quality that could be used in the hospital's home country. They should also meet the WHO guidelines for medicine donations[4]:

- medicines must have a remaining shelf life of at least one year
- medicines must have instructions written in a language that is understood in the host country and contain the international nonproprietary name
- medicines should appear on the host country EML
- medicines should come from a quality-assured source and comply with quality standards in both the donor and host countries
- medicines cannot have been returned by patients or be free samples

Medicines Licensing and Legislation

Every country has their own rules around the exportation and importation of medicines. In most countries, some medicines need approval in the form of a license before they can be imported or exported. These licenses generally need to be applied for in advance to allow processing. It is worthwhile contacting the licensing body to determine whether they will allow a multiple-use annual license. A license will also be needed for the host country. Assistance of host-country embassy staff may expedite this process.

The field hospital must maintain the pharmacy according to local host-country legislation and the legislation governing medicines in the team's country of origin. This includes medicine storage requirements, documentation requirements, and the pharmacist's scope of practice.

All practitioners within the field hospital need to have a valid "authority to practice" in the host country. They must also work only within their usual scope of practice and within the scope of practice of the profession in the host country. For example, if the pharmacist does not administer vaccines as a part of their normal scope of practice, it would be inappropriate to administer vaccines in the field hospital. In addition, if vaccine administration is part of the pharmacist's usual work in their home country, but not a permitted role of pharmacists in the host country, then their "authority to practice" will not cover this service and it should not be offered.

Australian Experience

The Australian government requires 30 days' notice to issue an import/export license, which is not feasible if you are to be deployed at short notice. The Australian Medical Assistance Team (AUSMAT) applies for a multiple import/export license from Australian customs at the start of each year listing the maximum amount of medicines an AUSMAT may take. The Australian government is not concerned if fewer are taken. AUSMAT does not apply for licenses to every possible host country for a deployment; rather, it relies on the Australian government's assistance in acquiring a permit at short notice. As we do not go without an invitation from the host country, this has been successful in the past.

Dangerous Goods Categories

Some medicines and ancillary products, such as hand cleaners and disinfectants, may be considered dangerous goods and therefore may have specific requirements regarding their suitability for travel and packaging requirements. There are explicit requirements for different modes of transport for pharmaceuticals, such as land, sea, and air. Transport and packaging information on pharmaceuticals and associated medical products can be found on safety data sheets. Ensuring these are always readily accessible with all products is essential. Safety data sheets identify dangerous goods information, which will assist with compliance and packaging requirements. To meet compliance requirements, packaging of dangerous goods should be done by qualified personnel or an agency.

Medicines Procurement

Consideration needs to be given as to how medicines will be sourced. Each method has its own challenges. There are three methods that can be used:

1. Import medicines with the team
2. Deliver medicines from an international supplier
3. Purchase medicines once in country

Import Medicines with the Team

The benefit of importing medicines with the team and field hospital is that work can begin as soon as the field hospital is set up. The medicines can also be set up in a system that makes locating items simple.

The disadvantages are that import/export license requirements for two countries need to be navigated: the home country's and the host country's. The packaging of medicines to ensure that they arrive intact and are not affected by heat falls to the team. There also needs to be a method to ensure that medicines are in date. This can be done either by finding a facility or supplier who is willing to rotate stock for the field hospital or by arranging for a medicines supplier to supply the medicines at short notice when a deployment is announced.

Deliver medicines from an international supplier

Premade, standardized emergency health kits designed by WHO, such as the interagency emergency health kit and the noncommunicable diseases kit, are available[5,6]. These kits are based on the WHO's EML and are designed to provide reliable and affordable medicines and supplies quickly. They are already located in strategic sites worldwide and can be purchased at the time of disaster. They are packed to be dangerous-goods compliant and only one import license is necessary. A potential problem is the lag time in receiving medicines. There can be a significant wait time for goods to be cleared through customs. This is often extended after a disaster as customs may not be operating at full capacity and an increase in imports can quickly overwhelm the local systems. This can mean that the hospital may not have medicines for a significant amount of time; in some cases, weeks to months. This may be the only method available if medicines in the team's country of origin are not labeled in a language understood in the host country or do not contain the international nonproprietary name.

Purchase medicines in the host country after arrival

Purchasing medicines once in country negates the need for any import/export licenses and ensures the medicines align with the host country's EML, but this method needs significant planning and will take time. The manufacturing sites may need to be inspected to ensure that the company follows good manufacturing practices and that counterfeit medicines are not purchased. This method is not feasible after a sudden-onset disaster (SOD), but may be suitable if long-term medicine supply is required or for resupply of a hospital.

Australian Experience

On a past AUSMAT deployment, there were lag times in receiving a standardized medicine kit. This led us to holding our own medicines for future deployments. We have a relationship with a local hospital and so purchase and rotate our medicines within this health service. This ensures medicines meet the donation requirements. It ensures the medicines are packed in an acceptable way. We monitor heat exposure in transit and ensure medicines are easily located. We also have the flexibility to make small changes to tailor our medicines to the deployment.

Medicine Choice for Deployment

Consideration needs to be given on the choice of medicines and their quantities. The EML is a good starting point. It is then useful to consider the health demographics of the likely deployment areas, including the age ranges and common diseases of the population. Diseases, such as malaria, which may be rare in the team's country of origin and that require specific medicines, may be common in the host country, but the medicines may not be readily available in the team's country of origin.

Medicines that require refrigeration should be substituted for medicines that can be stored at room temperature, if possible. This includes powdered mixtures, which require refrigeration after reconstitution. Many children's preparations on the EML include tablets in strengths suitable for children, rather than liquids. If a child cannot take tablets, consider crushing and suspending tablets or opening capsules as an alternative to refrigerated products. Consider how well the medicines will transport. For example, plastic is more robust and lighter than glass.

The use of clinical assumptions is one method to double-check your quantities and is used in the example below.

Australian Experience

In the AUSMAT model, we use clinical assumptions to decide on suitable quantities. The following assumptions have been used to determine the amount of metformin to be carried:

- Per day, 150 patients will attend the emergency department for the first 14 days' deployment.
- The split is 40% (60) children, 60% (90) adults per day.
- Of the adults, 20% will have diabetes (20% of 90 = 18 diabetic patients per day, so 252 patients over the 14-day deployment).
- All the diabetic patients are taking metformin at an average dose of 2 g per day and each patient receives 7 days' supply (252 patients × 2 g × 7 days = 3528 g of metformin required for the first 14 days' deployment).
- The most common strength of metformin tablet is 500 mg (3528 g ÷ 0.5 = 7056 tablets of 500 mg metformin will be required). This is rounded up to whole packets (100 tablets per packet), so 7100 tablets or 71 packets.

Medication Storage in the Hospital

Storage of medicines in the field hospital needs to be secure and held in a way that assures the quality of the medicines, but still allows access by approved staff members only.

Temperature monitoring is essential for all medicines, both during transit and in the field hospital, for both cold-chain and room-temperature medicines. Temperatures need to be checked regularly to ensure storage conditions are being met. Accredited vaccination refrigerators should be used. "Strive for 5"[7] is a useful guide to packing portable coolers for transport and, in an emergency, converting a domestic refrigerator for short-term use if the vaccine fridge malfunctions. Programmable data loggers with spare batteries should be carried, being aware that batteries are dangerous goods and there are issues with their disposal.

Room-temperature medicines are tested for stability up to 25°C or 30°C. Temperatures are likely to go above this in transit and in the field hospital. There are a lack of data about the effect of sustained exposure, so medicines need to be monitored and assessed as to their usability according to their exposure.

Medicines need to be stored so that they can be easily located and stock usage easily monitored. Items with longer expiry dates should always be placed behind shorter-dated stock to minimize stock expiring before use.

Medicine storage requirements may change according to the deployment type. Storage of medicines in an outreach setting or for retrievals is more appropriate in soft backpacks and storage on the ward in a sturdy lockable container. Most countries have extra storage and monitoring requirements for dangerous drugs such as opioids and ketamine. It is important this is adhered to.

Australian Experience

In the AUSMAT field hospital, medicines are packed into large space cases with shelves. Space cases and shelves are numbered to allow easy location of the medicines. On arrival, the space cases are placed upright and are used as lockable cupboards. Two different-colored padlocks are used for security. Keyed-alike green padlocks are used to limit pharmacy access to the pharmacist, head nurse, and doctor. Keyed-alike purple padlocks are used for cupboards that the health professionals on the team should have access to. Purple keys are given to all health professionals to ensure medicines are not accessible by the public.

The hospital needs to have a process in place for the use of medicines that have not been sourced by standard means. For example, other organizations may offer donations, patients' own medicines may be left behind, and there may be requirements to buy local medicines. These medicines should be quarantined and approved before circulation and use to ensure their integrity.

The pharmacy also needs to have access to other equipment to assist in services. These may include a laptop with dispensing and logistical software, a label printer, calculators, references, stationery, and cautionary and advisory labels.

Pharmacy Personnel

A field hospital is often operational for long hours with minimal trained pharmacy staff. This is not unique to pharmacy, but to all the specialist roles where coverage by others is difficult such as laboratory staff.

Consider the best way to prevent burnout in staff. Ensure time is rostered off and these breaks are taken. Consider which roles could be outsourced to other hospital staff, even if training needs to occur to allow this. For example, the nurses could be tasked with ordering and restocking of the ward imprest cupboard.

Develop a method for after-hours access to urgent medicines, which does not involve recall of pharmacy staff unless complex advice is required. Clearly outline which pharmacy tasks should take precedence if the pharmacist finds themselves overwhelmed.

Local staff are very valuable and can assist in many ways in the pharmacy such as translating and counselling patients, ensuring local cultural brokerage, and promoting continuity of care.

Closing Down a Field Hospital

After a SOD, a field hospital is set up for a short time (not more than a few months) to ensure it does not disrupt local services. For this reason, it is important to consider the tasks required to close down the field hospital. Some of these tasks should be planned at the start of the deployment. Donation of medicines takes planning and approval and so needs to be considered from the start. Firstly, the medicines need to be suitable for donation, as mentioned earlier[4]. Additionally, the quantity should be such that they can easily be used before their expiry. All donations should go through the host country's ministry of health (MoH) for approval.

Waste cannot be transported across international borders. Therefore, any medicine that is to be destroyed needs to be safely destroyed before leaving, either by concrete slurry, chemical inactivation, or another approved method.

Review of Pharmacy Operations

On returning home, a review of pharmacy services should be completed:

- medicine usage
- medicines needed that were missing
- clinical questions
- problems relating to pharmacy services and suggestions for improvement
- heat exposure of medicines

- survey of staff asking about adequacy of service

This review should then be used to determine any changes needed before the next deployment.

Diagnostic Imaging

Background

The main medical use of imaging on the battlefield took place in 1914 at the beginning of World War I, when the famous physicist Marie Curie joined the French war effort and began to build dedicated vehicles with portable X-ray machines, designed to provide a diagnostic response on the battlefield. For this purpose, Madame Curie trained some 150 nurses who actually performed these X-rays [8].

Today, over 100 years later, the imaging department within a field hospital operates as an autonomous unit, providing investigative and diagnostic services. As a significant operational element within the hospital, the mobile imaging systems enable high-quality imaging tests, whether located in the imaging department tent, a dedicated container unit, or on the various hospital wards for patients who cannot be transferred due to their medical conditions (bedside X-rays).

The imaging department also includes a documentation and archival system, and the ability to send results through the field hospital internal network using picture archiving and communication system (PACS) and radiological information system (RIS) technologies.

The Field-Hospital Imaging Department: Capabilities (Table 11.2)

A field-hospital imaging department is expected to carry out the following:

- conventional X-rays using portable digital X-ray systems with computerized radiography (CR) and direct radiography (DR) technologies
- diagnostic ultrasound tests, including general tests, gynecological tests, and cardiac tests
- X-rays in operating rooms and ICUs
- radiological interpretation of tests on demand
- remote diagnosis and interpretation using teleradiology technologies (optional)
- documentation and archiving of imaging tests in the RIS and PACS (optional)

X-ray Imaging

The X-ray imaging needed in a field hospital includes:

- spine
- lower extremity
- upper extremity
- head
- chest
- pelvis
- abdomen

Personnel Needed to Run an Imaging Department

The imaging department should be able to provide round-the-clock imaging and interpretation services. Work should be divided into three shifts. The recommendation is for each shift to have one radiologist for interpretation and two to three radiology technicians.

The Radiology Technician

The duties of the radiology technician are to:

- perform X-rays, medical imaging, and ultrasound scans at the request of the doctor; performed both in the imaging department and on the various hospital wards for patients who cannot be moved
- document and feed results into PACS

The Radiologist

The duties of the radiologist are to:

- interpret imaging examinations on demand and feed results into the RIS
- provide radiology consultation and support to all hospital functionaries
- provide consultation and diagnosis via the teleradiology system

The Principal Operational Systems

As a rule, the nature of activity in the imaging department should be fully computerized and digital. The workflow should be as follows (Figure 11.2):

1. A referral from the department physician is received, which includes a detailed request for the type of imaging examination required. The referral is entered into the department's computer system and includes patient medical history, instructions for the radiology technician, and any relevant medical question for the radiologist who will interpret the imaging.

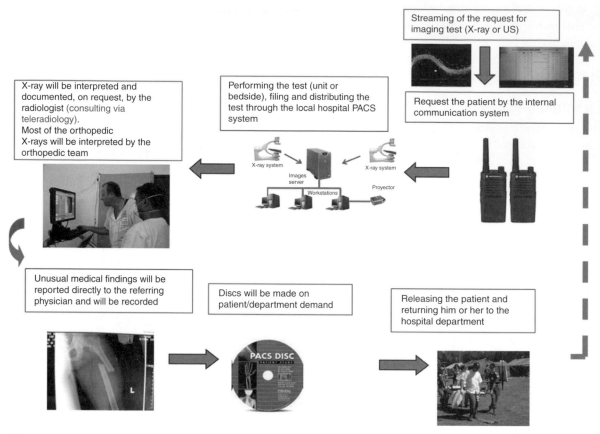

Figure 11.2 The imaging chief operational system

2. The imaging department summons the patient (whether ambulatory or by stretcher) via the hospital's internal communication system.

3. The examination is performed either in the imaging department or on one of the hospital wards (usually intensive care, operating room, or recovery).

4. The radiology technician will perform radiographic and photographic control and input the image into the hospital's PACS if available.

5. The radiologist then interprets the results. If needed, remote diagnosis and interpretation is performed and entered into both the RIS and the patient's computerized medical file.

6. If necessary, and depending on the department's request, the radiology images are copied to a disc.

7. Unusual medical findings are reported directly to the referring physician and documented.

8. The patient is discharged from the radiology department and returned to the ward.

Radiation Safety Principles in a Field Hospital

Operating X-ray machines in tents made of fabric or any other durable plastic material has significant implications for radiation safety and potential exposure of patients and staff to ionizing radiation. The radiation safety officer must take these into consideration (Figure 11.3).

We recommend both the planning and imaging teams familiarize themselves with the unique radiation safety guidelines available for operating X-ray machines in tents to protect staff and patients and ensure minimum exposure to ionized radiation.

These guidelines were developed based on the International Atomic Energy Agency instructions and they relate to X-rays taken in the imaging department tent or on the wards (mainly operating rooms, emergency room, and intensive care).

The guidelines define how the tests are carried out, with reference to the physical location of the imaging

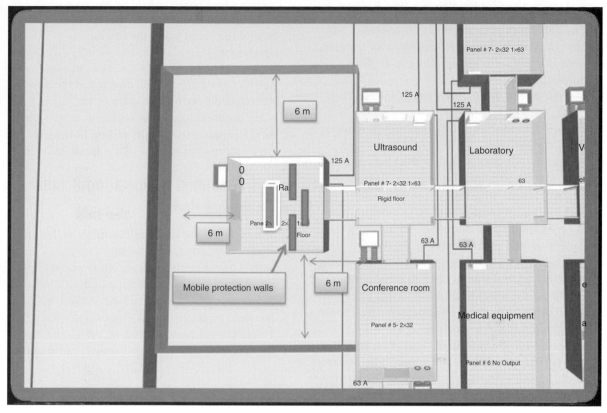

Figure 11.3 The imaging department: radiation safety zone

tent in the field hospital and its isolation, safety distances, how to place lead partitions, the use of protective gear (such as lead aprons), and the monitoring of staff by way of a dedicated radiation dosimetry badge.

The team of radiologists and hospital staff should be briefed by the radiation safety officer on the guidelines and safety precautions of field-hospital radiation conditions as part of their preparations for possible deployment. A printed summary of the guidelines should be prominently displayed on all hospital wards.

These guidelines and safety precautions have been implemented in real time by the Israel Defense Forces (IDF) field hospitals with the humanitarian-aid missions sent to disaster areas such as the earthquake in Haiti in 2010, the tsunami in Japan in 2011, the typhoon in the Philippines in 2013, and the earthquake in Nepal in 2015.

The radiation safety officer must also address new safety guidelines regarding the use of X-ray machines in a tent scenario if the hospital intends to equip with mobile X-ray machines for use in the operating rooms.

Radiation Protection Considerations

The principal radiation protection guidelines for the imaging department include the following:

- correct positioning of the X-ray shelter (connected tents)
- proper placement of the portable lead walls in the X-ray shelter
- maintain a 6 m safety zone on each side of the shelter (using a fence)
- for radiographs in vertical positioning, the patient will stand near the side of the tent, where people are not intended to be
- place portable lead walls in all ICUs, recovery rooms, and operating rooms
- reduce the use of bedside X-rays: these should only be used with patients whose health would be compromised if moved
- ensure anyone in the area is at least 3 m away from the X-ray machine before using it
- use lead aprons and thyroid gland protection

General Instructions for Imaging in a Field Hospital

- The field hospital deployment site is made up of connected tents. Allocate the end tent for imaging.
- Only use mobile X-ray machines in the field hospital.
- Use the mobile X-ray machine in the operating room or the ICU.
- Reduce the radiation to a minimum before using the X-ray machine.
- Protect the patient's genitals with a lead apron. Do not use the lead apron if it impedes diagnosis.
- Do not allow anyone near the patient being X-rayed except those who must be present.
- Where possible, use accessories for assisting the patient instead of using another person.
- If the assistance of another person is necessary during the X-ray, provide him or her with a lead apron.
- While the X-ray machine is operational, staff must stand behind a protective wall or wear a lead apron and thyroid-gland protection.
- When X-raying a woman during her reproductive years, make sure she is not pregnant. If there is any doubt, contact the referring physician for a review.
- The X-ray machine should only be operated by personnel authorized by the unit officer.
- Before turning the X-ray machine on, make sure it is intact and not missing any parts.
- Turn the X-ray machine off at the end of the imaging session.

The Dosimetry Badge

- The dosimetry badge records the radiation exposure of the wearer.
- Badges should be given to all personnel who will be in close proximity to the patient.
- Personnel must wear the badge on their upper chest areas.
- If lead aprons are used, the badges must be placed under the apron on the neck area.
- While not in use, store the badges in a closet as far away as possible from the radiation source.

X-Rays Performed in the Dedicated Tent Area

- Most X-rays should be performed in this tent.
- Lead protection boards should be placed at both tent openings.

- Another lead board should be placed a small distance from the entrance. The technician stands behind the board when the machine is operational.
- When taking across-table X-rays in the horizontal position, the beam will be directed at the position where people are not intended to be.
- Mark the area close to the tent with warning tape.
- At the entrance to the tent and on its outside edges, place signs that state: "Caution: Radiation".

X-Rays Performed in Operating Rooms or Emergency Rooms

- Minimize the use of X-ray machines in the operating or emergency room.
- Only X-ray patients in these rooms whose transfer could cause a severe worsening of their condition.
- Before using the X-ray machine, make sure everyone in the vicinity is at least 3 m away.
- To use the machine, the technician should extend the operating cable to its full length and stand at

Table 11.2 Imaging equipment for a field hospital

Item	Remarks
Mobile X-ray machine	
Field X-ray machine pack	
Tabletop CR scanner	
Tabletop DR scanner	
Mobile ultrasound	Can be used for gynecology and echocardiography
Fluoroscopy system	Optional
CT system	Optional
Lead apron	
X-ray cassettes	
Mobile lead wall	
Lead aprons of varying sizes	
Position book	
Set of lead letters	
Chest X-ray stand	
Examination bed	
Dosimetry badge	
PACS	
RIS	

the end of the cable before pushing the start button.

- As stated earlier, all personnel must wear lead aprons and thyroid-gland protection.
- Provide instructions to all staff involved who might be near the X-ray machine.

The recommended imaging equipment for a field hospital is listed in Table 11.2.

Clinical Laboratory

Background

The clinical medical laboratory performs tests to obtain information about the patient's health and provides crucial information, which enables diagnosis and treatment. This is done by using dedicated equipment. The laboratory provides multidisciplinary clinical diagnostic services to the hospital in the fields of biochemistry, hematology, and microbiology.

Clinical specimens are collected from the hospital wards and brought to the laboratory. The results of the tests are received within a short period of time to improve the therapeutic response. All results are recorded in the hospital's medical records, either manually or electronically if available.

The laboratory provides rapid diagnoses of the pathogens involved in infectious diseases: identifying the type of bacteria and their susceptibility to various antibiotics. Additionally, pathogens in the water and food are analyzed for the safety and protection of the treating staff. The laboratory also performs blood-type tests, Rhesus tests, and direct and indirect Coombs tests.

The laboratory uses automated analyzers: relatively small and portable automatic measuring devices, which measure and provide diagnostic results. They are based on the use of dry reactive methods, which mean the device is mobile and can be switched on and put into action quickly. The use of such equipment enables a diagnostic response, wherever required, 24 hours a day.

Personnel

The laboratory staff must consist of at least three qualified, certified, and experienced laboratory personnel, whose active occupation is in at least one of the following fields: hematology, biochemistry, microbiology, or the blood bank. All four disciplines should be covered, and in smaller teams, cross-training should enable multitasking. The team must be competent and receive training on the relevant machines, and they must know how to operate the machines and how to fix them if they break. Laboratory work in a field hospital is carried out in a difficult and vastly different work environment than a regular hospital laboratory, and brings many clinical and technological challenges. Therefore, the selection process of laboratory team members is essential and critical to the work process.

Equipment

We recommend that the basic list of equipment for the clinical laboratory includes a portable device for complete blood count (CBC), a coagulation device (PT, PTT, INR), basic blood chemistry (liver function, kidney function, glucose, CPK, amylase, electrolytes, and blood gases), and blood culture devices.

Due to the wide range of devices available today, several factors should be considered when choosing which portable equipment to purchase for a field laboratory. The most important features to bear in mind are the weight, dimensions, and stability of the device; the range of accompanying kits it comes with; and, of course, the operating protocol and reliability of its results. After the devices have been selected, a comprehensive list of supplies (and quantities) should be drawn up, which includes all the relevant kits, manual test kits, disposables, and personal safety equipment. The equipment list should also include a refrigerator for preserving samples/reagents, an air conditioner, and an uninterruptible power source.

The laboratory equipment/furniture should be lightweight, tabletop models, which are easy to install without the aid of a technician. A general hospital will usually have 5–10 fully automated laboratories, equipped to run all tests. This is obviously not feasible for a field hospital.

Microbiology equipment should include a standard laboratory microscope; equipment for Gram staining; culture plates with blood agar for standard cultures, chrome agar for Gram-negative bacteria, MacConkey, and SS agar for fecal culture; agar tubes for biochemical identification; and Mueller–Hinton and XLD plates for sensitivity identification.

Incubation should be performed in an Imperial III incubator (Lab-Line). Standard urinalysis sticks include blood, glucose, nitrates, ketones, pH, bilirubin, and specifically leukocytes. They should also be dispensed to the departments. Minimal blood-bank services should be provided: Rhesus typing of mothers to decide whether anti-D immunoglobulin is necessary,

AB typing for cases where a fresh blood donation is considered necessary and type-specific blood is given without crossmatching. This is achieved with a standard typing set including anti-A, anti-B, anti-D, and antihuman globulin.

Additional equipment includes two desktop centrifuges, a standard household refrigerator, and automatic pipettes. The tubes necessary for these tests are plain (serum), EDTA (CBC), and sodium citrate (coagulation). Equipment not mentioned, but also requiring detailed preparation, includes slides, gloves, tubing, and so on.

Dismantling the Field Hospital and Preparing for the Journey Home

When taking the decision to end the field hospital's activities, all medical staff must first be instructed on how to clean the medical devices, with emphasis on disinfecting them thoroughly (this is done to protect the technicians at home who will be receiving the equipment for testing). The staff must also receive instructions on how to pack the equipment.

A list should be compiled of all equipment being returned home. Equipment is sometimes left at the disaster site, for various reasons, and therefore a final list must be drawn up and organized for transport according to availability of the transport aircraft. As mentioned earlier, equipment should ideally be packed according to department, but nevertheless all crates should be clearly marked.

Any equipment that is broken or out of order should be packed separately and marked accordingly (preferably with a description of the problem). This will ease the transition of the equipment to the repair workshop on reaching home.

Preparing for the Next Mission

On returning home, broken equipment should be sent for repair and all the remaining equipment needs to undergo safety testing. Any equipment with rechargeable batteries must be recharged and any equipment left at the disaster area should be repurchased. This ensures each department is ready and up to standard for the next mission.

A debriefing session must be held regarding the field hospital's performance throughout the mission. Personnel should confirm whether any additional or new equipment needs to be purchased to maintain the standards required of the mission delegation, and whether existing equipment should be replaced with alternatives in keeping with the lessons learned.

Repurchasing of equipment that was left behind in the disaster area must be completed and new equipment purchased in accordance with the lessons learned at the debriefing session.

References

1. Norton I, von Schreeb J, Aitken P, Herard P, Lajolo C. *Classification and minimum standards for foreign medical teams in sudden onset disasters.* Geneva: World Health Organization; 2013.

2. World Health Organization. WHO model list of essential medicines. 20th edn. 2017.

3. World Health Organization. WHO essential medicines list for children. 6th edn. 2017.

4. World Health Organization. Guidelines for medicine donations: revised 2010. 2011.

5. World Health Organization (2017). Interagency emergency health kit. Online article. http://www.who.int/emergencies/kits/iehk/en

6. World Health Organization (2016). Non communicable diseases kit. Online article. https://www.who.int/emergencies/kits/ncdk/en

7. Australian Government Department of Health and Ageing (2013). National vaccine storage guidelines: strive for 5. Version 2.

8. Jorgensen TJ. Marie Curie and her X-ray vehicles' contribution to World War I battlefield medicine October 11, 2017.

Information and Communication Technologies in a Field Hospital

Gad Levy and Dror Yifrah

Information Technologies

The Role of Information and Information Needs in a Crisis Event

Accurate and timely information providing a detailed description of a disaster zone is a significant prerequisite to an efficient relief operation. A large-scale crisis situation following a natural or man-made disaster event immediately creates information demands by all those involved while concurrently disrupting the means that are usually available to obtain and distribute information. The decreased ability to provide and receive information following a crisis event is the combined result of several joint factors, including the disruption of telecommunication infrastructures, an overwhelming demand that remaining functional infrastructure is unable to sustain, as well as the effect on the human factor responsible for maintenance of vital infrastructure systems, and the provision of information. The discrepancy between the growing information needs and the ability to supply them creates a situation that can be termed an "information crisis," which has to be quickly resolved to enable effective disaster response planning and relief efforts: activities that heavily rely on information.

This chapter focuses on the information needs and the means of information provisioning within a field-hospital operation, and so a broad coverage of the "information crisis" and its mitigation among all involved parties in a disaster event is beyond the scope of this chapter. However, following is a brief classification of information needs that immediately arise during a crisis event. At the time of writing, there is still a considerable way to go in terms of the abilities to effectively fulfill these information needs at the time of a mass disaster.

Different groups have divergent information needs during the acute phase of a crisis event.

Information Needs of Victims and the Affected Population

Individuals, families, and communities affected by a disaster event have an immediate need for information and guidance regarding how and where to receive assistance, shelter, food, and medical care. Trapped or hurt individuals may need to be able to signal relatives or authorities on their whereabouts and situation. All members of the population in an affected area will typically require information concerning the whereabouts of relatives and friends.

Information Needs of Authorities

Local, state, and other authorities are the sum of personnel, equipment, establishments, and systems. A large-scale disaster event has the potential to severely affect each one of these components, reducing the ability of authorities to function. This occurs just at the moment when the demand for the functions provided by authorities is in its peak. Moreover, authorities need timely and accurate information at the time of disaster to provide their functions. These initial information needs will typically include numbers and geographic distribution of victims, severity and types of injuries, status of vital infrastructure components, and the location, capacity, and abilities of rescue and medical teams, both local and foreign, whether deployed or on the move to the disaster zone. Authorities need to be able to quickly communicate and distribute this vital information to other authorities, both local and foreign, so that an effective collaborative response effort may take place.

Information Needs of Responders and Caregivers

Responders and caregivers in a disaster event are a diverse group, ranging from single volunteers up to fully equipped field hospitals. They may be local or foreign, inexperienced or professional. However, the first decision any responder or caregiver needs to make is where to go, and, in the case of a field hospital where to deploy. This decision, if possible, should be guided by authorities in charge of the disaster zone and be based on accurate information concerning the geographic distribution of victims, severity and types of injuries, and the numbers and abilities of currently deployed responders and medical teams. This information is crucial if an efficient allocation of available resources is to be made, maximizing potential benefit to the affected population while minimizing overlap. Information remains a vital commodity throughout the relief operations following a disaster. Deployed medical teams, as well as authorities, need to be constantly aware and updated regarding numbers, abilities, and capacities of other deployed teams within the disaster zone to effectively coordinate the flow of affected individuals to and from the different available facilities in a way that maximizes each facility's abilities. In addition to the large-scale information needs and roles, when it comes to a field hospital, comprised of various departments with diverse medical teams operating within it, an internal flow of information is vital to its proper function, as the following section describes.

Information as the Driving Force of Successful Field Hospital Operations

Acquiring and managing the information required for a successful field-hospital operation are the goals of deploying an information system within a field hospital. Information should be timely acquired, accurate, and comprehensive enough to serve the higher goal of contributing to the efficiency and effectiveness of the field hospital mission. It is important to remember there may be a multitude of means, systems, and technologies involved in the process of acquiring and managing information, but all these are meant to facilitate the achievement of the goal; they are not the goal itself. It is a fact that field hospitals have been deployed in the past without the use of electronic information systems, but information itself has always been an important asset. With an electronic system or without it, certain subgoals and principles in the acquisition and management of information and its flow within a field hospital should exist.

The Namespace: Putting a Stop to Outside Chaos

Disaster may cause levels of dysfunction and, depending on its severity, may be an inherently chaotic situation. This chaos is fed by the disruption of the normal fabric of life and an overwhelming number of individuals in need of acute care in the face of a struck infrastructure. Affected individuals, more often than not, will be separated from their families, their belongings, and their identifying documents. Victims in large numbers, hurt or not, may be roaming the streets after having lost their homes. Food and clean water may be in shortage. It is within this chaos that a field hospital is expected to function and provide high-quality medical care. One of the first objectives that need to be achieved is putting a barrier to the outside chaos and preventing its continuation within the field hospitals' facilities. Good clinical practice cannot be provided in the face of chaos. An essential ability in the initial stages should be a basic internal and external communication means.

One of the first and most important anti-chaos measures a field hospital needs to apply is the creation of the *namespace*. The namespace is a predetermined system that should be strictly enforced to provide a unique and constant identity to each patient within the field hospital. An unidentified patient within the facility should not be allowed under any circumstance, including acute trauma care. Such a namespace can be based, for instance, on a unique alphanumeric identification in combination with a passport-style photograph. The primary namespace system of identification should be provided by the field hospital itself. Relying on local identification systems and numbers as the primary identification means is not recommended because, depending on the deployment area, such local systems may be partial (there may be individuals who do not possess a local identification at all) and identifying documents normally used to assert an individual's identity may be lost or missing. Local identification numbers, if available, should be registered, but they should not be relied on as the main means of identification.

Patient Flow Management and Tracking

Allocating a unique identification to every patient is the first step and a prerequisite for a well-organized field medical caregiving system. Once patients are identified, their information may be gathered and kept under this identification tag in all stations of care. The required flow of patients within the facility may be guaranteed and whereabouts of patients may be tracked. Under such a system, it becomes possible to make sure that every patient is accounted for and that prescribed and planned treatments and procedures are actually being delivered and carried out. A large multidepartment field hospital might be difficult to navigate by patients, especially in the face of language discrepancies, and a personal escort for every patient is not always possible. It is not uncommon for patients to misunderstand their designated destination within the facility. For these reasons, it is advisable to register a designated destination (department or tent number) for every patient going through the triage area and track the whereabouts of patients by registering them on arrival to a certain department, including a timestamp. With such a system, the staff can be alerted in case patients do not make it to their designated department within a certain period of time. This also enables analysis of patient flow efficiency within the hospital and the identification of possible bottlenecks. If possible, the identification process should be implemented in the prehospital facilities.

Situational Awareness and Control

A disaster zone within which a field hospital is operating is a dynamic environment. A field hospital, as large as it might be, will typically have limited available resources in contrast to the needs, which may be overwhelming and changing with time. The allocation of those limited resources should be based on a clear and accurate picture of both the internal and the external situation at all times, which calls for a high situational awareness by hospital management and key personnel members. Such situational awareness is only possible if relevant accurate and timely information is available for decision-making. Departmental occupancy rates, next-day discharge predictions, numbers and percentages of inpatients versus outpatients, developing characteristics of the case mix, and the status of pharmaceutical and equipment stocks are some of the parameters that need to be evaluated timely by management for successful decision-making within a field hospital. For some departments within the hospital, daily aggregate reports may be enough. However, for some resources, a fine-grained situation analysis and awareness is required. An example of the latter is the management of intensive care beds.

Aggregative Data and its Role in Decision-Making within a Field Hospital

What exactly is situational awareness and how should it be defined in the context of a field-hospital operation? The extent of information that is required to achieve awareness depends on the level at which the term is applied. For example, the extent of information that is required by the hospital's management team to be "situational aware" is quite different from that of a certain caregiver within the hospital or that of a logistics team member. So, perhaps it is best to define situational awareness as a state in which every official within the hospital has timely access to accurate and comprehensive information that is required for decision-making by that official. For example, personnel at the pretriage and triage areas need to be aware of departmental occupancies before making a decision to admit a new patient. A decision on admission of a patient that will require ventilation during the course of his or her treatment has to be made knowing whether and when a ventilator is made available. The hospital's pharmacy personnel should keep track of critical pharmaceuticals inventories, laboratory staff need reports of the number and types of studies performed to predict reagent consumption rates, and so on. Therefore, it is quite clear that, to achieve the desired state of situational awareness by all hospital personnel, it is not enough to have information available at the level of a single patient, but rather information should be aggregated and presented as dashboards or reports to hospital officials on demand.

Aggregative information is also needed for reporting purposes and regulatory compliance. An EMT working within a disaster zone is usually required by local authorities to provide daily information summarizing the activity within the facility, as well as pointing out cases that may have a special significance for public health and safety such as certain communicable diseases.

The World Health Organization (WHO) EMT initiative has compiled a minimum data set (MDS) platform as a means of data collecting and reporting between the EMTs and the EMTCC (Figure 12.1). Due to the large variability in the size, staffing, and technical capabilities of the various teams, the MDS is based on symptoms rather than on diagnoses. It includes 50 reportable criteria regarding patient demographics, health events, procedures and outcomes, and context. These criteria are then aggerated into a tick box and tally sheet, and reported daily to the EMTCC. The system enables overall assessment of the situation and medical activity in the disaster zone, enhancing resource utilization, and alerting to significant events such as disease outbreaks and violent activity. The MDS forms will be available on the WHO EMT website[1].

(Example) MDS tickbox on medical record

			MDS - Check all that apply
Demographic	Age		☐Month ☐Year
	Sex	1 ☐	Male
		2 ☐	Female non-preg.
		3 ☐	Female pregnant
Health Events	Trauma	4 ☐	Major head / spine injury
		5 ☐	Major torso injury
		6 ☐	Major extremity injury
		7 ☐	Moderate injury
		8 ☐	Minor injury
	Infectious disease	9 ☐	Acute respiratory infection
		10 ☐	Acute watery diarrhea
		11 ☐	Acute bloody diarrhea
		12 ☐	Acute jaundice syndrome
		13 ☐	Suspected measles
		14 ☐	Suspected meningitis
		15 ☐	Suspected tetanus
		16 ☐	Acute flaccid paralysis
		17 ☐	Acute haemorrhagic fever
		18 ☐	Fever of unknown origin
	Additional	19 ☐	
		20 ☐	
		21 ☐	
		22 ☐	
	Emrg.	23 ☐	Surgical emergency (Non-trauma)
		24 ☐	Medical emergency (Non-infectious)
	Other key diseases	25 ☐	Skin disease
		26 ☐	Acute mental health problem
		27 ☐	Obstetric complications
		28 ☐	Severe Acute Malnutrition (SAM) *
		29 ☐	Other diagnosis, not specified above
Procedure & Outcome	Procedure	30 ☐	Major procedure (excluding MDS32)
		31 ☐	Limb amputation excluding digits *
		32 ☐	Minor surgical procedure
		33 ☐	Normal Vaginal Delivery (NVD)
		34 ☐	Caesarean section
		35 ☐	Obstetrics others
	Outcome	36 ☐	Discharge without medical follow-up
		37 ☐	Discharge with medical follow-up
		38 ☐	Discharge against medical advice
		39 ☐	Referral
		40 ☐	Admission
		41 ☐	Dead on arrival
		42 ☐	Death within facility *
		43 ☐	Requiring long term rehabilitation *
Context	Relation	44 ☐	Directly related to event
		45 ☐	Indirectly related to event
		46 ☐	Not related to event
	Protection	47 ☐	Vulnerable child *
		48 ☐	Vulnerable adult *
		49 ☐	Sexual Gender Based Violence (SGBV) *
		50 ☐	Violence (non-SGBV) *

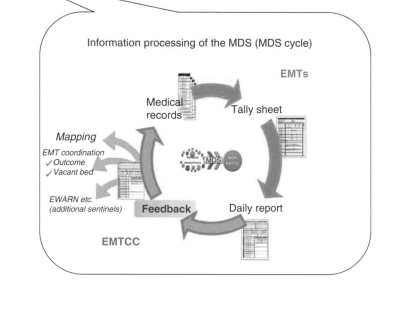

Figure 12.1 The WHO EMT initiative MDS

Clinical Information and Documentation

Ethical, Legal, and Regulatory Considerations

A proper documentation of care is both an established ethical requirement of the modern medical practice and a legal requirement in many countries in the developed world, as well as elsewhere. Moreover, court rulings throughout the Western world emphasize the importance of medical recordkeeping and regard medical records as legal evidence-of-care documents and therefore often hold care providers responsible in case records are missing or incomplete. For instance, the American Medical Association Code of Medical Ethics state that "medical records serve important patient interests for present health care and future needs as well as insurance, employment and other needs[2]."

Although in most countries the physical record does not belong to the patient, the information contained in the record is usually considered as belonging to the patient, who has a right to obtain a copy of everything that is contained within the record.

The WHO publication *Classification and Minimum Standards for Foreign Medical Teams in Sudden Onset Disasters* lists the keeping of a medical record as one of the "core standards" for all types of EMTs operating within a disaster zone, not just field hospitals[3]. WHO requires that medical teams "will undertake to keep confidential records of interventions, clinical monitoring, and possible complications." Moreover, the WHO standard requires that EMTs "will undertake for the individual patient, to have record of treatment performed."

Clinical Documentation as a Practical Necessity Within a Field Hospital

Legal and ethical considerations aside, keeping a comprehensive and updated "living" document of care is a necessity in any multipatient and multicaregiver environment and perhaps even more so in the extremely dynamic setting of a field hospital. With multiple patients pouring through the gates of a field hospital, many of them requiring care from multiple caregivers within the hospital, it is practically impossible to ensure the provision of adequate care, including the timely administration of medications at the appropriate dosages and the timely performance of procedures, as well as physician orders, in the absence of a well-kept medical record and chart.

Moreover, medical records are known to improve the quality of patient care by contributing to consistency and by providing a detailed description of a patient's status and a logic for treatment decisions, which can be reviewed, analyzed, and acted on at any time. Moreover, electronic medical record (EMR) systems improve patient outcomes and safety through improved management, reduction in medication errors, reduction in unnecessary investigations, and improved communication and interactions among providers involved in care[4,5].

The returning patient is another challenge that cannot be dealt with without a proper medical record. During the time course of a field-hospital deployment, it is not unusual to encounter patients who are returning to the hospital for additional treatment or follow-up. Adequate care of these patients requires a correct identification and review of their prior encounter.

Ethical, legal, and international standards, and practical considerations should make the presence of a comprehensive and well-kept medical record a standard of care within a modern field hospital.

Enabling the Continuity of Care (Intra- and Inter-organizational)

Perhaps the most important role of a clinical medical record in a disaster zone setting is to enable the continuity of care, both within the field hospital itself and following discharge to the community or transfer to other medical facilities within the zone or elsewhere. Continuity of care may be defined as the ability of a caregiver to provide medical aid that takes into account care that has previously been administered, including performed procedures and prescribed medications, as well as the ability to rely on results of previously performed diagnostic tests in a way that minimizes resource usage and maximizes patient comfort and safety. A comprehensive medical record is the most important means of achieving continuity of care. For this means to be effective, medical records should be organized in a way that facilitates the creation of a structured medical care summary document, which can be provided to the patient and passed onto future medical facilities and caregivers. Imaging studies performed within a medical facility should also be made available to the patient and future caregivers on discharge or transfer, either in a hard copy or a digital format. There may be an advantage for hard copies over digital formats in a disaster zone due to the uncertainty regarding the availability of electronic equipment and electricity required for viewing imaging stored in digital formats.

As one may appreciate, when information is managed to the full extent (recorded, gathered, analyzed, collated, transmitted, and selectively made available to consumers), it becomes a driving force, which streamlines field hospital operations and facilitates mission accomplishment.

Lessons Learned from Past Experience

Medical literature that deals with medical record keeping in a setting of a disaster zone field hospital is scarce. However, existing publications demonstrate that medical record keeping has been an important issue since the early days of humanitarian medical aid. Jafar and colleagues[6] carried out an extensive literature review and analysis on the subject of medical record usage by foreign medical teams (FMTs) in sudden-onset disasters (SODs), and yielded just 15 publications in which a reasonably adequate description of the medical record keeping system that had been used was provided by authors. Publication years ranged from 1983 to 2011. The earliest paper from 1983 was about the 1979 Tumaco earthquake in Colombia[7]. The authors suggested that a quick "card" system for recording information will improve data collection.

The term "medical records" in those early days referred solely to paper charts, obviously. A paper-based medical record is still in use in many disaster-response medical teams. At the single patient level, an elaborate paper chart can be an acceptable solution even today. However, when all requirements are considered, including the need to produce aggregative data for management decision-making and reporting purposes on the fly, there is a clear advantage to the use of electronic (computerized) records.

One of the first descriptions of the feasibility of implementing a computerized medical-records system on a large scale within a field hospital is our own experience from the Israeli field hospital that had been deployed in Port-au-Prince, Haiti, following the 2010 earthquake[8]. In the course of this deployment, which lasted 10 days, the electronic medical system registered more than a thousand patients, and hundreds of procedures and surgeries were documented, as well as follow-up information, pharmaceutical therapy, imaging studies, laboratory results, and lists of diagnoses. The clinical record also included a patient digital media album in which passport-like images and photos of injuries were documented. This deployment served as proof that it is possible to use a computerized system as the main means of care documentation, while at the same time demonstrated some of the possible risks and difficulties including developing a dependency on technology in a harsh and demanding environment in which technology can sometimes fail; a fact that highlights the importance of built-in redundancies, routine backup procedures, and a detailed fallback plan.

Currier and colleagues (from the Haiti aid project, Medishare), in a paper describing aid following Hurricane Katrina[9], and Burnweit and Stylianos (from the American Red Cross), in a paper describing aid following the Haiti 2010 earthquake[10], state that they had no adequate record-keeping method in place and that such a method had to be devised during the relief efforts. Additionally, Burnweit and Stylianos emphasize that the medical record system should allow for modifications based on specific needs encountered during the mission. This is an important

lesson, which should impact the way medical record systems for disaster response are developed.

Many publications describe the changing case mix of patients over time. It is a recognized pattern to encounter patients with afflictions directly related to the disaster early on in the course of the deployment, with the ratio of these patients diminishing over time, and the ratio of patients with general ailments unrelated to the disaster increasing[11,12]. Again, this is an important lesson mandating that field hospital medical record systems be tailored to suit the documentation of various types of diseases, including chronic conditions, not just trauma or disaster-related cases.

Callaway and colleagues described their experience with an off-the-shelf modified mobile health record iPhone application (iChart) at a field hospital in Fond-Parisien, Haiti, following the 2010 earthquake[13]. Their experience is important in several aspects. Firstly, the EMR app was put to use seven days following the hospital deployment so that patients initially admitted were being treated without a record-keeping system in place. Thus, the authors were able to appreciate the effects of the lack of such a system within a busy field hospital:

> This resulted in many directly observed and anecdotal adverse outcomes. For example, unaccompanied minors initially were not identified and monitored. Patients missed scheduled surgeries because they could not be located, prosthetic care was suboptimal because dates of surgery were not recorded, and care plans were fragmented as medical teams frequently transitioned.

Following the introduction of the iChart app, the authors state the observed benefits: the triage process became more accurate. The majority of providers felt that a handheld, electronic patient tracking system and medical record could reduce workload, improve patient care, and prove valuable in the postdisaster care setting. The iChart app improved provider hand-offs and continuity of care within the facility. Patient information was standardized. Patients could be tracked within the facility and those who needed special postsurgical care, such as amputees and patients with external fixation devices, were flagged and easily searched and located within the database and the facility. Information on amputation patients was made available to UN-sponsored registries to facilitate postoperative treatment, short-term wound care, rehabilitation, and prosthetic planning. Aggregative reports prepared following data export from the app assisted hospital administration in planning logistic support, operations, and staffing requirements. Another important aspect of their experience is the successful use of mobile handheld devices as the major means of interaction with the medical record; no doubt a marker for the future.

Planning, Development, and Preparations

Deployment Plan

A successful deployment of an IT solution within a field hospital begins with an elaborate planning process, which should be undertaken prior to and without relation to any certain mission. An IT plan can be created only as a derivative of a more general hospital deployment plan. Only after key operational parameters are known can a suitable IT plan be produced. These parameters include the deployment scheme, types of departments, expected hourly and daily flow of patients, and possible characteristics of patients, numbers and types of personnel, housing types, and types and quantities of certain medical equipment such as laboratory devices and radiology machines, as a minimum. Prior to an actual deployment, additional mission specific planning should be carried out going all the way down to the most basic details.

Skills and Personnel Considerations

Staffing is a resource in shortage in a field hospital. There is only a certain limited number of staff members that can be transported and supported. Taking into account that the mission is to care for patients, it may be counterintuitive for hospital decision-makers to opt for including IT professionals in the team at the expense of more medical team members. However, experience shows that the benefits associated with having a large-scale IT solution operating within the hospital outweighs this perceived disadvantage. Nevertheless, as high as the benefit from an IT solution be, the number of IT professionals on the team will be very limited. In fact, by our own experience in prior missions from recent years, the IT team included two people in smaller deployments and up to four people in larger ones.

The very small number of IT personnel expected to be available during a deployment necessitates careful consideration as to the desired mix of professional skills IT team members should possess. In any deployment, there will likely be a great demand for simple IT support such as setting up printers, connecting equipment to the network, operating the applications, and solving various common problems. More complex ethernet and wireless issues may be encountered during a deployment and, although serious server faults should not occur, they are still possible and may have a fatal effect on the IT operation. Taking into consideration the challenges the IT team may face many miles away from home base and with no backup personnel to assist, based on a four-person team, the following professional composition is recommended as minimum:

- one server administration specialist
- one network specialist
- two general IT support personnel

All team members must be familiar with the applications being deployed and be willing to provide general IT support and application specific support to users.

Materials and Equipment

Software

Requirements

The software for a field hospital is the tool that manages information and should be constructed in such a way that will enable information to become a driving force toward a successful deployment, as described above. Following is a set of requirements, which should be considered for inclusion in a field-hospital software application. This is by no means a complete set nor should it be considered mandatory to support each and every feature. Items that we feel are key and should be included in every field hospital software solution are marked by an asterisk.

- namespace creation with generation of unique patient IDs*
- barcoded patient identification tags/bracelets support
- patient identification and demographic information entry, including a photo identification (a quick method of registering patients and their demographic information should be developed suitable for use in a busy triage environment)*
- patient tracking, including past trail within the hospital*

- patient search and browsing capabilities*
- clinical information documentation by patient, including:
  - chief complaint and history*
  - body systems survey
  - physical examination*
  - injuries documentation, including mechanism of injury and severity category or score
  - follow-up notes*
  - surgical and other procedure reports*
  - anesthesia notes
  - coded diagnoses
  - multimedia patient album
  - medical document scanning capabilities
  - informed consent documentation*
  - nursing notes
  - pharmaceutical physician prescriptions*
  - physician order entry*
  - drug administration and physician order execution monitoring and alerting
  - evacuation readiness monitoring
- lab tests ordering and results display
  - imaging studies ordering and report display
  - alerts for newly received imaging and lab results.
  - summary of care document creation*
- dashboards, displaying summarized data to enable situational awareness at a glance
- reports suitable to the needs of the various officials within the hospital and as demanded by regulatory bodies and authorities*
- hospital inventory management
- system asset tracking

Emphasis Points for Field Hospital Software Development

- Software within a field hospital will be used in a demanding environment by users who may be unfamiliar with it. Special emphasis should be given to *ease of use* and *user friendliness*. Navigation within the application should be clear and obvious with the number of clicks needed to achieve a certain goal kept to a minimum.

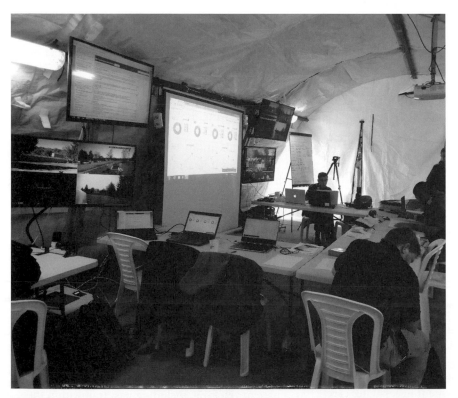

Figure 12.2 Situational awareness: display screens at the Israel Defense Forces (IDF) field-hospital headquarters presenting a dashboard depicting departmental occupancy data from the hospital information system, as well as feeds from internet protocol (IP) surveillance cameras

- A field hospital is a medical facility operating in extremely demanding conditions with patients receiving critical care while their lives are often at stake. The software solution for such a hospital should be *robust* and *medical grade*. Information elements should be signed and timestamped to allow for an accurate depiction of the course of care provision and caregiver *accountability*.

- A field hospital is an environment in which many caregivers are involved in the care of a single patient and they often do so simultaneously or in quick succession. Software should *avoid enforcing any kind of locks* at the patient file level. Simultaneous atomic updates should be supported.

- Workstation availability within a field hospital may be limited, with many users sharing available stations. Therefore, software should support *quick user switching* without complicated login and logout procedures.

- Patient data *confidentiality* should be maintained. However, in the tradeoff that may exist between privacy and usability, we feel that in the setting of a field hospital operating within a disaster zone, *usability and system throughput* should be preferred.

- A field hospital is not a stable environment as far as computer networks go. Software should be *tolerant* to transient network shortages or server unavailability and be designed to reduce the incidence of data loss due to such events.

- A field hospital network may quickly become congested, especially if it is used by additional consumers such as radiology machines and unified communication systems. Software should be designed to reduce network load. *Just-in-time* loading of data elements is preferred over prefetching large amounts of data in case it is needed.

- A field hospital is a diverse and dynamic environment with aid being delivered in multiple points of care, including bedside. Software should support the use of *mobile and handheld devices* with specially crafted interfaces suitable for use on such devices.

- At the time of writing, there is no assurance that a stable internet connection will be available at a certain disaster zone. Therefore, cloud-based solutions cannot be relied on. A fully *self-sufficient local* implementation is required.

Interfaces

A complete EMR solution should be able to receive and transmit data. This is achieved by the implementation of software computer interfaces which can be divided to inbound and outbound interfaces based on the main direction of data flow. Inbound communications include the receipt of imaging studies from radiology machines (usually performed using the digital imaging and communications in medicine [DICOM] protocol[14]) and lab results from laboratory diagnostic equipment. Outbound interfaces may include broadcast of data to remote systems for backup and distant monitoring purposes.

Computer Hardware

Users' End Units

These devices should be given careful consideration because they are the primary means of interacting with the system and, as such, they determine the way users perceive the system and their willingness to use it. Experience from prior field hospital deployments shows that it is best to have several form factors deployed including stationary workstations as well as mobile handheld devices. Stationary devices will typically be used to enter large volumes of clinical data such as daily follow-ups and preparing detailed discharge summaries. Mobile devices can be carried around during rounds and will typically be used to review patient information at the bedside, enter quick notes, and order lab and imaging studies.

The last few years have brought a myriad of new computer designs, which question the traditional classification of devices to either stationary or mobile. One of these form factors that has been deployed in recent field hospital missions is the "two-in-one" design. These devices typically resemble a laptop in their stationary state and can be separated into a keyboard part and a slate part, which can be carried around. According to the chapter authors' own experience, these are happily received by users and may fulfill the requirements for both stationary and mobile devices as one(Figure 12.3).

It is important for end units to have an internal battery to prevent data loss as a result of transient power shortages and ensure operational continuity. The use of desktop computers is not recommended due to the lack of internal power supply and display, in addition to weight and space considerations. Devices should be kept plugged in whenever possible. Mobile devices should be in sufficient amounts to allow part of the stock to be charged while the other part is being used so that charged devices are available to users at all times. Depending on the type of device, the use of spare batteries may be another option in this regard.

Servers

Usually the term "server" brings up a mental picture of a big computer data center complete with cooling, fire elimination systems, and racks filled with big humming computing machines. However, in the context of a field hospital, this is definitely not the case. A modern well-equipped laptop computer (at the

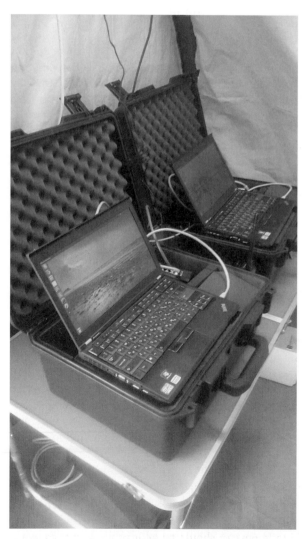

Figure 12.3 "Two-in-one" devices being used for clinical data entry during a field hospital deployment in Bogo, Cebu, Philippines, following Typhoon Haiyan, 2013

time of writing, an Intel i7 processor or equivalent with 8 GB to 16 GB of RAM can be considered to be well equipped) is more than capable of handling the workloads associated with running the backend of an efficiently constructed hospital information system serving a large field hospital with several dozens of connected end devices without maximizing the machine's resources.

Simplicity is of extreme importance and in our past experience we have opted to have the entire server software stack installed on one machine, including database, application, and web server. Fewer machines means a shorter setup time, reduced maintenance, and a diminished chance of faults related to inter-server communication issues.

The choice of server software, starting with the machine's operating system, depends on the specific solution being deployed, and many options are available, details of which are beyond the scope of this text. Whatever the chosen solution may be, it is crucial that the team's server administration specialist be experienced and well familiar with every component of the installed stack, setup process, and troubleshooting procedures. The required level of expertise from the server specialist is to be able to reinstall and configure all software stack components from scratch up to achieving a working application.

Network Gear

Wired Network

At the time of writing, ethernet networks and transmission control protocol (TCP) (and for some applications, user datagram protocol [UDP], TCP/IP or UDP/IP) are the mainstays of computer communications. A backbone of a wired network grid is important within a field hospital and, according to our experience, cannot totally be replaced by wireless solutions at this time. Wired networks are still faster in comparison with their wireless counterparts, are more robust, and are immune to radio spectrum interference, which can be a real problem in a disaster zone packed with various relief teams all using some form of radio communication. The radio signature emittance off a field hospital can also cause potential problems for neighboring facilities, such as airports, and may be completely banned by authorities. These reasons make it crucial for a field hospital to have a wired computer network solution in place.

Wired network topography should be thought over and planned in advance, taking into consideration the hospital's deployment scheme. The plan will determine the numbers of needed network equipment components such as switches and routers, as well as the total length of cables required. A choice needs to be made whether to prefer a "star" topology, which is probably more resilient to equipment failures but may be heavy on cable demands, versus a "daisy-chain" topology, which is prone to malfunctions due to single points of failure, but requires much less cabling. In our past experience we have opted for a mixed topology, with critical points within the hospital such as triage and intensive care served by a robust and redundant network infrastructure.

Wireless

Wireless network capabilities introduce the ability to have a system up and running within virtually minutes of arrival at the scene and enable the use of mobile and handheld devices within the hospital. Therefore, it is a welcome addition to a hospital IT solution. However, relying on wireless to serve as the only, or even as the main, computer communication platform is risky and inadvisable.

Achieving a reliable Wi-Fi coverage can be a challenging task within a field hospital depending on the deployment scheme and equipment used. Access point distribution within the facility should be planned in advance and take into consideration possible obstacles to Wi-Fi signal, especially if the deployment takes place in an urban area or inside buildings. When multiple access points are deployed, thought should be given to possible mutual interference between individual radios and multiple available channels should be used in a way that adjacent access points use different ones.

Various "mil-spec" network devices that can withstand rigorous weather conditions are available for purchase. However, an advantage over the use of multiple cheap household consumer grade routers in the setting of a field hospital is yet to be determined.

Accessories

Peripherals

Printing is a necessity even in a field hospital that strives to be "paperless," and has a big demand. Discharge documents, including imaging studies and lab results, are printed for every patient, as well as a multitude of other general printing needs. It is advised to plan for at least one printer per department and it is useful to have printers connected to the network so that they can receive print jobs from any network connected device.

Other recommended peripherals include barcode scanners. These should be used whenever feasible to read patient bracelet identification numbers instead of manually entering them to minimize entry errors and the risk of wrongfully ascribing information to patients. To support such a workflow, the information system is required to be able to produce such barcodes.

Electrical Independence

Past experience has shown that it is crucial for the IT department of a field hospital to be power independent. This means that a portable small generator should be on the packing list of IT equipment (various types of silent lightweight and low maintenance generators are available for purchase from various manufacturers). This need arises out of two possible situations: the first is to enable medical teams to be up and running and provide documented care within minutes of arriving at the deployment site. It is not uncommon for medical care to be provided even prior to erecting the hospital and operating the main generators. The second is a prolonged main AC power or hospital generator shortage, which may occur. This capability may also come in handy during the disassembly phase, as parts of the hospital (typically outpatient care) may still be going on as other hospital departments have shut down their operations and are being dismantled.

Packing Gear

IT equipment is sensitive by nature and expensive. As such, it should be suitably protected during storage and while on the move to a deployment site. While in storage, consideration should be given to keeping equipment batteries in good shape. This usually means keeping them partially charged and especially preventing a complete drainage. When it comes to dozens of different end units – including laptops, two-in-ones, and mobile devices – this can be quite a challenge. The use of specially crafted storage cases with built-in charging capabilities is recommended. Mobile devices should be kept in protective cases to reduce the risk of accidental breakage.

equipment redundancy and data backup (known as business-continuity plans or disaster-recovery plans). Many solutions to this problem are possible and a detailed review is beyond the scope of this chapter, but as a rule, such a plan needs to address at least the following issues:

- In case of a catastrophic server fault, a preinstalled backup server should be available. To allow for seamless operational continuity, all data that are entered by users should be replicated to the backup server as well (so-called "hot replication" or a similar solution, "active–active" or "active–passive" configuration).

- In addition, all data should be backed up at regular intervals to independent backup media, to protect against possible data corruption, which may affect both the main database, and the hot replica. The backup media should be kept away from system servers.

- The hardware plan (servers, network gear, end units, peripherals) should take into account possible hardware breakdowns that may occur during a deployment and backup devices should be made available.

Privacy and Security Issues

Medical information is highly sensitive and private by nature. Confidentiality is mandated by medical ethics as well as the law throughout the world. A field hospital environment is no exception and the hospital EMR should express this. However, a good balance should be sought between the protection of confidentiality and system usability, bearing in mind that a field hospital operating in a disaster zone with an overwhelming number of casualties first and foremost must be able to perform its role: to save lives. The EMR should support this main goal and allow for quick data access when and where needed by caregivers. Time-consuming user authentication and switching procedures within the application should be avoided. Physical limitation of system access should be employed if possible. For instance, In the "Haiti" EMR field hospital system (IDF), privacy and reliability of EMR data is ensured by the following means:

- Handheld devices, which allow access to the system, are allocated personally to medical team members according to their role within the hospital.

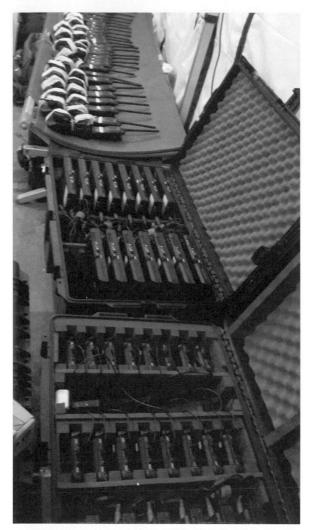

Figure 12.4 IT equipment storage and transport gear from the IDF field hospital; equipment is being charged while stored by special electricity fittings within the enclosures

Redundancy and Backup

The importance of safeguarding against possible malfunctions and data-loss events cannot be overestimated. This is the "primum non nocere" (first do no harm) directive of medical IT. Loss of ability to operate a field hospital information system or loss of operational and medical information stored in the system can have catastrophic implications for the mission as a whole and should not be allowed to happen. Nevertheless, technology can fail. Servers may break down, switches may stop functioning, and end units may become unresponsive; all with little or no warning. The answer to these risks is a well-thought-out plan for

- Stationary departmental workstations are located at places that are continuously monitored by departmental staff, so that the risk of unauthorized access is reduced.
- Updating the medical record requires the input of a personal unique identification code, which is kept secret. Viewing information does not require a code.

Cyber security is a growing concern to the well-being of medical information systems throughout the world. Although in the setting of a field hospital this risk may be lower compared with regular hospitals or other systems, it should still be taken into account and system development should be carried out with awareness of security issues. Professional penetration testing of the system is recommended. General internet access from within the system is best avoided, with access limited to dedicated interface servers secured behind an appropriate firewall where needed.

Training

Training and regular drills are key to deployment preparedness and should be carried out for two separate groups. The first group is the hospital IT team itself. After carefully handpicking the team members, they should undergo extensive training covering all components and functions of the system with a special emphasis on troubleshooting and problem solving. Critical malfunctions should be simulated and their remediation taught and exercised, keeping in mind the team will be required to handle such events in real time without the presence of additional experts. The second group requiring training is composed of all system users. They should be walked through the system and its functions, and data entry and extraction should be exercised using simulated patients. Exercises should be held at regular intervals (preferably at least yearly). Training materials both for IT personnel and system users should be produced and kept updated. These may include technical knowledge summaries, user manuals, presentations, and multimedia materials.

Field Testing

All system components should be field tested at regular intervals. (This can usually be accomplished at the same time as personnel training.) It is not satisfactory to test software and system components separately under lab conditions, but rather a comprehensive field test in which all system components are operated simultaneously is required. This should be repeated with every software version introducing new features and the introduction of new system components. System interfaces should also be tested.

Deployment

A field hospital deployment for an actual humanitarian mission is a climax toward which all efforts including planning, equipment procurement, system development, personnel training, field testing, and regular exercises are directed. Following is a description of an IT team involvement in a typical disaster zone relief mission based on recent IDF field hospital deployments.

Preliminary Phase

This phase relates to the period of time that begins with the decision to deploy the hospital and ends when equipment and personnel actually embark for the mission. These are "golden hours," which should be used wisely. IT personnel are gathered and quick refreshment of knowledge using training materials is advised. If time permits, all IT equipment should be checked and made sure it is in a working order. While loading IT equipment for ground, sea, or air transport, checklists should be used to ensure nothing is left behind.

En Route

The time spent en route to a deployment zone may be quite prolonged and last up to several days at times. Again, this is precious time that can be used to deepen users' knowledge and familiarity with system features, workflows, and procedures. This may be achieved using previously prepared training materials or standalone system stations, if applicable.

Deployment on Site

On arrival at the disaster zone and designation of a deployment site, a most strenuous effort of erecting the hospital begins. For the IT team, this means locating and gathering all IT equipment and setting up the IT headquarters, which houses system servers and main network equipment. In case care delivery begins simultaneously with hospital deployment, the basic EMR functionality should be enabled based on the independent IT power supply, system servers, wireless LAN, and mobile end units.

As the hospital is being built, the wired LAN network is gradually deployed in accordance with the previously prepared plan. Switches, routers, and additional wireless access points are distributed and connected, and network connectivity throughout the facility is established and tested. As medical equipment is hauled into departments, computer workstations, peripherals, and mobile units are allocated. Interface servers are brought online and communication with the radiology department machines and lab equipment is established.

Special attention is given to the organization of the triage area. A well-organized and functioning triage procedure, which includes patient registration, is crucial for a successful IT solution application and achieving information goals previously discussed. For a predetermined namespace system to be effectively enforced, the entry to a field-hospital facility should be controlled and guarded. All patients seeking medical care should be directed through this entry. A single point of entry is preferred. In addition to the enforcement of the namespace system, this type of setup also serves and enables the performance of effective medical triage, ensuring every admitted patient is met by a qualified triage physician, who makes an important decision as to which department within the hospital the patient is referred to.

At the point of entry, a unique identification, in accordance with the namespace system, is generated and allocated to every incoming patient. Once generated, the identification should be physically attached to the patient throughout their stay within the field hospital's grounds in a secure way that prevents an accidental loss. The use of a physical device such as a bracelet is compulsory.

Patient location tracking is usually achieved by updating a patient location on each entry to a certain hospital department or facility. (In the "Haiti" EMR, for instance, this is done by scanning the patient's bracelet barcode.)

Medical care is documented during the patient's stay in the hospital according to the EMR's capabilities and features. When a patient is ready to be discharged, a summary document is produced from the EMR and imaging studies are burned onto CD and/or printed on paper.

The actual discharge from the hospital is performed by a special discharge post within the hospital to make sure the discharge is properly marked in the information system and that demographic and contact information for the patient are known and recorded in case a need arises to contact them later on. Patient discharge destination is also noted.

Maintenance During Deployment

Once the hospital erection effort comes to an end and workflows within the hospital are established and running properly, a maintenance period begins for the IT team. This period is characterized by proactive activities designed to reduce the likelihood of system malfunctions and make sure that hospital information goals are met: systems maintenance includes periodic application checks, database status, and hot replication status checks. This also includes the performance of periodic data backups. Hardware maintenance includes server status checks, network equipment connectivity checks, and wireless signal quality checks throughout the hospital. Also of great importance is the performance of regular information maintenance and analysis. This relates to measures taken to ensure the quality of medical documentation is adequate and that all information deemed important to the establishment of situational awareness within the hospital is promptly registered by users. In case discrepancies are found, these are discussed in daily staff meetings. Another role of the IT team during this period is to produce the reports that may be required by hospital management and local authorities.

Asset Protection and Tracking

IT equipment should be monitored and protected, especially handheld devices that can be easily misplaced or stolen. It is advisable to have a built-in automatic function for this purpose within the hospital's application, which registers periodic "heartbeats" from connected devices. In the absence of such a feature, equipment should be properly labeled, regularly counted, and safely stowed away when not in use.

Termination and Debriefing

The information system is perhaps the last to be turned off when a field hospital's mission is over, and this is done only after the very last patient leaves the facility with their discharge document in hand and all documentation is done.

Every deployment is an excellent opportunity for the IT team to receive quality feedback from users, which should be sought in a systematic fashion, collated, and turned into actionable items, change requests, and new feature descriptions, which should then be prioritized and added to the system development plan. IT team members themselves need to be debriefed systematically following a mission. Their insight and experience gathered during the course of a mission usually proves to be very valuable.

Advanced Data Analysis and Usage

Following a mission, one of the most important advantages of having a computerized information system in the field hospital becomes apparent, as a large-scale academic effort usually ensues to summarize information and derive the lessons learned to improve patient care in future missions and contribute to disaster management and medical relief knowledge bases. This is achieved by applying computerized data analysis tools directly on a replica of the deployment database.

Future Considerations

We live at a time when internet access is becoming more and more ubiquitous and technology is constantly changing and influencing every aspect of our lives. Social network applications are connecting and enabling real-time interaction, communication, and collaboration between billions of human beings. However, at a disaster zone where countless human lives are at stake, somehow the power of these innovative internet-age technologies is not being harnessed to the full potential and information needs of the various parties involved in a disaster, which were briefly described at the beginning of this chapter, are only very partially fulfilled. Judging from experience in recent field hospital deployments, communication between different facilities was lacking, thus hampering collaboration between the various teams. A regional information platform is greatly missed. Such an information platform could connect all stakeholders within a disaster zone, including affected members of the population, authorities, and responders, and could even potentially create a single disaster zone namespace and medical registry of patients that can be fed by the different systems operating within the various facilities. Such a system is expected to greatly contribute to zone-wide continuity of care and facilitate collaboration and coordination of relief efforts. It seems that required technologies to implement such a regional disaster zone solution are available. Now is the time to harness them.

Communication Technologies

The Role of Communication and Communication Needs in a Crisis Event

As described above, accurate and timely information providing a detailed description of a disaster zone is a significant prerequisite to an efficient relief operation. The communication capabilities are the means for information exchange between all the stakeholders to achieve a successful deployment and maximize resource utilization.

The WHO publication *Classification and Minimum Standards for Foreign Medical Teams in Sudden Onset Disasters*[3] provides guidelines for communication capabilities during EMT deployment:

> All types of EMTs must consider robust communication systems, with redundancy, as mandatory. Without communication systems, EMTs will continue to be outside of any Ministry of Health or global health cluster (GHC) coordination framework. Technology used should be robust, appropriate for task and likely to still function in a SOD. EMTs must have more than one form of communication system (e.g. mobile and satellite phone). EMTs should consider telephone and data communication both to be priorities. EMTs should not focus purely on communication methods back to their countries of origin, instead ensuring they quickly establish means of communication with local MoH and emergency controllers, the cluster leads and through that cluster, local health facilities and EMTs to establish a functional health referral network. Reporting of activities to the MoH health cluster by e-mail, fax or other means is considered mandatory for EMTs. Use of communications equipment for expert opinion from either other EMTs, national or international specialists should be encouraged. Telemedicine in disaster response has the potential to develop further in the future to the benefit of beneficiaries.

Telecommunication represents a crucial component in a field-hospital operation. Careful consideration should be given to the types of communication equipment that are included and brought to the mission. In a mass-casualty incident, such as a devastating earthquake, some types of communication equipment might not be appropriate, whereas other types of gear originally thought to be superfluous could prove very useful. The greater the distance between the deployment site and the various disaster arenas, the greater the need for sophisticated means of telecommunication for use by different consumers. These needs include communication between stations and personnel inside the hospital, communication with teams out on peripheral missions, information exchange with local authorities, reporting and consultation with headquarters and various resources back at the homeland, and communication with the media[15].

Communication capabilities included in the mission should be derived from the needs of the EMT and all stakeholders involved in the operation.

Homeland Communications

These needs may include reporting, control, and management decision-making, logistic coordination, technological and scientific backup (such as online data analysis), and teleconsulting/telemedicine with experts. These needs are usually filled via telephone calls and broadband internet, capable of supporting video conference. It is advised to base these capabilities on independent satellite equipment, since usually, at least in the first days following the disaster, local networks will be down or severely impacted. End-user communication equipment, including phones, intercoms, and personal computers, should be set up in advance, as well as during the first phase of deployment, to support various types of communications, including email and video conferencing. The quantities of end-user equipment units taken to a mission should be derived from the number of users plus 20% surplus for backup and redundancy purposes. Establishing a robust wideband Internet service is key due to the fact that many communication channels may rely and be carried over the Internet. In case an Internet connection is not available, satellite-based end-user equipment, such as satellite phones, may be appropriate to establish initial communication capabilities. As is the case for the IT effort, it is advised that an independent power source, such as a portable generator, be available to charge the communication equipment in case of a power shortage. As a case study, in Port-au-Prince, Haiti, during the 2010 earthquake relief mission, the Israel EMT achieved international telecommunication capabilities during the first day of deployment based on the AMOS-3 satellite allowing an 8 GB bandwidth channel. This was split into several streams: telephone and fax, internet and email, and video conferencing. The satellite communications with all subsystems provided superb service to all

personnel, rescue, medical, and logistics, as well as to the many visitors to the camp such as other delegations and the media.

Communication with stakeholders in the disaster arena

On a SOD, the local MoH, with the assistance of WHO, will usually operate an EMTCC. Continuous communication with the EMTCC through all the deployment stages is a prerequisite for a smooth integration and an effective medical assistance operation. Communication with other EMTs (both local and international), local hospitals, pharmaceutical suppliers, evacuation agencies, and so on, is crucial. The means for these communication needs are usually the same as described above but may require some adjustments. Internet capabilities should also be used for local communications via emails, fax-mail, and video conference, and may make use of predefined data exchange protocols. In case the local cellular communication networks are available (it is not unusual for these networks to become available at some time following the disaster), it is recommended to stock up on mobile phones that support all local cellular networks. Multisim card support is beneficial and recommended.

Communication inside the EMT

As described above, information is the driving force of successful field hospital operations. The medical information inside the EMT is available through the EMR with its built-in wired and wireless communication system. Other means for communication inside the EMT should include wired and/or wireless telephones and two-way radio equipment ("walkie talkies") allowing interpersonal as well as group communication. Multiple communication channels are usually used; for example, a discrete channel for command personnel, another for hospital staff, and a third for the coordination of rescue services. A separate channel is usually allocated for logistic needs.

In addition, a public address system should be available to convey messages relevant for multiple staff members and broadcast important announcements. It is advised that this system supports multiple means of control and operation, including an interface with the in-hospital radio system allowing broadcasting announcements from mobile devices.

Considerations for a successful deployment

Communication capabilities are necessary means for command and control. The communications team should be involved in the planning and implementation process, from the first directive phase to the end of the mission. Communication equipment should be stored, arranged, and made ready to deploy in a specially allocated space within the field hospital, preferably in proximity to the EMT headquarters. It is important to appoint an official in charge of communications with the international and local agencies: telephone and fax numbers, email addresses, relevant Internet-site addresses, and communication officials' colleagues' details should be collected and made available. It is also recommended to conduct routine communication tests between the affiliates. Deployment and operation of communication equipment demands trained personnel. The communication team in an EMT operating and maintaining the communication means described above should consist of enough members – both in quantity and expertise – domains, and levels to support all phases of the mission. Some of the team members may be shared with the IT effort.

References

1. The WHO Emergency Medical Teams initiative. Website. https://extranet.who.int/emt/

2. American Medical Association Code of Ethics (2016). Chapter 3: opinions on privacy confidentiality and medical records. https://www.ama-assn.org/sites/defaul t/files/media-browser/code 2016-ch3.pdf

3. Norton I, von Schreeb J, Aitken P, Herard P, Lajolo C. *Classification and minimum standards for foreign medical teams in sudden onset disasters.* Geneva: World Health Organization; 2013.

4. Adams WG, Mann AM, Bauchner H. Use of an electronic medical record improves the quality of urban pediatric primary care. *Pediatrics* 2003: **111**(3): 626–32.

5. Manca DP. Do electronic medical records improve quality of care? Yes. *Canadian Family Physician* 2015: **61**(10): 846–7.

6. Jafar AJ, Norton I, Lecky F, et al. A literature review of medical record keeping by foreign medical teams in sudden onset disasters. *Prehospital and Disaster Medicine* 2015: **30**(2): 216–22.

7. Gueri M, Guerra ES, Gonzalez LE, et al. Health implications of the Tumaco earthquake, Colombia, 1979. *Disasters* 1983: **7**(3): 174–9.

8. Levy G, Blumberg N, Kreiss Y, et al. Application of information technology within a field hospital deployment following the January 2010 Haiti earthquake disaster. *Journal of the American Medical Informatics Association* 2010: **17**(6): 626–30.

9. Currier M, King DS, Wofford MR, et al. A Katrina experience: lessons learned. *The American Journal of Medicine* 2006: **119**(11): 986–92.

10. Burnweit C, Stylianos S. Disaster response in a pediatric field hospital: lessons learned in Haiti. *Journal of Pediatric Surgery* 2011: **46**(6): 1131–9.

11. Helminen M, Saarela E, Salmela J. Characterisation of patients treated at the Red Cross field hospital in Kashmir during the first three weeks of operation. *Emergency Medicine Journal* 2006: **23**(8): 654–6.

12. Kreiss Y, Merin O, Peleg K, et. al. Early disaster response in Haiti: the Israeli field hospital experience. *Annals of Internal Medicine* 2010: **153**(1): 45–8.

13. Callaway DW, Peabody CR, Hoffman A, et al. Disaster mobile health technology: lessons from Haiti. *Prehospital and Disaster Medicine* 2012: **27**(2): 1–5.

14. Digital Imaging and Communications in Medicine. (2016). Website. http://dicom.nema.org

15. Niemtzow RC, Yarbrough G, Harwood KL, et al. The amateur radio emergency service (ARES) and the national disaster medical system (NDMS). *Military Medicine* 1993: **158**(4): 259–63.

13

Advanced Triage Management for Emergency Medical Teams

Frederick M Burkle, Jr

Introduction

A mass-casualty incident (MCI) is an "event which generates more patients at one time than locally available resources can manage using routine procedures requiring exceptional emergency arrangements and additional or extraordinary assistance [1]." Direct MCI mortality and morbidity arise from natural disasters, human system failures, and war and armed conflict-based crises[2]. Additional indirect mortality and morbidity will occur from each of these crises when the public health system's essential infrastructure (water, sanitation, shelter, food, medical access and availability, and energy) are absent, destroyed, overwhelmed, not recovered or maintained, or selectively denied to populations[3].

Historically, both national and international MCIs have frequently resulted in the deployment of *field level hospitals* that are focused on civilians, the military, or both, and defined as a "mobile, self-contained, self-sufficient health-care facility capable of rapid deployment and expansion or contraction to meet immediate emergency requirements for a specified period of time [4]." These hospitals have served as the major frontline response capacity to MCIs for many decades and share the following characteristics:

- have capacity and capability to bring lifesaving care as close to the frontline of war or armed conflict, natural disaster, public health emergencies of international concern, or other humanitarian crises as possible
- operationally, are considered resource constrained facilities
- triage management will be practiced at every level of care on a daily basis
- standards of care impacting the triage process may vary depending on resources

The World Health Organization (WHO) Emergency Medical Team (EMT) System

In 2013, WHO published *Classification and Minimum Standards for Foreign Medical Teams in Sudden Onset Disasters*, with a trauma and surgical focus[5]. In 2014, over 40 organizations – including international NGOs, military, faith-based organizations, and governments – deployed FMTs throughout the Ebola response. Recognizing the important lessons gained from these events led to formalizing a global health workforce designed to improve coordination, quality, and predictability of clinical response teams deploying with surge capacity now referred to as EMTs. These teams, both I-EMTs and N-EMTs "serve as a deployment and coordination mechanism for all partners who aim to provide clinical care in emergencies such as tsunami, earthquake, flood, and more recently, in large outbreaks, such as the West Africa Ebola outbreak, which require a surge in clinical care capacity. It allows a country affected by a disaster or other emergency to call on teams that have been pre-registered and quality assured[6]."

Under this system, EMT type 1 facilities pertain to initial outpatient emergency care of injuries and other significant health-care needs. Traditional EMTs (field-level hospitals) fall under type 2 inpatient surgical emergency care facilities, which provide inpatient acute care and general and obstetric surgery for trauma and other major conditions, and type 3 inpatient referral care facilities, which provide complex inpatient surgical care, including intensive care capacity. Additional specialized care teams and specialized care cells will be placed within type 2, 3, or a local hospital. WHO serves as the deployment and coordination mechanism for all partners prepared to provide clinical care in emergencies. Through a global registration system, WHO provides preregistered, quality assured, verified, and classified EMTs, which meet minimum standards for deployment as a time-limited surge clinical capacity to affected populations[6].

Triage Guidance Under the WHO Classification and Minimum Standards for FMTs

The WHO publication *Classification and Minimum Standards for Foreign Medical Teams in Sudden Onset Disasters* provides guidelines starting with "initial and field level triage, assessment and first aid" at type 1 EMTs, stating that "staff should be experienced in those elements of initial trauma care that relate to triage on a mass scale, wound and basic fracture management, basic emergency care of pediatric, obstetric, mental health, and medical presentations." Surgical triage and assessment at type 2 levels calls for "ability to receive, screen, and triage new and referred patients, with ability to perform at least 7 major or 15 minor operations daily with at least 20 inpatient beds per one operating table and be able to perform 24 hours per day, seven days per week for at least 3 weeks but ideally longer." Type 3 EMTs are required to provide "complex referral triage[5]."

The WHO publication further recognizes eight different EMT classification systems worldwide, which have in common the three levels of EMT response teams with "escalating complexity and capacity for each level." It emphasizes that no one model is applicable to all EMTs functioning internationally. For example, the European Union European Civil Protection Modules call for triage of "at least 20 patients per hour stabilizing 50 patients in 24 hours, with supplies to treat 100 patients with minor injuries per 24 hours" at the equivalent of a type 1 EMT, and an "advanced medical Post with surgery providing similar triage numbers per hour" plus "surgical team capability of damage control surgery for 12 patients per 24 hours, working in 2 shifts, and supplies to treat 100 patients with minor injuries per 24 hours." Their EMT level equivalent calls for both initial and/or follow-up trauma and medical care with "10 beds for heavy trauma patients with possible capacity to expand with medical teams" for "triage, intensive care, surgery, serious but not life-threatening injuries, evacuation, specialist support personnel and at least covering the following: generalist, emergency physicians, orthopedist, pediatrician, anesthetist, obstetrician, health director, lab technician, X-ray technician[5]."

Mass-Casualty Incident Triage Management Requirements

Operational Levels of Triage

In MCIs, the practice of triage must occur to both sort and prioritize patients to meet unexpected circumstances traditionally using immediate, delayed, minimal, or expectant categories within minutes of arrival. Prehospital *primary triage* is practiced for all MCIs, at which point victims are assigned an acuity-level based on injury severity. The decision-making processes involved in primary triage and patient hospital distribution are influenced by both reactive (ad hoc) and proactive (based on situational awareness) factors[7]. The most commonly adopted triage systems used are sort, assess, lifesaving interventions, treatment/triage (SALT): a nonproprietary free system developed from available research, with widely accepted best practices of existing mass triage systems and consensus opinion, the simple triage and rapid treatment (START), which substitutes radial pulse for capillary refill[8], and coupled with a system of secondary triage termed "secondary assessment of victim endpoint (SAVE)."

The SAVE triage was developed to direct limited resources to the subgroup of patients expected to benefit most from their use. The START and SAVE triage techniques are used in situations in which triage is dynamic, occurs over many hours to days, and only limited, austere, field, advanced life-support equipment is readily available[9].

Secondary triage, or a reevaluation of the victim's condition after initial medical care, may also occur at the scene of the MCI following emergency medical services' (EMS) interventions or during transport to an emergency department or secondary collection station[7]. In EMTs, secondary triage is an ongoing process, which continues after the initial triage decisions are made, which move the first stage of victims to the operating rooms and others for delayed treatment or as stable candidates initially triaged for evacuation, as the patient's condition may change for the better or for the worse.

Many of the crises responded to by EMTs realistically exist where little or no effective prehospital care or triage occurs before victim arrival. This chapter restricts itself to *advanced triage* where some victims are triaged based on inclusion criteria but others –

those severely injured or ill who are triaged based on resource-poor or constrained settings (exclusion criteria) – may not receive the resources normally expected.

Minimal Qualifications for Survival

Based on collective knowledge of existing resource constraints, EMTs are held responsible to develop predetermined agreed-on criteria referred to as "minimal qualifications for survival" (MQS), which define what cases will *not* receive curative care but will receive pain relief, emotional care, and, if available, spiritual support[10]. MQS define who is triaged in the "expectant" category, which normally includes those moribund with multiple major wounds whose management would be considered wasteful of scarce resources including operating time and blood transfusions, those without vital signs regardless of injury or illness, transcranial ballistic wounds, multiple-organ failure from severe trauma, severe third-degree burns without reasonable chance of survival, open pelvic injuries with uncontrolled class IV shock, advanced respiratory failure, and dosimetry-confirmed lethal radiation doses[11].

Every disaster has its own contributing factors for MQS requirements, but the conditions influencing the MQS are not always immediately known and become more clarified as the nature of the crisis and state of the victims are better understood[12]. For example, in the 2010 Haiti earthquake, a significant number of neglected casualties presented with serious wounds and advanced infections, which progressed to multiple-organ failure resulting in higher-than-normal expectant triage category designations [13,14]. Triage officers (TOs) may seek reassessments of the triage protocols to ensure they remain appropriate to the MQS. For example, the traditional disaster medical assistance team (DMAT) triage system collapsed when it became evident on the first day of hurricane Katrina that thousands of evacuated seriously ill critical care patients with nontraumatic illness were being triaged using inappropriate DMAT trauma-related protocols[15,16].

Potential Injury/Illness Creating Event

Koenig and colleagues have developed a potential injury/illness creating event (PICE) nomenclature, which provides a method and framework for consistency in "crisis classification" based on the likelihood that outside medical assistance will be needed. Stage 0 means little or no chance, stage I means there is a small chance, stage II means there is a moderate chance, and stage III means local medical resources are clearly overwhelmed. As such, EMTs, both international and national, are deployed as assets for PICE stage III events[17].

Legal and Ethical Issues of Triage

Society recognizes that legal, ethical, and moral expectations and obligations exist during crises and that triage plans exist to treat as many victims as possible who have an opportunity for survival. When triage is performed in accordance with accepted medical practice, it is both sanctioned and recognized by law in most countries[18,19]. In fact, medical providers are held legally accountable for the triage process, but the process itself cannot ensure either treatment or survival [11,20]. Because unrealistic triage results in unacceptable death rates among those who should survive, triage plans must be well thought out and designed. The WMA asserts that "The physician must act according to the needs of patients and the resources available. He/she should attempt to set an order of priorities for treatment that will save the greatest number of lives and restrict morbidity to a minimum[21]."

Under- and Overtriage

The primary goal of triage is to identify the majority of field trauma victims at risk for life-threatening injuries. The accuracy of triage is the degree of match between the severity of injury and the level of care. Sensitivity and specificity of screening tests are useful indicators of accuracy[22]. In reality, casualty differences, occult injuries, and the complexities of assessment preclude perfect accuracy in triage decisions suggesting that, in practice, a "perfect" triage system is not possible[10,18,21].

Most triage protocols are based on physiological criteria and subject to under- and overtriage. Overtriage occurs when a casualty receives a high acuity triage assignment, is transported to the EMT, and unnecessarily consumes scarce resources. Undertriage occurs when a casualty receives a low acuity triage assignment and does not receive the specialized trauma treatment needed, resulting in inappropriate admission or death. Based on disaster experience, studies have sought a balance between over- and undertriage for a given set of triage criteria[23,24].

Designing a triage system that maximizes specificity (undertriage) to avoid delaying care for sick people, while maximizing sensitivity (overtriage) to avoid wasting resources, is a challenge for any EMT. Once this balance has been defined, triage guidelines can be modified to meet unique triage objectives. Standards set by the American College of Surgeons Committee on Trauma aim for overtriage rates less than 50% (i.e., a specificity of greater than 50%), considered acceptable to minimize patients who are undertriaged, and undertriage rates of less than 5–10% (i.e., a sensitivity of greater than 95%) considered acceptable for trauma patients[25]. A multisite assessment of the American College of Surgeons Committee on Trauma offers a field triage decision scheme for identifying seriously injured children and adults. Anything higher may lead to unnecessary morbidity and mortality in severely injured, but potentially salvageable, patients [26,27,28].

Studies suggest that triage can conflict with human rights legislation and even with humanitarian laws, but "accountability for reasonableness" can temper the disagreements on the setting of priorities[29]. After a comprehensive evaluation of the actions taken under the extraordinary circumstances during the Haitian relief experience, it was determined that the concept and triage policy used allowed the best chance of survival for the largest possible number of victims. At EMT levels of care, the triage systems must be flexible and reevaluated daily with "extensive adaptation to local condition[13]." For example, significant improvement of over- and undertriage rates and casualty severity predictability were accomplished across triage levels when the South African Triage Score (SATS) four-level system made modifications to make it more clinically and culturally sensitive[30,31]. Similarly, the chosen triage protocol (START) used in the Haiti earthquake was tailored to the local situation for surge capacity either by increasing resource availability or by reducing inpatient use. The process not only differentiated patients according to the severity of their injuries but also by the resources required and expected outcomes. The triage system must be flexible, reevaluated daily, and "requires extensive adaptation to local condition[13]."

Altered Standards of Care

The term "altered standards of care" generally means a shift in the provision of care and the allocation of equipment, supplies, and personnel in a way to ensure the greatest good for the greatest number. The majority of studies on altered standards of care pertain to emergency services triage management in developed countries. EMTs function daily in resource-poor or constrained settings where shortfalls are anticipated and standards of care maintenance strategies are best when planned for, ongoing, and steady, with the least observed consequences to avoid untoward, abrupt, or unethical consequences.

In EMTs, triage protocols need to be flexible enough to change as the size and speed of the crisis grows. Any change in triage decision tools must be understood by the entire medical staff. TOs first consider "reactive and proactive alterations" of the triage protocol process, but much can be done before alteration becomes an operational reality. Hick and colleagues list six key strategies: *prepare* with optimal stockpiling, *conserve* use of certain therapies, *substitute* equivalent medications, *adapt* existing devices for purposes they were not intended, *reuse* material resources, and as a last resort, the *reallocation* of resources to those most likely to benefit[32,33].

Triage decisions will affect the allocation of resources across all triage categories and the entire EMT. For example, the triage area may be reserved for immediate casualties only, intensive care areas may become surgical suites, and regular wards become isolation or other specialized units. Recovering casualties may be evacuated/transferred earlier than anticipated, nurses function as physicians and physicians function outside their specialties, disposable supplies reused, treatment decisions based on clinical judgment from physical exams without additional laboratory testing and X-ray resources, single person isolation units become group isolation units, and identifying safe alternate care sites from facilities not previously designed to provide medical care[32,33].

Reverse Triage

Geneva Convention (GC) medical protocols and ethicists are opposed to any system of triage prioritization other than medical need. The GC explicitly states "only urgent medical reasons will authorize priority in order of treatment to be administered [34]." However, under extreme battle conditions when the combat situation demands that soldiers be returned to combat as rapidly as possible, NATO may contradict this position, using "reverse triage", resulting in military personnel with minimal injuries treated first and returned to duty before more seriously injured casualties are managed[35]. The legal argument supporting reverse triage is that military physicians do not enter into a physician–patient relationship with the casualties. Therefore, this difference warrants that triage reversal should occur if the chain of command requires it.

Triage Officers

The placement of experienced civilian and military TOs at the EMT level is crucial to success. Burkle described the desirable characteristics of TOs as "surgically experienced, easily recognized, and respected, demonstrating good judgment and leadership, decisive, knowledgeable, familiar with resources, staff skills, and limitations, equipment and evacuation potential" and who "maintain control of the often unpredictable triage situation[36]." Others assert that few cases are sorted improperly where trained TOs exist, adding that while the "full extent of the disaster may not be fully known for several hours, the parameters of casualty flow, patient care, and rapid recognition of priorities require the continued attention of the TO.

International Committee of the Red Cross (ICRC) guidelines recommend that only one TO is required, a physician or nurse, with experience and understanding of war wounds, with an overview of all aspects of the functioning of the EMT and its resources, and the ability to make clear decisions under stress. The decisions made by the TO must be respected[37]. The TO decides when triage is implemented and ensures that all departments are informed. The clinical assessment and allocation of a triage category must be supervised or performed by the TO, who must see all the patients. The triage process is implemented and defined with specific roles of each member of the EMT and of each department as an extension of the normal hospital routines. The situation needs constant reassessment to determine the need for additional staff, supplies, and ward areas. The ICRC cautions that, while a surgeon can make an accurate surgical assessment of each patient, they might give preference to those cases corresponding to his or her own specialty. An anesthesiologist may be able to leave the operating theater to help the TO with clinical assessment. The TO has the responsibility to ensure that the EMT is "a safe place" by being aware of outside events, any security situation, and maintaining control of the number of people entering the EMT[37].

Baker, with extensive experience in war surgery, maintains that the ideal triage officer needs "exceptional leadership skills, strong clinical expertise, and good communication abilities that requires constant situational awareness, tactical understanding, adaptability, and decisiveness." Additional expectations are that the TO prevents confusion, fear, competition among staff members, prevents bottlenecks at critical locations, and ensures that critical casualties are not passed unnoticed and a contaminated casualty is prevented from entering the wrong staging area[38,39].

Triage Teams

TOs are dependent on clinically strong, knowledgeable, and trusted team members who, at a minimum, have triage experience (nurse or medic/corpsman) and with immediate access to other triage team members from logistics and communications. The triage team for a public-health emergency requires multidisciplinary expertise emphasizing public health skills, infectious disease, field epidemiology, and cultural anthropology, which was especially relevant during the Ebola epidemic in West Africa when the native population resisted treatment out of fear of the motives of foreign aid workers[40].

Triage Tagging

Tagging is important to continuity of care and often serves as the only ongoing medical record of the casualty. The purposes of tags are to (1) identify the victim, (2) identify to which triage category the victim belongs, and (3) provide some space to document details about the victim and their management[41]. Among the numerous varieties available, the most useful are those easy to read and interpret, having space for instructions and vital signs. Colored tapes and more permanent plastic tags are also available. Tags are usually attached to the large toe or wrist. If the casualty is retriaged to another level, the new tag is attached over the original tag, providing evidence of a change in clinical status[36].

Tags may be unavailable or destroyed. A system using "Xs" marked on the forehead with indelible pens is acceptable. X indicates minor injury, XX indicates serious injury but some delay in treatment possible, and XXX indicates serious injury requiring immediate attention.

There is no published evidence that indicates triage tags improve management of incidents involving more than 24 people[41]. Alternative systems demand adherence to the "daily routine doctrine," an expansion of normal services to accommodate the new patient load, and emphasizes that "geographical triage" of victim separation on urgency pertains only to the pre-EMT incident scene[42,43]. This outcome may be helpful in that all "immediate" category victims will arrive together at the EMT. It is dependent on a well-organized pre-EMT system, a state that is not normally available for most EMT situations[43].

The Triage Process

The first round of decisions in the triage area is often where the most decisive, collective, efficient, and agreed-on stage of the triage process occurs in directly moving casualties to the operating rooms[44]. The initial triage exam, and those that follow, should focus equally on physiological and anatomical parameters. Physiologic parameters, with a prehospital triage sensitivity of 0.7, provide only a brief "snapshot" of the physiologic stability at the time of the triage exam and may initially lead to undertriage. Anatomical criteria alone have a prehospital sensitivity of 0.5 and a 20%–30% yield for identifying major trauma victims. When both parameters are combined, the triage sensitivity becomes 0.8[45]. This information, along with attention to mechanism of injury of the chest, head, upper abdomen, face, and amputations, represents for the first triage performed at the EMT, the combination of information that best determines casualties triaged as "immediate" for emergency lifesaving surgery. Additionally, focused exams and tests performed in the triage area better clarify the extent of organ injuries, including occult fractures.

The second round of triage for remaining casualties begins automatically and is often more challenging, complex, and unpredictable, especially when an unexpected influx of new casualties occurs. During the Vietnam War, this stage of triage was referred to as "the triage dance." The singular actions of the TO become more demanding as each casualty is reassessed by the triage team process, which is constantly updated and performed in an orderly and consistent manner. The TO monitors and supervises the physiological information provided by trusted team members, which depict an increasingly accurate picture of how casualties are maintaining their stability[46]. Additional focused exams and tests performed in the triage area better clarify the extent of organ injuries including occult fractures. This continuous triage flow of information and decision-making confirms that

basic and advanced procedures are being carried out despite the continuous decision challenges.

Knowledge of the larger system of resources and security beyond the EMT is required, including trusted relationships with outside resources and authorities. The TO needs to know and be updated on the status of crucial resources in medical logistics, blood products, staffing, evacuation potential, expected time to an open operating room, and additional security risks for the wounded and EMT staff, while preparing for the arrival of additional casualties, to name but a few. Scarce items that impacted ongoing triage decisions during the 100-hour 1991 Persian Gulf War were blood products, surgical sutures, lap pads, stretcher straps, blankets, and surgical gloves: any one of these had the potential to disrupt the entire triage process and the functional capacity of the EMT[47,48,49].

These second-stage decisions directly impact the priority list for surgery and may prompt the triage team to consider other options, including immediate evacuation if such a calculated decision provides an opportunity for survival without additional risks that compromise safety or vital resources. These decisions are often difficult to make, always debated, second-guessed, and learned from when discussed during the post-event evaluation.

Decoding Vital Signs

Over the generations, there have been multiple attempts to improve triage scoring systems and correlation with outcomes. Unfortunately, they are a poor substitute for good clinical judgment and experience. Vital signs are routinely monitored and reported as numbers either electronically or by medical professionals other than physicians or experienced nurses. The number values alone of vital signs provided verbally to the triage officer, triage team, or written on a triage tag fail to provide the needed sensitivity and specificity desired for expeditious decisions required in triage. The numbers alone may or may not properly alert the triage officer and team to pending physiologic failure. Properly "decoding the vital signs" and attention to their physiologic meaning can discover subtle worsening of the physiologic state by incorporating visual alerts such as subtle mental status changes, especially in an otherwise quiet but increasingly anxious or apprehensive casualty, and delayed capillary refill, first on the distal extremities and moving up to the core of the body, which reveals physiologic attempts to maintain the central blood flow[46,50].

Parameters for Decoding Vital Signs

- mental status: anxious, apprehensive
- resting tachycardia
- pulse: soft, nonexpansive, nonvibratory
- systolic BP < 100 mm Hg
- pulse pressure < 30 mm Hg
- narrowing pulse pressure: absent or faint diastolic
- resting tachypnea or bradypnea
- regions: head, chest, upper abdomen, amputation, face

Triage Protocols in Deployed EMTs

A large number of triage protocol systems are available to prehospital emergency medical systems in the developed world. Few are relevant to EMT resource-poor or constrained settings where triaged victims include those unlikely to survive. Despite all the current technological advances, the basic skill of disaster triage of large numbers of injured to optimize available resources remains a vital tool.

This section describes advanced triage protocols currently in use for:

- sudden-onset disasters
- complex humanitarian emergencies
- public health emergencies of international concern
- war and conflict

Sudden Onset Disasters (SODs)

Weather-related disasters increased by 50% between 2005 and 2014, along with a dramatic intensification of natural disasters from earthquakes, typhoons, cyclones, wild fires, and floods, which are often exacerbated by climate change, severe droughts, rapid unsustainable urbanization, biodiversity crises, and national scarcities of food, water, and energy. Over 20 million refugees have been displaced by these disasters[51].

Surgical Need

At baseline, only 15% of the world's countries are able to provide a minimum of 5000 surgical procedures per 100 000 persons[51]. Countries most at risk of climate-related natural disasters frequently have among the lowest surgical procedure rates. The 2010 Haiti earthquake killed or injured 5% of the population and internally displaced 19%, drawing the deployment of over 300 governmental and nongovernmental EMTs; more than any previous SOD.

EMTs remained operational from one week to over a year. But most operations were unrelated to the earthquake. Studies demonstrated that outside support improved short-term recovery, but it is unclear how long surgical capacity changed or what role volunteer surgical relief efforts played[52].

Triage Categories

Médecins Sans Frontières (MSF) used ICRC triage categories, but added the color codes listed:

- Category I/red: serious wounds: resuscitation and immediate surgery for those with a good chance of recovery. ICRC experience that most of these casualties have abdominal, thoracic, and peripheral vascular wounds.
- Category II/yellow: second priority wounds: can await surgery; not on urgent basis. Majority of casualties triaged; most with compound fractures and penetrating head injuries.
- Category III/green: superficial wounds: ambulatory management. Minor wounds managed under local anesthesia. Are often frightened, in pain, and may be the most problematic to manage.
- Category IV/black: severe wounds: supportive treatment. Likely to die. Management considered wasteful of scarce resources including operating time and blood.

MSF cautioned that the triage process clashed with local factors such as cultural (e.g., the deceased take priority in evacuation), emotional (e.g., preference given to adults, not children), ethical (e.g., sorting considered unacceptable), logistics (e.g., lack of security, in sufficient medicines, stretchers, mattresses, traction pins), and medical management factors (e.g., lack of ear, eye, nose, and throat expertise)[53,54].

Complex Humanitarian Emergencies

1989 heralded in the post-Cold War era where cross-border wars had all but disappeared and were replaced primarily by the emergence of intrastate complex humanitarian emergencies (CHEs), which frequently overflowed into regional political crises, armed conflicts, and war. CHEs are defined by the UN as:

> Humanitarian crises in a country, region, or society where there is total or considerable breakdown of authority resulting from internal or external conflict and which requires an international response that

goes beyond the mandate or capacity of any single and/or ongoing UN country program[55].

With the absence of an adequate national medical care system, the ICRC under protections of the GC and international humanitarian law (IHL) were the first to provide surgical care to both civilians and combatants in multiple post-Cold War CHEs in the former Yugoslavia, Afghanistan, Cambodia, Chechnya, Congo, Somalia, and Sudan, to name but a few. The ICRC's presence and security was guaranteed under existing IHL and GC legal provisions to ensure a "right to humanitarian assistance" for all victims – civilian and military – with providers bound to the policy and practice of the humanitarian principles of neutrality, impartiality, universality, and independence[56]. Under the same international legal protections, additional field hospitals were developed by health-related NGOs, such as MSF in 1970 and IMC, Mercy Corps, UK-MED, the Israel Defense Forces (IDF), and hundreds of others representing multiple nations and academic surgical centers.

Many CHEs are ongoing: Afghanistan since 1979, Somalia since 1991, and unrelenting conflicts in Iraq, Syria, Yemen, Libya, and South Sudan, which currently see no viable conclusion. Additional insurgencies continue in southeast Turkey, Egypt's Sinai Peninsula, and north-east Nigeria.

Health Consequences

CHEs have proved devastating, resulting in large numbers of civilians suffering both direct and indirect mortality and morbidity as public health infrastructure and protections disappear. EMTs serving CHEs are challenged by intrastate displaced populations (e.g., internally displaced, refugees, migrants, asylum seekers), unattended trauma, malnutrition and starvation, infectious diseases, severe exacerbation of noncommunicable diseases and relapses of untreated mental illness, and severe war-witnessed psychological impairments and abuses (e.g., post-traumatic stress disorder [PTSD], rape), especially impacting the most vulnerable populations of women, children, the elderly, and disabled.

Impact of Triage on EMTs

Although triage as a medical sorting process was originally developed and applied to echeloned military field medical systems dealing with mass casualties, the term has now permeated most aspects of

EMT practice, especially in CHEs. Among the limitations directly impacting EMTs are: the enormous numbers of civilians of all ages injured, ill, and dying; indigenous medical care is rarely available; EMTs are frequently overwhelmed and inaccessible; first aid and transport are haphazard; water and electricity are nonexistent; EMT facilities are often threatening and hostile; personnel, equipment, and evacuation are often compromised; it is difficult to import both surgical skills and equipment, which may not be usable under dangerous conditions; and triage decisions are based primarily on exclusion criteria.

At no time in recent history have so many aid projects, including health clinics and EMTs, closed or suspended because of insecurity or danger to staff. In Syria, over 757 indigenous medical personnel, as of June 2016, have been killed, 90% by the Syrian government and its allies, and an additional 15 000 have fled. Over 346 attacks on 246 separate medical facilities including permanent and field hospitals have occurred as a widespread and systemic policy[57]. Syrian indigenous EMTs must be small and mobile or face certain destruction. Basic health care has all but disappeared in north-east and west Syria. Triage training has occurred, but organized triage is, at most, an ad hoc practice.

The unique characteristics of CHEs directly impact decisions whether or not to launch an I-EMT and where it could safely provide the best care. Currently, the only deployed I-EMTs are in Turkey along the Syrian border. In Yemen, health facilities, including I-EMTs, have been attacked over 100 times, resulting in MSF closing their EMT in 2016 when aerial bombing on their hospital killed 16 and continued despite the fact that they systematically provided GPS coordinates with the parties in the conflict as required under international law. Similar attacks have taken place in 19 additional countries[57].

Refugee Camp-Specific Triage Requirements

Refugee camp EMTs are more commonly type 1 and are deployed rapidly and rarely have equipment, personnel, or evacuation capabilities. Exclusion criteria are the daily norm. The triage process must seek out severe treatable cases, cases at risk to the refugee camp (e.g., measles, cholera, tuberculosis) and exclude chronic nonrisk patients.

Public Health Emergencies of International Concern

Mass illness management of public health emergencies of international concern (PHEICs) is challenging. Planning for specialized public health EMTs that meet operational requirements is vital. Tasks facing responders to the 2014 Ebola epidemic were described as "large and difficult requiring countries, complex international systems (UN, the WHO, and others) to scale up, coordinate, and interact operationally at speeds that proved extremely difficult[58]."

A triage team approach is favored. The knowledge base for triage decisions requires multidisciplinary team guidance, including anthropologists, social scientists, epidemiologists, and logisticians. Successful triage management is, at any one time, patient, community, and organizational resource centered. Most important is that resource constraints and how they impact clinical decisions must be immediately transmitted to a central authority to mitigate the threat it exposes. Even slight breaches in protocol will lead to transmission, the very action that proper triage management is supposed to prevent[59].

Population-based Triage Systems

Public-health skill sets are not widely known nor distributed among the traditional EMT provider population, especially emergency physicians who were dispatched to triage the massive patient population. This was considered a major educational and training priority during the entire Ebola epidemic [60]. Global legal triage supports the mobilization of public health infrastructure through which governments can adequately detect, declare, and address these PHEICs, as well as unique triage requirements.

Popular triage systems that depend on anatomical or physiological criteria are not relevant in PHEICs. Population-based triage categorization is essential to determine individual victim disposition and serve as markers in the evolving epidemic, such as distribution of infectious contacts within the population, the rate of spread, and as a predictive value in anticipating the outcome of the disease. The ultimate magnitude of the epidemic/pandemic will determine required resources and resource allocation. Population-based triage management under a central authority is vitally indicated to control the transmission and ensure fair and decisive resource allocation across all triage categories.

Any bioevent triage must reflect exposure, duration, and infectiousness, not necessarily the severity of presentation. *The goal of triage is to prevent transmission measured as secondary infections.* With this, the epidemic or pandemic will cease. MQSs guiding triage must be sensitive and specific enough to seek out severe treatable cases, seek out cases at risk to populations, and exclude nonrisk patients. Initially, triage management questions will be driven by case definition (which changes daily), differences in lethality, incubation, age, and gender vulnerability, and physical diagnostic and laboratory criteria of the offending agent. For example, in the 2014–2015 West African Ebola epidemic, the initial triage was based only on clinical signs and case definitions, resulting in alarming false-positive rates exposing those patients to transmission[61]. Control was established only when triage was based on reliable and accurate point-of-contact confirmatory testing[62,63].

Patient demand far exceeds the capability to provide critical care services in all epidemics: a fair and just system to allocate limited resources will be essential[64]. Expectant categories have been based, in part, on independent predictors of death: (1) age of > 65 years, (2) altered mental status, (3) respiratory rate of > 30 breaths/min, (4) low oxygen saturation, and (5) shock index of > 1 (heart rate/systolic blood pressure)[65].

Five suggested biologically sensitive triage categories aligning with the acronym SEIRV can be modified depending on the biological and epidemiological nature of the agent[67]:

- category 1: susceptible but not exposed, making up the majority of the population (where applicable, it includes those with incomplete or unsuccessful vaccination)
- category 2: exposed individuals who are infected, incubating without signs or symptoms, and not contagious
- category 3: infectious individuals experiencing signs or symptoms listed in the case definition and contagious; includes those who died, but whose remains are contagious
- category 4: removed individuals who are no longer a source of infection, including bodily remains that are no longer contagious and those geographically evacuated to a different resource profile
- category 5: vaccinated-protected: those recovered and protected either by vaccination or prophylactic medication

SEIRV is an appropriate tool for fixed and mobile EMTs in the first days and weeks of any epidemic, but risks exposing large numbers of the population who seek medical assistance out of fear becoming exposed in waiting and treatment areas to those who do have the disease. Other layers of triage screening are necessary to prevent that exposure, but mitigation is best obtained when these triage categories are applied to population broadcasts or as a telephone tool.

The *pandemic influenza triage algorithm (PITA)* is a standardized triage tool algorithm for use by professionals for face-to-face encounters. Health-care professionals use the PITA to determine patient acuity and estimate resource needs (e.g., intravenous fluids or ventilator) and to predict the complexity of care required to adequately treat patients. Health-care professionals who use the PITA are expected to be experienced or otherwise trained in patient triage specific to their site of practice. The PITA uses a valid, five-level triage scale to determine patient acuity and estimate resource needs to predict complexity of care required. Patients are classified on a scale from 1 to 5[67]:

- PITA level 1: resuscitation
- PITA level 2: emergent
- PITA level 3: urgent
- PITA level 4: semiurgent
- PITA level 5: stable, discharge

Military Triage in War and Conflict

As of writing, global war battle deaths per 100 000 people have declined since the 1980s[68]. Conflict is considered as deaths below 1000 per year[69]. Traditionally, the ultimate goals of combat medicine and military-led EMTs are the return of the greatest number of war fighters to combat and the preservation of life, limbs, and eyesight. MQS commitment of resources is decided first based on the mission and immediate tactical situation, and then by medical necessity, irrespective of a casualty's national or combatant status. Casualties are divided into three categories:

- emergent
- nonemergent
- expectant

These categories are useful in dividing casualties into those requiring further immediate surgical treatment (emergent), and those that are less injured and still require care in the near term (6–12 hours) but have low expected mortality (nonemergent). It is anticipated that 10–20% of casualties presenting to a forward-placed casualty-receiving facility will require urgent surgery, but this is incident dependent[11]. Most of the wounded will not require intensive decision-making, intervention, and care. Military triage is a fluid process at all levels, with altered standards of care situations and resources requiring a change in category at any time. In the extreme example, a casualty may be triaged from emergent to expectant during surgery, abruptly terminating the operation ("on-the-table triage")[11].

The USA military mass-casualty triage categories comprise:

- immediate
- delayed
- minimal
- expectant
- urgent surgical

The USA/NATO system, also referred to in the military as "conventional triage," added a fifth "urgent surgical category" used to describe surgical patients who need an operation, but can wait a few hours[70]. Casualties who receive the appropriate initial categorization (e.g., urgent surgical) and intervention may be sufficiently stabilized and retriaged to a lower subsequent category (e.g., delayed). This is similar to the NATO triage system, which is partly based on medical emergency triage tags methodology. There are five levels of care, previously referred as echelons of care by NATO and USA doctrine. Level 1 care is by self or buddy care level. Level 2 care occurs at forward surgical centers where life- and limb-saving surgery is done. Level 3 is the highest care in the combat setting for the USA forces, while in the host country it would mean treatment at a large general or zonal hospital. Level 4 is treatment outside combat zone. Level 5 is the highest care in civil or military setup[71].

These levels are not to be confused with the American College of Surgeons designated civilian trauma centers, where level 1 is the highest and the best facility and level 5 the least[72]. The USA/NATO triage categorization should also not be confused with MEDEVAC precedence categories (urgent, urgent surgical, priority, routine, and convenience), which are used to determine evacuation priorities[70].

Persian Gulf War

At the outset of the Persian Gulf War in 1991, triage was considered the most important single factor in combat casualty management of an expected 1500–3000 casualties in the first 24 hours[47]. It was the first war where potential for biologic and/or chemical use was feared. Triage plans included triage preparations for neuropsychiatric patients driven in part because of the threats and fears of biological and chemical weaponry contamination[71,72]. Trauma-center staff began the war in protective gear and all casualties were questioned rapidly on possible exposure and screened by vesicant and nerve-gas detection devices at a safe distance: first at the helicopter pad, the weapons search area, and again at the triage area. No gas exposures were confirmed.

The triage area for assessment and stabilization contained 28 stations prepared to manage immediate and delayed category casualties. The TO formed two small triage teams made up of a general surgeon, orthopedic surgeon, and anesthesiologist to supervise the prioritization to the 17 operating rooms and confer with the TO on any matters affecting overall triage decisions. A contingency area with an anesthesiologist in charge was developed for monitoring of the highest priority delayed casualties and to provide vital information to the TO for the surgical priority list[47].

The revised trauma score (RTS), a physiological scoring system, was used, consisting of the Glasgow Coma Scale, systolic blood pressure, and respiratory rate. The RTS has a high inter-rater reliability and demonstrated accuracy in predicting death. Using a retrospective analysis of conventional triage and RTS data, 461 coalition and Iraqi military casualties were compared against expected NATO triage casualty estimates. The positive influence of the RTS on triage sensitivity was considered useful, but it failed to provide significant triage sensitivity. Triage categories for coalition and Iraqi forces were remarkably similar, but deviated significantly (P <.001) from expected NATO triage casualty estimates. Medical diagnoses were 6% and 11% of these forces, respectively. Only 7% of Iraqi casualties and 2% of coalition casualties required retriage[48]. Had the anticipated number of casualties actually occurred in this war, the triage process would have benefitted from additional information, probably physiologic information, to improve the sensitivity and specificity of the findings.

In previous wars, approximately 10% of combat casualties were classified as neuropsychiatric. To properly triage the anticipated large numbers of neuropsychiatric casualties, a psychiatrist or psychologist was placed in the triage area and used neuropsychiatric triage algorithms to modify conventional triage categories. An "NP" boldly printed on the face of the triage tag ensured that psychological and social support followed each casualty through the treatment process after evacuation. This triage identified 16 immediate casualties at risk for acute or delayed post-traumatic stress[48].

Afghanistan and Iraq Wars

In these wars, the USA military deployed one of the world's most complex trauma systems. Excellent outcomes (ratio of killed in action to those surviving with wounds of severity) are attributed to medical advances, especially in hemostatic resuscitation, extremity injury care, traumatic brain injury, effectiveness of protective equipment, improved and rapid echelon I care and equipment, and rapid evacuation[73]. All advances eventually impacted the triage process and expectations for future triage management.

- Level I echelon of care: combat medics at battalion aid stations provide immediate first aid and transport. Focusing on exsanguinating hemorrhage and pneumothorax and airway control, they are trained to use early tourniquet (not used in Vietnam), topical hemostatics, needle angiocatheter, and oral intubation or cricothyroidotomy. Triage consisted simply of return to duty or rapid evacuation[74].
- Level II echelon of care: this field-hospital forward surgical team is staffed from 5 to 20 personnel, trained to perform lifesaving resuscitative surgery, 10 operating room cases/day and 30 operations within 72 hours. Evacuation to level III care occurs as soon as possible after treatment to CSHs, Navy hospital ships, or Air Force theater hospitals where casualties are retriaged, resuscitated, transfused, and obtain initial to reconstructive surgery. Strategic evacuation to level IV military medical centers occurs within 48–72 hours[74].
- Bellamy cautions that, while mortality has been reduced to 16.1% from Vietnam levels at 21.1%, without more appropriate data analysis, it is "difficult to separate the effects of medical care on mortality from battlefield factors such as weapon lethality[75,76]."

Summary

The goal of triage is to treat as many victims as possible who have a chance of survival. Triage does not exist in isolation, but represents a complex process that balances clinical requirements with resource allocation and system management where the decision operatives are the likelihood of medical success and the conservation of scarce resources.

References

1. World Health Organization (2007). Mass casualty management systems: strategies and guidelines for building health sector capacity. Health Action in Crises, Injuries and Violence Prevention. http://www.who.int/hac/techguidance/MCM_inside_Jul07.pdf

2. GreenIII WG, McGinnes SR (2006). Thoughts on the higher order taxonomy of disaster. Notes on the science of extreme situations, paper no. 7. https://www.researchgate.net/profile/Walter_Green_Iii/publication/241053862_thoughts_on_the_higher_order_taxonomy_of_disasters/links/593af7540f7e9b33170df543/thoughts-on-the-higher-order-taxonomy-of-disasters.pdf

3. Burkle Jr FM, Greenough PG. Impact of public health emergencies on modern disaster taxonomy, planning, and response. *Disaster Medicine and Public Health Preparedness* 2008: **2**(3): 192–9.

4. WHO–PAHO Guidelines for the use of foreign field hospitals in the aftermath of sudden-impact disasters (2003). International meeting: Hospitals in Disasters: Handle with Care, San Salvador, El Salvador. http://www.who.int/hac/techguidance/pht/FieldHospitalsFolleto.pdf

5. Norton I, von Schreeb J, Aitken P, Herard P, Lajolo C. *Classification and minimum standards for foreign medical teams in sudden onset disasters.* Geneva: World Health Organization; 2013.

6. World Health Organization. Humanitarian Health Action. Emergency Medical teams. http://www.who.int/hac/techguidance/preparedness/emergency_medical_teams/en

7. Klein KR, Burkle Jr FM, Swienton R, et al. Qualitative analysis of surveyed emergency responders and the identified factors that affect first stage of primary triage decision-making of mass casualty incidents. *PLOS Currents* 2016: **19**: 8.

8. Federal Interagency Committee on EMS (2011). National Implementation of the Model Uniform Core Criteria for Mass Casualty Incident Triage. A Concept Paper for FICEMS consideration. https://www.ems.gov/pdf/2011/December/10-MUCC_Options_Paper_Final.pdf

9. Benson M, Koenig KL, Schultz CH. Disaster triage: START, then SAVE – a new method of dynamic triage for victims of a catastrophic earthquake. *Prehospital and Disaster Medicine* 1996: **11**(2): 117–24.

10. Burkle Jr FM. Triage. In Antosia RE, Cahill JD (eds.), *Handbook of bioterrorism and disaster medicine.* New York: Springer Science; 2006: 12.

11. *Emergency war surgery.* Fourth United States revision, Falls Church, Virginia. Borden Institute, US Army Medical department Center and School, Office of the Surgeon General; 2013.

12. Merin O. The evolution of surgical humanitarian missions. In Roth R, Frost EAM, Gevirtz C, Atcheson C (eds.), *The role of anesthesiology in global health, a comprehensive guide.* Springer Science+Business Media; 2015.

13. Merin O, Miskin IN, Lin G, et al. Triage in mass-casualty events: the Haitian experience. *Prehospital and Disaster Medicine* 2011: **26**(5): 386–90.

14. Merin O, Ash N, Levy G, et al. The Israeli field hospital in Haiti – ethical dilemmas in early disaster response. *The New England Journal of Medicine* 2010: **362**(11): e38.

15. Klein KR, Pepe PE, Burkle Jr FM, et al. Evolving need for alternative triage management in public health emergencies: a Hurricane Katrina case study. *Disaster Medicine and Public Health Preparedness* 2008: **2** Suppl 1: S40–4.

16. Klein KR, Nagel NE. Mass medical evacuation: Hurricane Katrina and nursing experiences at the New Orleans airport. *Disaster Management & Response* 2007: **5**(2): 56–61.

17. Koenig KL, Dinerman N, Kuehl AE. Disaster nomenclature – a functional impact approach: the PICE system. *Academic Emergency Medicine* 1996: **3**(7): 723–7.

18. Winslow GR. *Triage and justice.* Berkeley: University of California Press; 1982: 1–23.

19. Domres B, Koch M, et al. Ethics and triage. *Prehospital and Disaster Medicine* 2001: **16**(1): 53–8.

20. Raynaud L, Borne M, Coste S, et al. Triage protocol: both undertriage and overtriage need to be evaluated. *The Journal of Trauma and Acute Care Surgery* 2010: **69**(4): 998.

21. World Medical Association (Stockholm, Sweden 1994, revised South Africa 2006). Statement on Medical Ethics in the Event of Disasters. Forty-sixth WMA General Assembly. https://www.wma.net/policies-post/wma-statement-on-medical-ethics-in-the-event-of-disasters/

22. Sasser SM, Hunt RC, Faul M, et al. Guidelines for field triage of injured patients. *MMWR Recommendations and Reports* 2012: **61**: 1–20.

23. Davis T, Dinh M, Roncal S, et al. Prospective evaluation of a two-tiered trauma activation protocol in an Australian major trauma reference hospital. *Injury* 2010: **41**: 470–74.

24. Cook CH, Muscarella P, AC Praba, et al. Reducing overtriage without compromising outcomes in trauma patients. *The Archives of Surgery* 2001: **136**: 752–6.

25. Mohan D, Rosengart MR, Farris C, et al. Assessing the feasibility of the American College of Surgeons' benchmarks for the triage of trauma patients. *The Archives of Surgery* 2011: **146**(7): 786–92.

26. Newgard CD, Zive D, Holmes JF, et al. A multisite assessment of the American College of Surgeons Committee on Trauma field triage decision scheme for identifying seriously injured children and adults. *Journal of the American College of Surgeons* 2011: **213** (6): 709–21.

27. Rapsang AG, Shyam DC. Scoring systems of severity in patients with multiple trauma. *Cirugía Española* 2015: **93**(4): 213–21.

28. O'Laughlin DT, Hick JL. Ethical issues in resource triage. *Respiratory Care* 2008: **53**(2): 190–7.

29. Society of Critical Care Medicine Ethics Committee. Consensus statement on the triage of critically ill patients. *JAMA* 1994: **271**: 1200–3.

30. Rosedale K, Smith ZA, Davies H. The effectiveness of the South African triage score (SATS) in a rural emergency department. *South African Medical Journal* 2011: **101**(8): 37–40.

31. Mullan PC, Torrey SB, Chandra A. Reduced overtriage and undertriage with a new triage system in an urban accident and emergency department in Botswana: a cohort study. *Emergency Medicine Journal* 2014: **31** (5): 356–60.

32. Hick JL, Hanfling D, Cantrill SV. Allocating scarce resources in disasters: emergency department principles. *Annals of Emergency Medicine* 2012: **59**(3): 177–87.

33. Altevogt BM, Stroud C, Hanson SL, et al. (2009) Guidance for establishing crisis standards of care for use in disaster situations, a letter report. Board on Health Sciences Policy. Institute of Medicine. Washington DC: The National Academies Press; https://www.nap.edu/read/12749/chapter/1#ii

34. Geneva convention I. Wounded and sick in the field. https://ihl-databases.icrc.org/applic/ihl/ihl.nsf/7c4d08 d9b287a42141256739003e636b/ fe20c3d903ce27e3c125641e004a92f3

35. Pollaris G, Sabbe M. Reverse triage: more than just another method. *European Journal of Emergency Medicine* 2016: **23**(4): 240–7.

36. Burkle Jr FM. Triage in Burkle Jr FM, Sanner PH, Wolcott BW. *Disaster medicine: application for the immediate management and triage of civilian and military disaster victims.* Elsevier; 45–80.

37. Giannou C, Baldan M. *War surgery: working with limited resources in armed conflict and other situations of violence.* Volume 1. Geneva, Switzerland; 2010.

38. Baker MS. Creating order from chaos: part II: tactical planning for mass casualty and disaster response at definitive care facilities. *Military Medicine* 2007: **172** (3):237–43.

39. Baker MS. Creating order from chaos: part I: triage, initial care, and tactical considerations in mass casualty and disaster response. *Military Medicine* 2007: **172**(3): 232–6.

40. Burkle Jr FM. Operationalizing public health skills to resource poor settings: is this the Achilles heel in the Ebola epidemic campaign? *Disaster Medicine and Public Health Preparedness* 2015: **9**(1): 44–6.

41. Garner A. Documentation and tagging of casualties in multiple casualty incidents. *Emergency Medicine Journal* 2003: **15**(5–6): 475–9.

42. Nocera A, Garner A. An Australian mass casualty incident triage system for the future based upon triage mistakes of the past: the Homebush Triage Standard. *ANZ Journal of Surgery* 1999: **69**(8): 603–8.

43. Vayer JS, Ten Eyck RP, Cowan ML. New concepts in triage. *Annals of Emergency Medicine* 1986: **15**(8): 927–30.

44. Martin M, Izenberg S, Cole F. A decade of experience with a selective policy for direct to operating room trauma resuscitations. *The American Journal of Surgery* 2012: **204**(2): 187–92.

45. Sasser SM, Hunt RC, Faul M. Centers for Disease Control and Prevention (CDC). Guidelines for field triage of injured patients: recommendations of the National Expert Panel on Field Triage. *MMWR Recommendations and Reports 2011.* 2012: **61**(RR-1): 1–20.

46. Burkle Jr FM.Triage and the lost art of decoding vital signs: restoring physiologically based triage skills in complex humanitarian emergencies. *Disaster Medicine and Public Health Preparedness* 2017: **21**: 1–10.

47. Burkle Jr FM, Orebaugh S, Barendse BR. Emergency medicine in the Persian Gulf War – part 1: preparations for triage and combat casualty care. *Annals of Emergency Medicine* 1994: **23**(4): 742–7.

48. Burkle Jr FM, Newland C, Orebaugh S. Emergency medicine in the Persian Gulf War – part 2. triage methodology and lessons learned. *Annals of Emergency Medicine* 1994: **23**(4): 748–54.

49. Burkle Jr FM, Newland C, Meister SJ. Emergency medicine in the Persian Gulf War – part 3: battlefield casualties. *Annals of Emergency Medicine* 1994: **23**(4): 755–60.

50. Burkle Jr FM. Advances in the methodology of the triage of disaster related casualties. *The Japanese Journal of Acute Medicine* 1991: **15**(13): 1767–72.

51. Meara JG, Greenberg SL. The Lancet commission on global surgery 2030: evidence and solutions for achieving health, welfare and economic development. *Surgery* 2015: **157**(5): 834–5.

52. Gerdin M, Wladis A, von Schreeb J. Foreign field hospitals after the 2010 Haiti earthquake: how good were we? *Emergency Medicine Journal* 2013: **30**(1): e8.

53. van Berlaer G, Staes T, Danschutter D, et al. Disaster preparedness and response improvement: comparison of the 2010 Haiti earthquake-related diagnoses with baseline medical data. *European Journal of Emergency Medicine* 2016: (Epub ahead of print).

54. Herard P, Boillot F. Amputation in emergency situations: indications, techniques and Médecins Sans Frontières France's experience in Haiti. *International Orthopaedics* 2012: **36**(10): 1979–81.

55. Center for Disaster Philanthropy. Complex Humanitarian Emergencies. http://disasterphilan thropy.org/issue-insight/complex-humanitarian-emergencies

56. International Committee of the Red Cross. International review of the Red Cross. Volume 93, Number 884, December 2011. https://www.icrc.org/fr e/resources/international-review/review-884/review-8 84-all.pdf

57. Physicians for Human Rights. Anatomy of a crisis: a map of attacks on health care in Syria: findings as of June 2016. https://s3.amazonaws.com/PHR_syria_ma p/findings.pdf

58. Centers for Disease Control and Prevention. 2014-2016 Ebola Outbreak in West Africa. Online article. https://www.cdc.gov/vhf/ebola/history/2014-2 016-outbreak/index.html

59. Burkle Jr FM, Burkle CN. Triage management, survival, and the law in the age of Ebola. *Disaster Medicine and Public Health Preparedness* 2015: **9**(1): 38–43.

60. Burkle Jr FM. Operationalizing public health skills to resource poor settings: is this the Achilles heel in the Ebola epidemic campaign? *Disaster Medicine and Public Health Preparedness* 2015: **9**(1): 44–6.

61. Senga M, Pringle K, Ramsay A, et al. Sierra Leone Kenema district task force and Kenema Government Hospital. Factors underlying Ebola virus infection among health workers, Kenema, Sierra Leone, 2014–2015. *Clinical Infectious Diseases* 2016: **63**(4): 454–9.

62. Broadhurst MJ, Kelly JD, Miller A, et al. ReEBOV antigen rapid test kit for point-of-care and laboratory-based testing for Ebola virus disease: a field validation study. *Lancet* 2015: **386**(9996): 867–74.

63. Walker NF, Brown CS, Youkee D, et al. Evaluation of a point-of-care blood test for identification of Ebola virus disease at Ebola holding units, Western Area,

Sierra Leone, January to February 2015. *Eurosurveillance* 2015: **20**(12).

64. Lin JY, Anderson-Shaw L. Rationing of resources: ethical issues in disasters and epidemic situations. *Prehospital and Disaster Medicine*. 2009: **24**(3): 215–21.

65. Talmor D, Jones AE, Rubinson L, et al. Simple triage scoring system predicting death and the need for critical care resources for use during epidemics. *Critical Care Medicine* 2007: **35**(5): 1251–6.

66. Burkle Jr FM. Population-based triage management in response to surge-capacity requirements during a large-scale bioevent disaster. *Academic Emergency Medicine* 2006: **13**(11): 1118–29.

67. Pandemic Influenza Triage Tools. Pandemic Influenza Triage Algorithm. http://www.cdc.gov/phpr/health care/pan-flu-app/desktop/pita.html.

68. Roser M (2016). War and peace after 1945. https://ou rworldindata.org/war-and-peace-after-1945

69. Hegre H, Sambanis N. Sensitivity analysis of empirical results on civil war onset. *Journal of Conflict Resolution*. 2006: **50**(4): 508–35.

70. Gerhardt RT, Mabry RL, De Lorenzo RA, et al. Mass-casualty-incident management. In fundamentals of combat casualty care in Lenhardt MK, Savitsky E, Eastridge B (eds.), *Combat casualty care. Lessons Learned from OEF and OIF*. Office of the Surgeon General, Department of the Army, USA; 2012: 110.

71. Emergency War Surgery, 4th US Revision, Chapter 3 (Mass Casualty & Triage) P.3.1–3.10. https://quizlet .com/123921745/emergency-war-surgery-4th-us-revision-chapter-3-mass-casualty-triage-4-aeromedi cal-evacuation-flash-cards

72. Katoch R, Rajagopalan S. Warfare injuries: history, triage, transport and field hospital setup in the armed forces. *Medical Journal Armed Forces India* 2010: **66**(4): 304–8.

73. Gabriel RA. *No more heroes: madness and psychiatry in war*. New York: Hill and Wang; 1987.

74. Military health system echelons of care. In Nessen SC, Lounsbury DE, Hetz SP (eds.), *War surgery in Afghanistan and Iraq: a series of cases, 2003-2007*. Washington DC: Department of the Army, Office of the Surgeon General, Borden Institute; 2008: 3–6.

75. Bellamy Combat trauma overview. In Zaitchuk R, Grande CM (eds.), *Anesthesia and perioperative care of the combat casualty. Textbook of military medicine*. Washington DC: Department of the Army, Office of the Surgeon General, Borden Institute; 1995: 1–42.

76. Holcomb JB, Stansbury LG, Champion HR, et al. Understanding combat casualty care statistics. *The Journal of Trauma and Acute Care Surgery* 2006: **60**(2): 397–401.

Medical Aspects in a Field Hospital

Ian Miskin and Eliezer Schwartz

Introduction

Even though most of the disaster situations in which international help was needed were related to trauma events (earthquakes, floods, and so on), all the missions that were deployed have shown a need for the deployment of a nonsurgical (i.e., medical) ward and medical staff. This is due to several reasons:

1. A high rate of wound infections among the casualties due to delay in treatment and lack of working hospitals, leading to treatment in suboptimal conditions. Treatment of these infections requires specialists in surgery, infectious diseases, and in wound care.

2. Within a short time, the team will have to deal with routine medical problems of the local population who will turn to them for help. On many occasions the international team has replaced local medical facilities, which, even before the event, were only able to provide a basic level of treatment. Thus, any treatment started must be sustainable after the departure of the mission.

3. These events usually occur in resource-poor countries where there is a high risk of the international team itself being infected by endemic diseases. Outbreaks of infectious diseases are liable to occur in the aftermath of the disaster due to the breakdown of the existing medical infrastructure and damage to homes necessitating transfer of the population to refugee centers.

Preparing the Team

Caring for the caregivers is highly important and should include vaccinations tailored to the area and conditions of deployment, together with lectures on relevant medical recommendations. These should cover at least the following areas and should be part of pretravel briefings[1]:

Food and Water Precautions

Ideally, the team should be self-sufficient, carrying supplies of food and water for the first 48–72 hours with capacity for food preparation from local supplies or continuous resupply from abroad.

A ready supply of potable water is a major priority to be addressed by the advance team. Clean, nonpotable water (for personal hygiene and so on) must be requisitioned from local sources, often requiring disinfection by team personnel.

Kitchen managers must be well versed in all aspects of setting up and operating food services under extreme conditions. Food and water will be purchased as available, often from unregulated suppliers. Food must be prepared according to strictest hygiene standards. Local kitchen workers, if employed, should be constantly supervised especially as to personal and hand hygiene. The manager must head a team including not only cooks but also hygiene specialists as food safety is critical for the continuing functioning of the whole unit. The level of functioning of foreign medical teams (FMTs) is notoriously prone to be affected by gastroenteritis caused by noncompliance of team members with simple guidelines followed by all travelers.

In some situations, the team may be allowed to experience local cuisine. In this case, the team members must observe the basic rules of travelers' hygiene ("boil it, cook it, peel it, or forget it").

Arthropod-Borne Diseases

Mosquito- and other vector-borne diseases are widespread. The field hospital team will rarely be working in an air-conditioned environment, and available sleeping accommodation will often preclude use of efficient mosquito nets. Mosquito and bug repellents must often be continuously applied.

Since different mosquitoes have different feeding times (Table 14.1), the team has to be instructed

Table 14.1 Common arthropod-borne infections and their time of activity

Vector	Activity time	Common diseases transmitted
Anopheline mosquitoes	Dusk to dawn	Malaria
Culex mosquitoes	Dusk to dawn	West Nile fever, Rift-Valley fever, lymphatic filariasis
Aedes mosquitoes	Daytime (mainly early morning and before dusk)	Dengue, Zika, yellow fever, chikungunya
Sandflies	Dusk to dawn	Leishmania (cutaneous and visceral)

according to their destination. Aedes-related diseases (such as yellow fever, dengue, West Nile, Zika, and others) are widely spread around the globe, requiring daytime preventive measures. Anopheline mosquitoes carrying malaria are night feeders and therefore applying nighttime repellent and sleeping under mosquito nets are important for prevention of disease. If required, malaria prophylaxis must be taken starting before departure using one of the available regimens tailored to local conditions and *Plasmodium* resistance.

Animal Bites

Historically, field hospitals have been deployed in areas endemic for rabies, and this is the scenario expected in the future. The team should be aware that the risk is not only from dogs and that, in these regions, most of the mammals are not vaccinated, and therefore contact must be avoided. Since rabies preexposure vaccine takes three to four weeks before deployment, in most scenarios the team will not have been vaccinated. This will require not only designated personnel to ensure the hospital is free of animals but also the transport of passive and active vaccination to enable treatment of team members, and, if possible, of locals exposed to animal bites.

Exposure to Human Body Fluids

All members of the team must be fully vaccinated against hepatitis B. HIV postexposure prophylaxis has to be carried by the infectious disease members.

Vaccines

Vaccines are a highly important measure in protecting the team, but in some instances the operation timeline does not allow the proper time recommended by the vaccine schedule; in others vaccine recommendations require a repeat dose after few weeks' interval, which does not always exist. In any case, last-moment vaccination is preferable to no vaccine.

Ideally, team members should have received basic travel vaccinations in advance, with additional specific vaccines (such as meningococcal and cholera) available for relevant destinations.

Vaccines before departure must include hepatitis A vaccine as this is the most common vaccine-preventable disease in most of these countries. Since the team often originates from highly industrialized countries, their chance of having natural immunity is very low.

Typhoid vaccine should be considered, especially when the target destination is in a highly endemic area for typhoid such as the Indian subcontinent. The current typhoid vaccine gives protection mainly against *Salmonella typhi* infection and does not cover *Salmonella paratyphi* infection, which has a similar clinical course.

To update tetanus toxoid, using diphtheria, tetanus, and acellular pertussis (dTaP) is recommended. For team members who last received the vaccine more than five years previously, a booster dose is advisable; tetanus exposure during the operation will not require a further dose during deployment.

Hepatitis B is indicated for all members of the medical team; a booster dose should be administered to all those without evidence of adequate cover.

Recommended Vaccines

Predeparture Vaccine

- hepatitis A (highly recommended for all missions; on-call personnel should be vaccinated)
- yellow fever (a must for missions in sub-Saharan Africa and South America)
- dTaP (recommended after five years from last dose)
- typhoid (for missions in endemic countries)
- meningococcal vaccine, preferably conjugate; consider group B vaccine
- cholera (in specific settings)
- Japanese encephalitis vaccine (to be considered in missions to South and East Asia)
- tick-borne encephalitis (in specific settings)

Carry-on Vaccines

These might be needed for the team and for local demands:

- tetanus vaccine
- tetanus immune globulin (TIG)
- rabies vaccine
- human rabies immune globulin

Vaccines must be transported under refrigeration and refrigerators must be available immediately on arrival.

Medicine During the Field Hospital Mission

The role of the nonsurgical side of the field hospital depends not only on the setting where the hospital is deployed but also the time of the deployment relative to the catastrophic event. Hospitals deployed into purely trauma events (such as earthquakes) find that the emphasis of treatment moves from emergency and urgent surgery to dealing with the medical requirements of surgical patients, but within a matter of days the balance again changes with the nonsurgical personnel being called to treat unknown and uncontrolled medical conditions by virtue of the field hospital hosting the only available medical services[2,3,4]. At this time, although only days after the defining event, the flow of patients requiring urgent surgery slows to a trickle. Most of those presenting at the hospital gates will at this stage require ambulatory care, with only a minority needing admission for overnight treatment and monitoring[3,5].

Thus, the role of the medical team in these situations can be grossly divided into two aspects:

1. Shoulder to shoulder with the surgical team – especially at the peak of surgical/orthopedic admissions – performing all nonsurgical tasks to free the surgeons to operate, then performing ambulatory follow-up together with the surgical team
2. A purely medical mission

Backing Up the Surgical Team and Treating Infections Associated With the Trauma Event

The medical ward, or more correctly the inpatient ward, will be mainly occupied at the early stage of the situation by postsurgery/post-trauma patients. Nonsurgeons will staff the ward, performing rounds together with a senior surgeon. In the first days, those hospitalized will be those requiring postoperative care, treatment of the nonoperable results of trauma, and those with conditions treated and stabilized in the operating room; some requiring further surgery. Most of the first wave of patients will be discharged within days, leaving those with severe infections, those requiring a second operation and those with other conditions such as crush injuries to be treated on a longer-term basis[4]. Pediatric patients show a similar pattern: inpatients comprising those with earthquake-caused injuries together with children suffering from non-trauma-caused infections [3,6].

In this setting, daily rounds must be done by the collaborative teams of the surgery and medical teams; the changing composition reflecting the lowering of the surgical burden and increase in medical inpatients and ambulatory workload.

One of the responsibilities of the nonsurgical team is treatment of infections. Antimicrobial treatment must be tailored to the individual patient, requiring daily refining, preferably by infectious disease specialists. Microbiology capacity as part of the hospital laboratory is often limited, but even limited data can be invaluable in identifying the local pathogens and antibiotic resistance. The circumstances of major traumatic events create conditions unlike any that physicians are likely to have met during regular hospital work, so the inclusion of physicians with experience of these scenarios is to be encouraged.

Even though wound infections complicate most injuries, it is not possible to treat empirically using nondisaster guidelines. These presume infection with Gram-positive species, which typically cause skin and soft tissue injuries in nonhospitalized patients. Pathogens causing wound infections are indeed traditionally considered to be Gram positive, but all those reporting culture results taken from infected wounds in the field have found that most are Gram negative. This fact must be taken into consideration when deciding which antimicrobials to use as empirical therapy, and which to include in the procurement list (Table 14.2).

Antibiotic resistance is found across the globe and has been shown to be worse in developing countries, albeit in many countries no reliable information exists [8]. This is caused by both a lack of requirement that all antibiotics be prescribed by qualified medical personnel and poor infection control in hospitals. The authors' experience in Haiti and Nepal has shown the existence of highly resistant Gram-negative bacteria

Table 14.2 The breakdown of bacterial isolates from victims of various disasters[7]

Place and year	No of isolates	No of patients	Gram staining		Polymicrobial	Nonfermenting species	Aeromonas spp.	Enterobacteria total	Staphylococcus aureus
			positive	negative					
Marmara, Turkey, August 1999	134	53	11.9%	87.3%		67.2%		20.1%	7.5%
Marmara, Turkey, August 1999	48	41	18.8%	81.3%		56.3%		25.0%	18.8%
Marmara, Turkey, August 1999	67	38	17%	79%		50.7%		9.0%	13.4%
Tsunami, December 2004	641	305	4.5%	95.5%	71.8%	17.6%	22.6%	54.6%	1.7%
India, Pakistan, October 2005	108	56	11.0%	89.0%	59.6%	46.3%		42.7%	5.6%
Wenchuan, China, May 2008	464	330	24.4%	73.2%		23.9%	3.4%	36.3%	16.4%
Wenchuan, China, May 2008	99	50	16%	82%	67.7%	40%		26%	5.0%
Wenchuan, China, May 2008	257	148	20.6%	77.8%					13.6%
Wenchuan, China, May 2008	169	123				32.6%		34.4%	11.8%
Spitak, Armenia, December 1988	130	88	20%	80%					
Haiti, January 2010	48	26	10.4%	89.6%	76.9%	22.9%	2.1%	64.6%	4.2%
Total	2165	1258							
Median			16.5%	81.6%	69.4%	40.0%	3.4%	34.4%	9.6%
Range			4.5–24.4%	73.2–95.5%	59.6–76.9%	17.6–67.2%	2.1–22.6%	9.0–64.6%	1.7–18.8%

Source: Miskin et al.[7]. Reproduced with permission.

even before contact with hospital-prescribed antibiotic therapy, which precludes empiric therapy with, for example, first-generation cephalosporin.

Decisions on antibiotic policy must be taken early in preparations for the mission. Policy will be determined by endemic diseases, the mission scenario (earthquake, tsunami, storms, floods, and so on), baseline antibiotic resistance, time elapsed from the event, and planned mission duration. A search must be performed for all available information on antibiotic resistance rates, vaccination policy and coverage, and endemic diseases.

Tetanus is an important pathogen, which may not be easily recognized by teams from Western countries. Tetanus has often been reported in patients wounded during earthquakes. This could be caused by a lack of childhood vaccination policy, poor vaccination rates, or a waning of protection caused by poor or nonexistent adult vaccination policy. The level of vaccine coverage is liable to be inadequate, especially among the elderly. Active tetanus vaccine should be offered to all those with wound infections, and TIG should be available for selected cases.

Missions arriving in the late phase of the disaster should consider including teams to vaccinate the local population, as routine vaccination capacity is likely to have been affected.

Pure Medical Mission

The role of the nonsurgical side of the field hospital depends not only on the setting where the hospital is deployed but also the time of the deployment relative to the catastrophic event. Hospitals deployed into purely trauma events (such as earthquakes) find that the emphasis of treatment moves from emergency and urgent surgery to dealing with the medical requirements of surgical patients, but within a matter of days, the balance again changes, with the nonsurgical personnel being called to treat unknown and uncontrolled medical conditions by virtue of the field hospital hosting the only available medical services[2,3,4]. At this time, although only days after the defining event, the flow of patients requiring urgent surgery slows to a trickle. Most of those presenting at the hospital gates will at this stage require ambulatory care, with only a minority needing admission for overnight treatment and monitoring[3,5]. An ambulatory capacity must be readied for this stage, utilizing physicians well versed in this type of care.

During the second wave, patients may present with acute medical conditions such as respiratory, digestive, ophthalmological, and infectious problems[3,9,10]. Others will present with chronic conditions or exacerbation of chronic diseases, which have become unstable due to loss of medications and access to medications, owing to losing shelter, housing, other nursing, and medical care[11,12]. Examples of this are exacerbation of congestive heart failure and uncontrolled diabetes mellitus or hypertension. Interruption of treatment for HIV and tuberculosis will require reinstating antimicrobials with repeated clinic visits to follow response to treatment and possible side effects[13]. Short-term admissions to treat previously untreated and neglected chronic conditions may be considered at this time[10], but continuation of care is of the utmost concern: long-term treatment should not be started if there is no possibility of the patient receiving medications after the field hospital leaves the area. For further details see "Approach to chronic illnesses management" in the Ambulatory Care chapter.

The nonsurgical personnel have a wide range of subspecialty areas to cover, and all members of the team must be able to function in a general setting in the wards and ambulatory clinic, as well as advising in the areas of their specialty when called on. The number of experts in different fields depends on the ability of the deploying agent and the specific aspects of the mission. The basic needs are of specialists in internal medicine, infectious diseases, gynecology and obstetrics, and pediatrics. In addition, foreign field hospitals (FFHs) should include public-health professionals, epidemiologists, hygiene/sanitation experts, and mental-health experts, who have proven to be valuable assets[14].

Altogether, versatility is of the utmost importance: the ambulatory service must also be able to shoulder the heavy burden of surgical patients who will be discharged early to ambulatory care to make way for other patients requiring urgent surgery: often limb saving or other procedures hugely important for future quality of life. These patients, who in a normal course of events may have been hospitalized for several weeks, will be treated in an ambulatory setting receiving intravenous antibiotics, wound debridement, and dressing changes – sometimes receiving daily treatment – handled mainly by nonsurgeons, with surgical backup as needed[15,16].

Infectious Diseases

Public-health professionals are needed throughout the mission, from planning stages up to and including health monitoring and continuing prophylaxis well after the team has returned and dispersed. Vaccination planning begins as soon as the general area of deployment is known. They will then monitor local endemic disease; to advise on treatment capacity and team protection. Their responsibilities include all levels of disease prevention for the entire delegation [17], personal protection, food and water safety, waste handling, and transfer of bodies and body parts for burial or cremation. These include:

- personal protection: pest, animal, and mosquito control, and providing insect repellent and bed nets
- food safety: sources, food preparation areas, refrigeration capacity
- water safety: safe drinking water (usually bottled); drinking water has to be purchased locally or be constantly transported from outside the area
- waste: latrine placing, safe disposal of contaminated and other hospital waste, kitchen waste
- transfer of bodies: some delegations will delegate this to an accompanying chaplain

Infection control personnel: other members of the team will be responsible for infection control throughout the hospital itself. These services must be up and running even before the first patient is admitted, and the equipment must be easily identified so as not to delay opening of the facility. The first hours after arrival will usually involve setting up the surgical capacity, as this is the raison d'être of the whole hospital. The number of surgical procedures performed in the first hours will put pressure on the sterilization capacity[18], with no relaxation of strict attention to procedures. Infection-control personnel will supervise all aspects of disease prevention, far more than their responsibility in normal settings:

- hand hygiene: ideally based on alcohol gels with > 70% ethanol
- sterilization versus steam autoclaving of equipment[17]
- team exposure to body fluids: including the provision of postexposure prophylaxis
- antibiotic stewardship: necessary even in field hospitals, especially in later stages
- cohorting of infectious patients: especially to prevent the spread of tuberculosis[13]

As tuberculosis is endemic or hyperendemic in most developing countries, arrangements should be made for the cohorting of patients with a high suspicion of tuberculosis or proven disease. This is typically performed by separating these patients using a dedicated space or tent[17]. Respiratory protection must be provided for those providing medical care. If the Mantoux status is known, it may be preferable for only those with positive tests to enter this area.

Infectious diseases specialists have overall responsibility for all aspects of their field, even when other personnel are performing the day-to-day work. They will be responsible for writing local antibiotic guidelines (working together with the other physicians) and implementing them. Antimicrobial planning should be based on existing guidelines, preferences, and experience in similar situations[7].

Their workload will comprise planned (daily rounds) together with unplanned consultations concerning patients (ambulatory as well as inpatients) on an as-needed basis. Infectious-disease physicians will be able to update treatment based on culture results from the microbiology lab (if available), together with patients' clinical responses to antimicrobial treatment. In many cases, a shortage of advanced antibiotics will require hands-on stewardship together with inventory updates from the pharmacy. In the second phase of the mission, when a large proportion of the presenting complaints are due to infectious disease, the infectious-disease physician will often find he or she spends a large part of the day in the clinic treating ambulatory patients. At this stage, a high rate of infectious disease was also reported among pediatric patients[2,6] and in diabetic patients with foot injuries[9].

The *laboratory* – a field lab with basic hematology and biochemistry tests – is indispensable. Laboratory personnel must be well versed in working with their equipment, under extreme conditions with only irregular electrical supply. A microbiology service should be included as part of this laboratory with the capacity for performing wound and blood cultures, antibiotic resistance, and Gram stains, as well as testing water supplies. The laboratory will allow identification of pathogens and local antibacterial resistance and enable the infectious-disease physicians to better tailor antimicrobial treatment. Results from blood and wound cultures taken from patients as they enter the hospital provide invaluable information on the true pathogens prevalent in disaster scenarios, allowing adapting of treatment guidelines and enabling future missions to provide better empiric therapy, even if they lack their own laboratory.

The caseload and patient breakdown of a field hospital changes rapidly in the days and first weeks following the traumatic event. The medical team must be able to deal with these changes, requiring versatility as one of the most important qualifications, especially in the first days after the event.

The composition of successive teams dispatched to the hospital must take into account the changing caseload[5,13]; for example, now requiring a basic rehabilitation capacity together with plastic surgery to enable optimal recovery [3,4,9].

When the field hospital remains in place for several months, attention must be paid to the livelihood of local medical teams. If all treatment and medications are provided without cost, the local practitioners will find themselves without income. This may cause them to leave the area, leaving the community without medical care on departure of the field hospital.

References

1. Erlich T, Shina A, Segal D, Marom T, Dagan D, Glassberg E. Preparation of medical personnel for an early response humanitarian mission – lessons learned from the Israeli defense forces field hospital in the Philippines. *Disaster and Military Medicine* 2015: **1**: 5.

2. Wang J, Ding H, Lv Q, et al. 2015 Nepal earthquake: analysis of child rescue and treatment by a field hospital. *Disaster Medicine and Public Health Preparedness* 2016: **10**: 716–9.

3. van Berlaer G, Staes T, Danschutter D, et al. Disaster preparedness and response improvement: comparison of the 2010 Haiti earthquake-related diagnoses with baseline medical data. *European Journal of Emergency Medicine* 2016: [Epub ahead of print].

4. Centers for Disease Control and Prevention. Post-earthquake injuries treated at a field hospital – Haiti, 2010. *Morbidity and Mortality Weekly Report* 2011: **59**: 1673–7.

5. Bar-On E, Abargel A, Peleg K, Kreiss Y. Coping with the challenges of early disaster response: 24 years of field hospital experience after earthquakes. *Disaster Medicine and Public Health Preparedness* 2013: **7**: 491–8.

6. Farfel A, Assa A, Amir I, et al. Haiti earthquake 2010: a field hospital pediatric perspective. *European Journal of Pediatrics* 2011: **170**: 519–25.

7. Miskin IN, Nir-Paz R, Block C, et al. Antimicrobial therapy for wound infections after catastrophic earthquakes. *The New England Journal of Medicine* 2010: **363**: 2571–3.

8. The Center for Disease Dynamics, Economics, and Policy (2015). The state of the world's antibiotics. Washington DC and New Delhi. Online article. https://cddep.org/wp-content/uploads/2017/06/swa_edits_9.16.pdf

9. Read DJ, Holian A, Moller CC, Poutawera V. Surgical workload of a foreign medical team after Typhoon Haiyan. *ANZ Journal of Surgery* 2016: **86**: 361–5.

10. Lin G, Marom T, Dagan D, Merin O. Ethical and surgical dilemmas in patients with neglected surgical diseases visiting a field hospital in a zone of recent disaster. *World Journal of Surgery* 2017: **41**: 381–5.

11. Dulski TM, Basavaraju SV, Hotz GA, et al. Factors associated with inpatient mortality in a field hospital following the Haiti earthquake, January–May 2010. *American Journal of Disaster Medicine* 2011: **6**: 275–84.

12. Redwood-Campbell LJ, Riddez L. Post-tsunami medical care: health problems encountered in the International Committee of the Red Cross Hospital in Banda Aceh, Indonesia. *Prehospital and Disaster Medicine* 2006: **21**: s1–7.

13. Pape JW, Rouzier V, Ford H, Joseph P, Johnson WD Jr, Fitzgerald DW. The GHESKIO field hospital and clinics after the earthquake in Haiti – dispatch 3 from Port-au-Prince. *The New England Journal of Medicine* 2010: **362**: e34.

14. World Health Organization, Pan American Health Organization. Guidelines for the use of foreign field hospitals in the aftermath of sudden-impact disasters. Area on emergency preparedness and disaster relief. International meeting. Hospitals in disasters – handle with care. San Salvador, El Salvador, 8–10 July 2003.

15. Merin O, Ash N, Levy G, Schwaber MJ, Kreiss Y. The Israeli field hospital in Haiti – ethical dilemmas in early disaster response. *The New England Journal of Medicine* 2010: **362**: e38.

16. Kreiss Y, Merin O, Peleg K, et al. Early disaster response in Haiti: the Israeli field hospital experience. *Annals of Internal Medicine* 2010: **153**: 45–8.

17. Lichtenberger P, Miskin IN, Dickinson G, et al. Infection control in field hospitals after a natural disaster: lessons learned after the 2010 earthquake in Haiti. *Infection Control and Hospital Epidemiology* 2010: **31**: 951–7.

18. Zheng W, Hu Y, Xin H. Successful implementation of thirty-five major orthopaedic procedures under poor conditions after the two thousand and fifteen Nepal earthquake. *International Orthopaedics* 2016: **40**: 2469–77.

Chapter

15

Pediatrics in a Field Hospital

Vladislav Dvoyris and Tarif Bader

Introduction

Natural and human-made disasters – earthquakes, tornadoes, floods, hurricanes, wildfires, and drought, as well as wars, massacres and genocides – have been afflicting humankind since the dawn of time. Although recent advancements in science and big data analysis enable the prediction of some of these disasters[1], most of them remain unpredictable and challenging to combat.

In 2005–2015, a total of 3853 natural disasters occurred, affecting about 1.7 billion people, 85% of whom were in Asia[2]. Extreme climate events represent 80% of these disasters and, while most of these disasters occur in rather developed countries, the small share occurring in lower-income countries and impacting an already impoverished population are the ones bound to be most devastating.

Disasters occur suddenly. However, they tend to have a long tail of collateral events and damage[3], bringing patients to seek medical help long after the disaster occurred and rendering recovery (contrary to relief) from the disaster a long and difficult process, impacting the local health-care system, economy, and quality of life for years.

Therefore, careful coordination between international relief agencies and emergency medical responders is critical to manage disaster victims both immediately and on a long-term basis. In this context, multiple agencies at national and local levels, including nongovernmental organizations (NGOs) such as the Red Cross and Médecins Sans Frontières (MSF), and military medical corps, are deploying their personnel in areas of disasters with a defined set of priorities aimed at disaster relief for the general population.

It has been reported that 50% of the population affected during natural or human-made disasters are children[4]. Moreover, in low- and middle-income countries, which contribute to the largest share of disasters, children are most likely to suffer from malnutrition, communicable diseases (CDs),

psychological illnesses, and family disruptions[5]. It is estimated that more than 200 million children are affected by disasters worldwide, disrupting their physical, socio-emotional, and cognitive abilities[6,7].

Children have unique vulnerabilities in such disasters or emergency situations, and require unique and specific management as they have limited communication skills and different physiological and psychological responses to stress. In this regard, it is vital to understand the optimal management in pediatric emergencies and to consider efforts regarding pediatric preparedness and response in humanitarian situations, including pediatric experts in all levels of disaster management[5].

This chapter aims at reviewing the necessary means of pediatric care that must be an integral part of any medical relief delegation in humanitarian situations, disasters, and mass-casualty events. A suitable structure of a dedicated medical team will be proposed, as well as necessary logistic considerations for medical teams that do not treat children on a day-to-day basis.

Field Hospitals Acting as Medical Relief Facilities

Military medical corps of armed forces around the world maintain airborne military field hospitals, which can be transported to different areas to treat soldiers during warfare and emergency. The Geneva convention (GC) has specified that military field hospitals must take care of the civilian population of the area to the maximum extent possible[8], and it has been agreed that military field hospitals are responsible for humanitarian civilian medical care where security risks exist for civilian health-care staff and where inadequate medical facilities are available. In times of peace, these hospitals are deployed in areas of disasters and mass-casualty events, together with humanitarian hospitals operated by NGOs and relief agencies.

To deal with a pediatric population during a disaster, most common causes of morbidity and mortality should be recognized. Common causes of pediatric morbidity and mortality include diarrheal diseases, infections, malnutrition, burns, trauma, and poisoning[9]. Various studies have suggested having pediatric surgical care in humanitarian settings, as pediatric surgical interventions account for more than a third of all surgeries[10]. Among these surgeries, trauma and burns are the most common.

In this regard, Edwards and colleagues have documented more noncombat pediatric trauma and illnesses as compared to those of combat-related injuries in the Iraq and Afghanistan wars[11]. In the Iraq and Afghanistan wars, pediatric admissions varied from 3% to 18% in military field hospitals, where thousands of sick, malnourished, and wounded children were treated[12]. Although the treatment outcome was satisfactory, it was a big challenge at all levels of military hospitals and health-care agencies.

In January 2010, a 7.0-magnitude earthquake struck Haiti, causing the death of an estimated 316 000 people, injuries to more than 300 000, and more than 1 million people were left homeless. Numerous relief agencies, military, and search-and-rescue teams rushed to deploy their staff in Haiti. Despite the 6000-mile distance, an Israeli field hospital was deployed in Port-au-Prince within three days and started accepting patients 89 hours after the disaster[13]. Among the patients treated, 24% were children aged 0–16, only 57% of whom suffered earthquake-related injuries – the others suffering from infectious diseases or being newborns delivered in the hospital[14].

Thus, a medical-relief hospital deployed in an area of mass-casualty disaster should include a dedicated pediatric team, consisting of pediatricians, pediatric surgeons, pediatric nurses, and medics. A pediatric division with a dedicated hospitalization ward and an emergency department should be clearly marked, yet despite the physical separation, it must be fully coordinated with the general emergency, intensive care, surgical, and obstetric facilities.

Triage and Emergency Treatment of Pediatric Patients

To follow instant and accurate assessment of pediatric patients during a natural or human-made disaster, having a reliable triage system is of prime importance. As the children are the most vulnerable population following the disaster, immediate response through a proper triage system plays a key role in offering in-time care.

Critical-care capacity in a disaster area may be even further limited than general health care. The lack of facilities and equipment creates a resource-poor situation, necessitating the need for a so-called "resource triage[15]." Our triage algorithm considers three key parameters: urgency, due to patient condition, available hospital resources, and the likelihood of saving a patient's life.

Naturally, the above approach poses ethical dilemmas. In times of disaster, the principle of justice becomes dominant, and should be implemented per the utility principle: providing the greatest good for the greatest number possible[16]. An egalitarian distribution of resources, despite seeming more attractive and "fair," may lead to waste of scarce resources on a hopeless patient, while these resources could have been used to save others. According to Schultz and colleagues, following an earthquake, it is feasible to treat only patients with more than 50% probability for survival[17], and this approach can be implemented in other mass-casualty disasters.

Nevertheless, every effort should be made to maximize the availability of critical-care facilities and equipment. Only when these efforts are exhausted to the maximum, should the resource be allocated to those likeliest to benefit from it[18]. However, in a field humanitarian setting, the chances of survival are often difficult to estimate. The entire situation, and the patient's condition within it, should be looked on through a prism of uncertainty. Room should always be left for the unexpected, and decision-making according to a strict rule may deprive patients of a chance to survive that we might think they do not have – only to be proven wrong on the next day[15]. An individualized approach, combined with an ongoing assessment and discussion by the hospital's ethical committee, is the recommended approach to triage and treatment of pediatric patients in critical condition.

Pediatric patients are usually accompanied by a caregiver or a family member, who may be helpful in translating, and feeding and bathing the patient. However, after disasters, some children are admitted to a hospital without the attendance of relatives, who may be lost, wounded, or deceased. In this case, the ethical committee of the hospital will have to decide on the necessary treatment without seeking the parents' consent and considering the benefit of the patient. During hospitalization, these patients may be assisted by family members of other patients. Their discharge, however, should be coordinated with local or international relief organizations to secure treatment continuity[14].

Additional ethical dilemmas are posed by the lack of proper routine medical care. In areas where the overall access to medical care may be low or nonexistent, a humanitarian hospital is indeed a miracle; albeit, a short-term one. Thus, every treatment decision made within the hospital should take into account the ability of the patient to survive with the commonly available medical care. This led, for example, to a sparing, conservative approach to limb amputations following the Haiti earthquake. In this case, considering the poor rehabilitation situation in Haiti, amputations were performed only for nonviable limbs, while any salvageable limb was treated with debridement and subsequent follow-up procedures, leading to fast exhaustion of supplies, yet providing improved quality of life to the patients[19].

Orthopedic trauma is usually predominant in earthquake injuries[13,17,20,21], while in floods and droughts, infectious diseases predominate due to lack of access to clean water[2]. Inappropriate sanitary conditions, crowded camps, and contaminated water and food may result in gastrointestinal, skin, and respiratory infections. During the second week after the disaster, one should also expect a decrease in incidence of new trauma cases, and an increase in cases of infectious and chronic diseases. Lack of antibacterial medications may lead to exacerbation of infections, and thus a humanitarian-relief hospital should carry systemic antibiotics, including intravenous ones, as well as tetanus-toxoid vaccines.

Pediatric trauma patients must be classified on the basis of type and severity of injuries following triage protocol[5]. The Emergency Severity Index (ESI) is a reliable tool for pediatric triage[22]. Although ESI was first designed for an adult population, pediatric vital-sign criteria were added to it in 2000, making it applicable for all ages[23]. A large study by the pediatric ESI research consortium has found that ESI Version 4 is a reliable triage tool for the pediatric population[24]. The triage nurse and health-care providers must keep in mind the following key points while triaging the pediatric population:

1. Follow a standardized triage approach as described in Table 15.1.

2. Infants must be observed, auscultated, and touched to get the necessary information.

3. Approach children in a nonthreatening way to avoid stranger anxiety.

4. Allow children to have a trusted caregiver with them at all times. Thoroughly explain the procedure to the child's caregiver and get his or her help in ascertaining the chief complaint and other information as children have limited communication abilities, or are too shy or frightened. Caregivers may also be helpful in holding the children and removing their clothing. However, many children arrive at the hospital without a caregiver or a family member, thus posing additional dilemmas when surgical treatment is necessary.

5. In neonates and young infants, the signs of severe illness – poor feeding, irritability, and hypothermia – may be subtle, and thus require special attention. Children have a relatively larger body surface area than adults, and thus are at a higher risk of heat and fluid loss. Neonates, in particular, have not developed an ability to thermoregulate, and thus they should not be kept undressed longer than absolutely necessary.

6. Offer immediate lifesaving intervention to a hypotensive child. Hypotension is a late marker of shock in children.

7. Get actual weight of all the children. The actual weight is important for medication dosage and the safe care of the child. If a child is critically ill and cannot be weighed, weight can be estimated, but should not be guessed.

It is vital to act promptly to classify the patients immediately to respective triage levels to offer them definitive evaluation and management. ESI levels 1 and 2 include potentially unstable patients requiring urgent management[25].

ESI Level 1 includes high acuity patients or those who would die without urgent and intensive care. Available literature reports that triage nurses underutilize ESI level-1[26], except children who are intubated or in cardiac arrest. Assigning ESI level 1 acuity is based on the clinical condition of the patient, and the conditions included are respiratory or cardiac arrest, major head trauma with hypoventilation, active seizures, unresponsiveness, altered consciousness with petechial rashes, anaphylactic reactions, respiratory failure, shock, or sepsis with signs of

Table 15.1 Standardized triage approach

Steps	Titles	Comments
1	Appearance/ breathing/circulation: quick assessment	Listen to the chief complaint and rush for immediate management if required. Observe appearance from tone, interactivity, look, and speech or cry; assess breathing through airway sounds, positioning, retractions, and flaring; observe pallor, mottling, or cyanosis.
2	ABCDE[a]	Assess airway patency, respiratory rate and quality for airway and breathing; assess heart rate, skin temperature, capillary refill time, and blood pressure for circulation; assess neurological status for disability; undress the patient to assess for injury or illness.
3	Patient history	Proper history of the patient should be obtained, especially regarding onset of chief complaint, immunization, allergies, medications, past health history, events prior to arrival, and diet. Most children arriving at a hospital in the first days after the disaster will suffer from trauma, and their physical state may limit the triage ability. In addition, some of the children arriving at the care facility will not be accompanied by adults: their family members may be missing or dead, or taking care of other siblings. This, especially in small children, may result in lack of communication, greatly jeopardizing the ability to assess the patient's history.
4	Vital signs	The rigorous evidence or guidelines for vital signs measurement is still lacking. However, oxygen saturation must be assessed in all children. Blood-pressure measurement may depend on the triage nurse assessment.
5	Fever	Must assess fever in all children. Rate ESI level 2 to the children with 38°C.
6	Pain	Assess pain using a validated pediatric pain scale, or as part of PQRLS[b].

[a] ABCDE: airway/breathing/circulation/disability/exposure

[b] PQRLS: assessment of pain, quality, radiation, location, and severity

hypoperfusion, flaccid baby, and hypoglycemia with altered conscience level.

ESI level 2 includes the patients who are potentially at high risk. Examples of conditions included in ESI level 2 are syncope, hemophilia with acute bleed, immune-compromised status with fever, febrile infant (< 28 days; > 38°C), hypothermic infant, moderate-to-severe croup, suicidality, seizures, meningitis, and moderate-to-severe lower airway obstruction.

There are three more levels of ESI: 3, 4, and 5. ESI level 3 includes stable patients and should be approached in 30 minutes. In ESI levels 4 and 5, the patients can be seen nonurgently (Table 15.2). Moreover, ESI levels in pediatric settings may differ from those for the adult population. For example, lacerations in adults are included in ESI level 4, while in pediatric settings they require sedation and thus are kept in ESI level 3. The following conditions may require sedation:

- displaced fractures
- complicated lacerations: facial, vermilion, or requiring multilayered closure
- contaminated wounds requiring debridement or thorough wash
- chest intubation

Pediatric Traumatology Considerations

In times of peace, trauma is the most common mechanism of injury among preteen and teen groups (71% and 58.7% respectively)[27], and pediatric trauma patients are always challenging, especially if internal injuries without any external marks are present. More importantly, the compensatory mechanisms (vital signs) in the pediatric population may hide the actual situation. Thus, the inclusion of a pediatric trauma team in disaster management plans would reduce pediatric mortality and morbidity[28]. In this context, considering the significant number of pediatric populations affected by disasters, Barthel and colleagues have put forth comprehensive mathematical justification for aggressive inclusion of pediatric traumatologists in disaster management planning in humanitarian settings[29].

In the aftermath of the Haiti earthquake, 47% of children with traumatic injuries suffered fractures, and 33% of the fractures were open and infected. These patients were operated on under general or regional anesthesia. There was no significant difference in the percentage of fractures in children versus

Table 15.2 ESI levels

Category	Definitions	Statistics
ESI 1	Severely unstable patients; require immediate management; die if left untreated	2% of total patients 73% are admitted
ESI 2	Potentially unstable patients; must be seen within 10 minutes	22% of all patients 54% are admitted
ESI 3	Stable patients; require laboratory or radiological testing; must be seen within 30 minutes	Makes 39% of all ED[a] patients 24% are admitted
ESI 4	Stable patients; can be seen nonurgently; require minimal testing; may be discharged	27% of all patients 2% are admitted
ESI 5	Stable patients; can be seen nonurgently; require no testing; usually discharged	10% of all patients Everyone is discharged

[a] Emergency department

adults. However, significantly more children required surgery due to a higher percentage of open fractures. Closed fractures should be treated nonoperatively, even if some residual deformity might occur, due to the risk of infection as well as the high remodeling potential in children[19].

Every effort should be made to relieve pain and distress in pediatric victims of disasters, and the use of procedural sedation and anesthesia should be considered the standard of care[30]. However, due to natural limitations of operating room capacities, some minor surgical procedures may and should be performed in the pediatric emergency department (PED), under local anesthesia or deep sedation, including repairs of skin lacerations and soft tissue debridement. Deep sedation may be administered by the pediatrician even without the assistance of an anesthesiologist, provided that he or she has received proper training, with a combination of intravenous midazolam and ketamine: the latter can be widely used due to its high safety profile. This approach to minor surgery enables freeing operating rooms and anesthesiologists for more complex procedures, while having an anesthesiologist ready to come into the PED in case of a complication[14].

The Necessary Connection to Ob/Gyn

The need to include obstetrics and gynecology personnel among humanitarian medical relief teams is often overlooked, yet it is essential to bear in mind that any catastrophe, either human-made or natural, is a stressful situation leading to an increase in miscarriage, preterm labor, and births; especially in the developing countries[31,32].

The existence of proper medical facilities is oftentimes crucial for the survival of both the mother and the child. Miscarriages, premature deliveries, intra-uterine growth restriction, and low birth weight tend to increase after natural disaster. As many as 10% of the hospital's patients may be women seeking help from an ob/gyn, and naturally, the newborns delivered preterm, often in field conditions, require the presence of neonatologists to survive[33]. The neonatology ward and intensive-care facility should be placed adjacent to the ob/gyn department[34], even if it is separated from the general pediatric ward.

In Haiti, 5 out of 16 deliveries (31%) occurred at 30–32 weeks of gestation, with neonates born at severely low weight and in fetal distress, and requiring emergency neonatal care. In Nepal (April 2015), 6 out of 8 deliveries were performed through a cesarean section.

The medical-relief team should be ready well in advance for such scenarios, and if an ob/gyn division is planned as part of the relief hospital, a neonatology facility must be added to the pediatric division, including incubators and respirators, as well as specialty personnel[34]. However, in disaster areas, the survival rates of low-birth-weight neonates are dramatically diminished, and thus, if the hospital's resources are scarce – and they usually are – an ethical dilemma arises, and a minimum-weight threshold may be imposed to better allocate resources to newborns with higher chances of survival[15].

Structure and Function of a Field Hospital Pediatric Ward

A humanitarian field hospital planning to include a pediatric ward under its auspices should address several issues prior to its deployment. The selection of personnel is of utmost importance, as the pediatric medical team (Table 15.3) consists of several important players, and merely adding a pediatrician to the crew will not be sufficient.

Primarily, the pediatric ward should be staffed by pediatric general physicians. In addition, it is advisable to include a neonatologist, a pediatric surgeon, and an orthopedist specializing in children. If a neonatologist is unavailable, one must make sure that at least one of

Table 15.3 Dedicated personnel of a field-hospital pediatric ward

	Number
Pediatric physicians	4–6
Pediatric surgeons	1–2
Neonatology specialists	1–2[a]
Pediatric orthopedists	1–2[b]
Pediatric anesthesiologists/ intensive care physicians	1–2
Pediatric nurses	5–10[c]
Neonatology nurses	1–2
Medics	2–5[d]
Social workers	2–3[e]

[a] Can be replaced by experienced specialists in pediatrics.

[b] Can be replaced by general orthopedists experienced in treating children.

[c] Can be replaced by general nurses experienced in pediatric care.

[d] Will be used as auxiliary personnel, performing nursing tasks as well. It is advisable to choose medics who can communicate well with children.

[e] Can be shared with other hospital wards. Experience with children is advisable.

the pediatric specialists is experienced in neonatal care and capable of filling this important role. In addition, an anesthesiologist/intensive care specialist experienced in working with children would be a valuable asset for the pediatric intensive care facility.

Pediatric and neonatal nurses are vital to the continued provision of medical care. Nurses should at the very least be seasoned in working with children, as their communication with the patients is often key to improved mutual understanding and recovery. This is also the role of auxiliary medical personnel – including social workers or psychologists who would communicate the medical situation to children and their families, and will be able to provide support to the medical team as well – considering the difficulty of treating wounded children, particularly in mass-casualty scenarios.

At the Israeli field hospital in Haiti (2010), a dedicated pediatric medical team was composed of seven pediatricians, a pediatric surgeon, six registered nurses, and two medics. The entire team worked in shifts around the clock, in the emergency department, the ward, and the neonatal ward, thus maximizing the limited human resources[14].

In general terms, the effective ratio of physicians versus nurses and auxiliary personnel to be deployed should be 1:1. All members of the team should be motivated and capable of performing duties in addition to their main specialty[35].

A surprising, often unthought of, addition to the pediatric ward activities was the presence of medical clowns. In Nepal (2015), the Israeli field hospital received a delegation of five volunteer medical clowns from Israel, and it was unsurprising to find that humor plays an important role in the pediatric ward, even in field hospitals, greatly improving the spirit of patients and personnel alike[36].

The pediatric ward of a humanitarian field hospital should be divided into several distinct units.

PED

The PED should be separated, if possible, from the general emergency room. The department should be staffed by pediatricians and pediatric nurses, with orthopedic and general surgeons available on call.

Pediatric Hospitalization Ward

The pediatric hospitalization ward should include several regular hospital beds and a single intensive care bed, which may be used for resuscitation and performance of minor surgical procedures under sedation; thus saving valuable operating room resources that can and should be used for severe cases.

Pediatric Intensive Care Unit (PICU)

Optimally, the PICU should be adjacent to the general pediatric ward yet separate from it. The unit should consist of one to two beds. However, if space is constrained, it is advisable to allocate beds in the general ICU for pediatric cases.

Neonatal Ward and ICU (NICU)

The neonatal ward and NICU should include an incubator and ventilator, as well as one to two intensive care beds. Specialists in neonatology are essential for the operation of this unit, and thus should be included in the personnel required for the hospital. The neonatal ward should be located adjacent to the ob/gyn ward, providing convenient, covered, and clean access from the ob/gyn hospitalization ward and the delivery room to the NICU.

The above units and personnel, however, will not be able to function and provide quality care without proper equipment. Military emergency storage facilities do not usually hold supplies for pediatric care, and thus fast deployment of a military humanitarian mission may present a challenge in this regard. It is, therefore, necessary to stock emergency pediatric equipment and disposables sufficient for at least the first two weeks of field-hospital operation. This can be achieved by dedicating an internal storage facility. However due to budgetary considerations – since this equipment may not be used – it is advisable to outsource the pediatric equipment storage to an external supplier capable of just-in-time delivery.

The equipment necessary for a functioning pediatric care facility should include the following:

1. Surgical and orthopedic equipment in pediatric sizes, for example chest tubes, orthopedic implants, and external and internal fixation. In addition, it is advisable to prepare medical disposables in pediatric sizes, among which are airways, and intravenous and intraosseous needles.
2. Additional intensive-care equipment dedicated for pediatric use, including neonatal incubators, ventilators, and monitoring systems.
3. Medications, including common medications in pediatric dosages and in liquid forms (syrups), and specialty medications; for example, pulmonary surfactant replacements for preterm neonates.
4. Food supplies suitable for small children, including breastfeeding supplement formulas.

Summary

Every mass-casualty event has unique characteristics, and an independently operating comprehensive medical team must be equipped and prepared for every possible scenario. Early humanitarian response to mass-casualty situations can be performed successfully by a medical team capable of delivering a wide range of treatments, which should include pediatric and neonatal care due to the high number of wounded children and preterm births following human-made and natural disasters.

The field pediatric care facility should consist of specialized personnel and suitable medical pediatric equipment, and be backed by a strong logistic support. While immediately after the disaster a large number of trauma casualties will arrive at the hospital, a gradual shift to nonsurgical treatments and routine care should be expected within days, including infectious diseases, which may spread in the area due to lack of access to clean water and hygiene facilities.

References

1. Radinsky K, Davidovich S, Markovitch S, eds. WWW 2012. Learning causality for news events prediction 2012: Lyon, France.
2. Guha-Sapir D, Hoyois P. Estimating populations affected by disasters: a review of methodological issues and research gaps, in *Centre for Research on the Epidemiology of Disasters (CRED)*. Brussels, Belgium: Université catholique de Louvain; ed. 2015.
3. Nicholls S, Healy C. Communication with disaster survivors: towards best practice. *Australian Journal of Emergency Management* 2008: **23**(3).
4. *Emergency field handbook: a guide for UNICEF staff.* Geneva, Switzerland: UNICEF; 2005.
5. Rothstein DH. Pediatric care in disasters. *Pediatrics* 2013: **132**(4): 602–5.
6. Peek L, Stough LM. Children with disabilities in the context of disaster: a social vulnerability perspective. *Child Development* 2010: **81**(4): 1260–70.
7. Bennett CM, Friel S. Impacts of climate change on inequities in child health. *Children (Basel)* 2014: **1**(3): 461–73.
8. IV Geneva Convention relative to the protection of civilian persons in time of war. 1949: Geneva, Switzerland.
9. Young H, Harvey P. The sphere project: the humanitarian charter and minimum standards in disaster response: introduction. *Disasters* 2004: **28** (2): 99.
10. Wong EG, Trelles M, Dominguez L, Gupta S, Burnham G, Kushner AL. Surgical skills needed for humanitarian missions in resource-limited settings: common operative procedures performed at Médecins Sans Frontières facilities. *Surgery* 2014: **156**(3): 642–9.
11. Edwards MJ, Lustik M, Burnett MW, Eichelberger M. Pediatric inpatient humanitarian care in combat: Iraq and Afghanistan 2002 to 2012. *Journal of the American College of Surgeons* 2014: **218**(5):1018–23.
12. Idenburg FJ, van Dongen TT, Tan EC, et al. Pediatric surgical care in a Dutch military hospital in Afghanistan. *World Journal of Surgery* 2015: **39**(10): 2413–21.
13. Kreiss Y, Merin O, Peleg K, et al. Early disaster response in Haiti: the Israeli field hospital experience. *Annals of Internal Medicine* 2010: **153**(1): 45–8.
14. Farfel A, Assa A, Amir I, et al. Haiti earthquake 2010: a field hospital pediatric perspective. *European Journal of Pediatrics* 2011: **170**(4): 519–25.
15. Ytzhak A, Sagi R, Bader T, et al. Pediatric ventilation in a disaster: clinical and ethical decision making. *Critical Care Medicine* 2012: **40**(2): 603–7.

16. O'Laughlin DT, Hick JL. Ethical issues in resource triage. *Respiratory Care* 2008: **53**(2): 190–7; discussion 7–200.

17. Schultz CH, Koenig KL, Noji EK. A medical disaster response to reduce immediate mortality after an earthquake. *The New England Journal of Medicine* 1996: **334**(7): 438–44.

18. Hick JL, Rubinson L, O'Laughlin DT, Farmer JC. Clinical review: allocating ventilators during large-scale disasters – problems, planning, and process. *Critical Care* 2007: **11**(3).

19. Bar-On E, Lebel E, Blumberg N, Sagi R, Kreiss Y, Israel Defense Forces Medical Corps. Pediatric orthopedic injuries following an earthquake: experience in an acute-phase field hospital. *The Journal of Trauma and Acute Care Surgery* 2013: **74**(2): 617–21.

20. Bulut M, Fedakar R, Akkose S, Akgoz S, Ozguc H, Tokyay R. Medical experience of a university hospital in Turkey after the 1999 Marmara earthquake. *Emergency Medicine Journal* 2005: **22**(7): 494–8.

21. Xiang B, Cheng W, Liu J. Triage of pediatric injuries after the 2008 Wen-Chuan earthquake in China. *Journal of Pediatric Surgery* 2009: **44**(12): 2273–7.

22. Jafari-Rouhi AH, Sardashti S, Taghizadieh A, Soleimanpour H, Barzegar M. The Emergency Severity Index, version 4, for pediatric triage: a reliability study in Tabriz Children's Hospital, Tabriz, Iran. *International Journal of Emergency Medicine* 2013: **6**(1): 36.

23. Wuerz RC, Travers D, Gilboy N. Implementation and refinement of the emergency severity index. *Academic Emergency Medicine* 2001: **8**(2):170–6.

24. Hohenhaus SM, Travers D, Mecham N. Pediatric triage: a review of emergency education literature. *Journal of Emergency Nursing* 2008: **34**(4): 308–13.

25. Gilboy N, Tanabe P, Travers D, Rosenau A. *Emergency severity index (ESI): a triage tool for emergency department care.* Rockville, Maryland, USA: AHRQ – US Department of Health and Human Services; 2011.

26. Travers DA, Waller AE, Katznelson J, Agans R. Reliability and validity of the emergency severity index for pediatric triage. *Academic Emergency Medicine* 2009: **16**(9): 843–9.

27. Trudeau MO, Baron E, Herard P, Labar AS, Lassalle X, Teicher CL, et al. Surgical care of pediatric patients in the humanitarian setting: the Médecins Sans Frontières experience, 2012–2013. *JAMA Surgery* 2015: **150**(11): 1080–5.

28. Petrosyan M, Guner YS, Emami CN, Ford HR. Disparities in the delivery of pediatric trauma care. *The Journal of Trauma and Acute Care Surgery* 2009: **67**(2 Suppl): S114–9.

29. Barthel ER, Pierce JR, Goodhue CJ. Availability of a pediatric trauma center in a disaster surge decreases triage time of the pediatric surge population: a population kinetics model. *Theoretical Biology and Medical Modelling* 2011: **8**: 38.

30. Weiser G, Ilan U, Mendlovic J, Bader T, Shavit I. Procedural sedation and analgesia in the emergency room of a field hospital after the Nepal earthquake. *Emergency Medicine Journal* 2016: **33**(10): 745–7.

31. Goldenberg RL, Culhane JF, Iams JD, Romero R. Epidemiology and causes of preterm birth. *The Lancet* 2008: **371**(9606): 75–84.

32. Tucker J, McGuire W. Epidemiology of preterm birth. *The BMJ* 2004: **329**(7467): 675–8.

33. Bar-Dayan Y, Beard P, Mankuta D, et al. An earthquake disaster in Turkey: an overview of the experience of the Israeli Defence Forces Field Hospital in Adapazari. *Disasters* 2000: **24**(3): 262–70.

34. Pinkert M, Dar S, Goldberg D, et al. Lessons learned from an obstetrics and gynecology field hospital response to natural disasters. *Obstetrics & Gynecology* 2013: **122**(3): 532–6.

35. Dvoyris V, Kreiss Y, Bader T. Treatment capabilities of field hospitals at war and mass-casualty disasters, in Wolfson N (ed.), *Orthopedics in disasters: orthopedic injuries in natural disasters and mass casualty events.* Berlin, Heidelberg: Springer-Verlag; 2016: 37–46.

36. Efrati I. [Medical clowns want to be treated seriously]. *Haaretz.* 2016.

Chapter

16

Surgery in a Field Hospital

Seema Biswas and Harald Veen

The Global Burden of Surgical Disease

The global burden of surgical disease may be estimated to be as high as 30%[1]; yet less than 5% of all surgery is performed in the poorest regions of the world[2]. Low- and middle-income countries, with almost 50% of the world's population, have only 20% of the global surgical workforce. While high-income regions of the globe have approximately 14 operating theaters per 100 000 people, low-income regions have fewer than two theaters per 100 000 people[3]. The need for overseas surgical assistance in elective and emergency conditions, the development of surgical training programs, and building relationships with local health-care personnel and health ministries are crucial. Field hospitals are designed to fulfill each of these priorities and, while this chapter focuses on the resources needed to deliver surgical services in the most austere of environments, in particular where there is conflict and/or disaster, surgical care in the field may be delivered by military and civilian international organizations (including charities and nongovernmental organizations [NGOs] working independently or integrated within local health services.

Field Surgery

Modern field surgery describes long- and short-term missions for disaster relief, the treatment of war wounded, and the support and development of surgical services in low and middle countries. Shrime[1] developed a taxonomy for overseas charitable surgical missions, classifying temporary surgical platforms, the most common form of surgical assistance, in terms of *short-term surgical disease specific trips* with long-term follow-up left to local clinicians (typically plastic surgery – Operation Smile, for example, craniofacial surgery, orthopedics and ophthalmology missions); *self-contained surgical platforms* involving longer missions with organizations bringing with them their own infrastructure, such as Mercy Ships; and *specialty surgical hospitals* establishing a specialist

service within local health-care or community infrastructure – the Addis Ababa Fistula Hospital as an exemplary model.

The World Health Organization (WHO) Global Initiative for Emergency and Essential Surgical Care and the Global Burden of Surgical Disease working group further describe surgical needs that surgeons in these field hospitals are likely to encounter. These may be prioritized in terms of surgical conditions with a high prevalence; those easily amenable to surgical treatment such as trauma interventions, exploratory laparotomy for acute abdominal emergencies, external fracture fixation, caesarian section, and hernia repair; conditions with a moderate public health burden, which are moderately amenable to surgical intervention such as vascular trauma, open reduction and internal fixation of fractures; surgery related to the complications of pregnancy; surgery for common malignancies such as breast or colon cancer; and, finally, surgical conditions that exert a relatively low public-health burden, requiring specialized interventions or procedures, which may not result in successful control of disease such as surgery for advanced malignancy or transplantation[4]. This last category, comprising surgical procedures of advanced complexity, is not within the domain of field surgery. Indeed, the more complex the procedure, the more the unsatisfactory the surgical outcome[5,6]. Field surgery is, therefore, recommended for the simpler surgical interventions, which may be performed safely within the environment of a field hospital and with a high probability of successful short- and long-term outcomes.

Surgical assistance programs of large humanitarian organizations such as the International Committee of the Red Cross (ICRC) and Médecins Sans Frontières (MSF) deploy in conflict zones. The ICRC functions under a unique mandate provided by the states involved. The International Federation of Red Cross and Red Crescent Societies (IFRC) deploys emergency response units (ERUs) in response to

148

disasters[7]. This chapter focuses on typical surgical field hospitals supported or established by these organizations, describing the unique mandate, the surgical needs met, and the surgical resources necessary to initiate and maintain field surgery operations.

The Medical ERU of the IFRC

The IFRC comprises 190 National Red Cross and Crescent Societies. The IFRC deploys in disasters and health emergencies through medical ERUs. Each medical ERU includes a team of trained specialists, prepared for deployment at short notice in basic health-care ERUs or in rapid deployment or referral hospital ERUs. Urgent mobilization and deployment are made possible through the organization and preparation of prepacked sets of standardized equipment. ERUs work with field assessment coordination teams and are designed to be self-sufficient for one month, although they can operate for up to four months, and longer if the emergency continues. The ERUs are much like the emergency medical teams (EMTs) of WHO or MSF. Types of deployment are described below.

Basic Health-Care ERU

The basic health-care ERU is designed to provide immediate basic curative, preventive and community health care for up to 30 000 people. The ERU uses a modular approach adjusting to local needs and the WHO basic protocols. The unit deploys with the interagency emergency health kit (a standardized kit of essential medicines, supplies, and equipment deployed by UN agencies and WHO in response to emergencies where the local supply has become disrupted). One kit is designed to meet the basic health needs of 10 000 people for approximately three months. The approximate weight is 18 metric tons. The unit can deliver basic outpatient clinic services, maternal and child health (including uncomplicated deliveries), community health outreach, immunization, and nutritional surveillance. There is no surgical capacity; thus, there must be a mechanism for referral of more serious cases for hospitalization within a reasonable distance with transportation (ambulance) facilities. Although the basic health-care unit does not function as a hospital, there are 10–20 overnight beds for observation. There are 5 to 8 staff and the ERU requires the availability of local health staff and interpreters to support services with the agreement of the local ministry of health (MoH).

Rapid Deployment Hospital

The rapid deployment hospital is a specifically modified and lighter version of the referral hospital ERU, which can deploy within 48 hours of alert and offers medical and surgical interventions such as triage, first aid, medical evacuation, and limited medical and surgical care. There is 10-bed inpatient capacity and an outpatient department.

The rapid deployment hospital can function up to 10 days pending assessment and arrival of a more complete hospital or basic health-care ERU. The hospital has 8 to 10 staff and the equipment weighs approximately 10 metric tons. Being flexible and mobile, requiring no loading equipment, the team works with limited equipment and resources. The Rapid Deployment Hospital can also be used as mobile clinic if required at a later phase of an emergency deployment.

Referral Hospital ERU

The Referral Hospital ERU is a first level field hospital, providing multidisciplinary care to a population of up to 250 000 people. The inpatient capacity ranges from 75–150 beds, providing surgery, limited traumatology, anesthesiology, internal medicine, gynecology, obstetrics, and pediatrics. Prepacked equipment weighs approximately 60 metric tons.

The hospital typically has one or two operating theaters, a delivery room, inpatient wards and treatment areas, X-ray facilities, and a laboratory for blood and urine examinations. There is an outpatient department and an emergency room.

The referral hospital ERU is designed in a modular way to be adaptable to a given situation in the field and to best integrate into the existing local health system and structures. This type of ERU needs to be self-sufficient and, therefore, includes supporting modules such as administration, IT networks and communication, a water and power supply, and staff accommodation and vehicles. The setup may be in tents or move partly or entirely into existing buildings and the unit works based on an agreement with the local MoH. The referral hospital ERU comprises 15 to 20 staff members working with local health staff who receive in-service training in the ERU and work in an integrated way alongside expatriate staff.

Surgery in a Field Hospital

Surgical field hospitals must be equipped to deal with both direct and indirect surgical pathology resulting from conflict and disaster. It is, in fact, indirect injury and illness that results in greater morbidity and mortality in conflict zones, and in the long term, in disaster-affected areas[8]. The minimal capabilities of the surgeon must, therefore, include basic trauma care (visceral and orthopedic), comprising airway management, tube thoracostomy, emergency thoracotomy, the management of bleeding, laparotomy for bowel injury and hemoperitoneum, stoma formation, wound coverage and closure (including skin graft), fracture management (especially debridement, external fixation, fasciotomy and amputation), decompressive craniotomy, obstetric emergencies, and the management of general surgical and urological emergencies such as bowel obstruction, peritonitis, testicular torsion, and complications of hernia.

The Operation Theater and Essential Equipment for Safe Surgery

Equipment and furnishings in the operating theater vary according the facilities available. Both the ICRC and MSF may set up operations in existing health facilities or support well-established surgical units. Figure 16.1 shows what would be considered to be a well-equipped operating theater, but even more basic

facilities should enable surgeons to safely perform laparotomy, orthopedic, and debridement procedures. Although, whenever possible, procedures are performed under regional or ketamine anesthesia, general anesthesia with manual and, less commonly, mechanical ventilation is possible. Battery-operated pulse oximetry and manual sphygmomanometry permit perioperative monitoring.

The delivery of oxygen requires an oxygen concentrator, which, in turn, requires an electricity supply, usually from a portable generator powered by gasoline. The operating light, fan, and, rarely, air conditioner, also depend on electricity. A battery-operated headlight is of huge potential assistance to the surgeon. The operating table may be tilted or broken, but usually has no special adaptation for the treatment of fractures, nor for obstetric procedures. Arm rests, however, grant the surgeon and anesthetist important access. Intravenous fluids may be warmed in a bucket of hot water[9]. At 42°C, the water becomes cool enough to touch, and thus warmed crystalloid is available for intravenous administration or irrigation and lavage. Blood transfusion facilities are not available in a basic setup such as this. Blood tests, other than MalariaSpot tests, HIV tests, and syphilis serology (as per the WHO standards) are

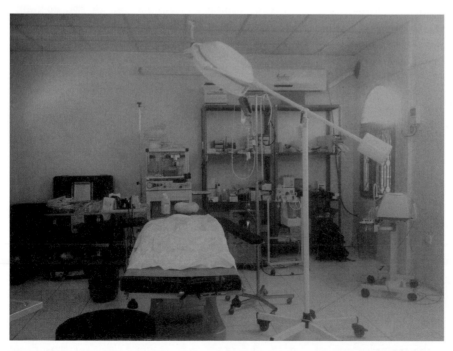

Figure 16.1 ICRC operating theater
Source: ICRC

not performed in these basic surgical hospitals. Clinical assessment and decision-making, therefore, must be sharp and fast. Treatment of hemorrhage relies on hemorrhage control with damage control resuscitation and surgery. Triage and judicial surgical decisions are necessary in dealing with an influx of wounded patients as a basic surgical facility is potentially overwhelmed without planning for mass-casualty scenarios.

Increasingly, ICRC field deployments take the form of mobile surgical teams working in tented facilities or ideally a makeshift building with solid floors, walls, and ventilation. One surgical team includes a surgeon, an anesthetist, scrub nurse, ward nurse, and physiotherapist. An operating theater assistant may be recruited locally and is invaluable not simply in the running of the surgical theater but in translation as the team communicates with each patient. A fully functional surgical setup should allow the team to perform up to 10 operations in 24 hours (60 per week including a rest day, comprising approximately 30 new patient admissions and 30 follow-up operations)[10].

Although mobile surgical teams work under basic conditions, the operating theater is supervised by the scrub nurse and remains clean and kept free of insects as far as possible. Sterile conditions are maintained in surgery through the use of disposable sterile drapes. Sterile disposable consumables are stored in clean, dry conditions, stocks monitored, and waste collected in large plastic bags within waste baskets. Sharps are collected in sharps bins and incinerated with clinical waste at a safe distance from the hospital buildings or tents.

Surgical instruments are cleaned in accordance with international standards including rinsing, disinfection, cleaning, drying, and autoclaving. Typical instrument packs include a basic surgical set with self-retaining retractor and bone nibblers used for minor procedures, debridements, and as an adjunct to external fixator kits; and split skin graft sets, which include a free-hand modified Humby-type knife; amputation sets; laparotomy sets; thoracotomy sets; vascular sets; and craniotomy sets. All surgery is open surgery.

Chest drainage is performed in the operating theater rather than the ward and employs a closed drained underwater-seal system. Major dressing changes (especially if sedation or morphine analgesia is required) are also performed in the operating theater. Dressings comprise gauze and bandages. Occlusive plastic dressings are not included in the standard list of consumables. Silver sulfadiazine covered with gauze and bandages are the dressings of choice for burns. Skin coverage is achieved with split skin grafts as soon as possible where appropriate. Plaster of Paris splints and casts are employed where limb immobilization is required. Debrided wounds remain bandaged until wound closure is performed two to five days after radical debridement and lavage under antibiotic cover. Steinmann pins for the management of femoral fractures in traction are inserted in the operating theater.

Surgical Care: The Realities in the Field: Dorein, South Sudan

As a field surgeon with ICRC, you find yourself with the mobile surgical team in a small field hospital. There are tents to sleep, to perform surgery, and care for your patients. It is raining: a lot. The mud is everywhere.

Life has not been easy since your arrival a week ago. Hot nights in a semiflooded tent prevented a good sleep. An ant attack did not help. However, the team spirit is good. You are the only surgeon. You have an anesthetist, a scrub nurse, and a ward nurse. You have no X-ray, and only simple laboratory tests (rapid malaria antigen test and hemoglobin spot tests), and pulse oximetry handled by the anesthetist.

The reason to deploy here was an outbreak of fighting in the region and the presence of wounded with no local treatment facilities. There are no roads. Airplanes cannot take off or land as all areas that can serve as landing strips are flooded. The only access is via helicopter.

Your tented hospital has a limited number of beds, and they are all occupied. There are more patients outside the hospital compound. The wounded are waiting with local patients and patients who have traveled for days on foot as news of an ICRC field hospital has spread. Expectations are high. Patients with a wide variety of pathologies are demanding elective procedures. You are feeling a little overwhelmed: the project specifies limiting your work to weapon-wounded patients and patients with other life-threatening conditions.

This morning you do a ward round, see new cases, documenting your findings as you go (Figure 16.2), and prioritize cases for theater:

ICRC

NAME: NUMBER:

COMING FROM: MALE/FEMALE   AGE:

DATE: TIME: GSW: MI: SHELL: BOMB: BURNS: OTHER:

TIME SINCE INJURY:
GENERAL CONDITION:
PULSE: BP: RESP: TEMP:
ANTIBIOTICS: ANTI-TETANUS:

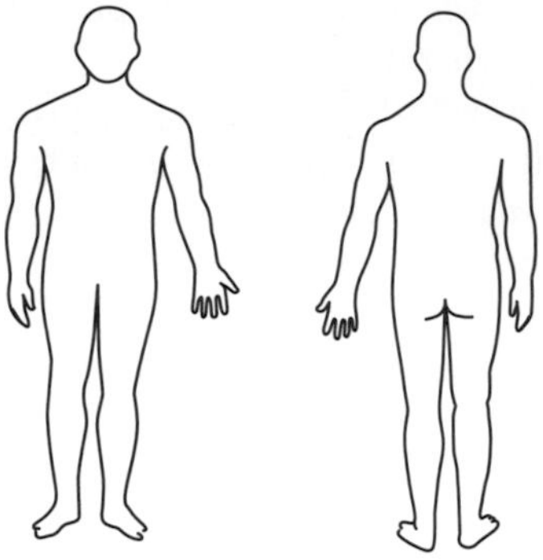

MEDICAL ASSESSMENT

Hb: MEDICAL ORDERS:
Hct: IV fluids:
X match: NPO from:

TRIAGE   Immediate surgery   No surgery   Wait for surgery

OPERATION NOTE   POST OPERATIVE INSTRUCTIONS
                                                                            Antibiotics:

                                                                            to stop:

                                                                            Position Physio/drains/traction

                                                                            By mouth: Food/fluids/nil

                                                                            Other:

                                                                            Next in OT:

PENETRATING WOUND SCORE   OTHER INFORMATION

E [   ]   X [   ] C [   ] F [   ] V [   ] M [   ]

E [   ]   X [   ] C [   ] F [   ] V [   ] M [   ]

Figure 16.2a The ICRC patient history sheet. Clinical and operative findings and postoperative instructions are documented
Source: ICRC[10]

- Surgical debridements for patients with infected gunshot wounds of the limbs, several days old, due to the delay in reaching the hospital. They will also need fracture fixation with plaster, traction, or external fixation.
- Drainage of an infected hemothorax.

- Laparotomy for a patient who survived an abdominal gunshot wound, and who has developed a colonic fistula.
- One patient has been the subject of discussion within the team. This boy has a cerebral gunshot wound. The entrance of the gunshot wound is

E   entry wound in centimetres
X   exit wound in centimentres
     (X=0 if no exit wound)
C   cavity   Can the cavity of the wound take two fingers before surgical excision?
                         C0 = no
                         C1 = yes
F   fracture   Are any bones fractured?
                         F0=No fracture
                         F1=Simple fracture, hole or insignificant comminution
                         F2=Clinically significant comminution
V   vital structure   Are dura, pleura, peritoneum, or major peripheral vessels injured?
                         V0=no vital structure injured
                         VN=(neurological) penetration of the dura of the brain or spinal cord
                         VT=(thorax or trachea) penetration of the pleura or of the larynx/trachea in the neck
                         VA=(abdomen) penetration of the peritoneum
                         VH=(haemorrhage) injury to a major peripheral blood vessel down to brachial or popliteal arteries, or
                         carotid artery in the neck
M   metallic body   Are bullets or fragments visible on X-ray?
                         M0=no
                         M1=yes, one metallic body
                         M2=yes, multiple metallic bodies

Figure 16.2b The ICRC wound classification. Mechanisms of injury and wound scores are documented for monitoring, evaluation, and research

Source: ICRC[26]

through the eye. There is no exit. The neurological prognosis is dubious. As he is still alive, with a Glasgow Coma Scale of 11, and the wound is purulent, he is now scheduled for debridement.

- The next patient has osteomyelitis of the mandible months after a gunshot wound. He is drooling, cannot eat, and is losing weight. You plan to refer him to a specialist working in the capital, but he needs to fly there and planes have not been able to land near the field hospital since you arrived,

- Several patients are ready for delayed primary closure. It is now five days since initial debridement of their wounds. ICRC protocol is to perform a radical initial debridement, bandage the wound, continue antibiotics (usually penicillin), and perform delayed primary closure of a clean wound, usually on the second to fifth postoperative day. Hopefully, these patients have clean wounds, otherwise they will undergo re-debridement. If the wounds can be closed, most of them will require a split skin graft. The battery-powered dermatome has just arrived.

- One patient with an exposed proximal tibia will require a muscle flap. This has to be scheduled for a quiet moment – you are not used to performing this procedure.

- Halfway during the morning, a patient with closed head injury and signs of lateralization is brought to the hospital. There is no CT scan, and the decision for craniotomy must be taken on clinical grounds.

- There may be a caesarian section to do. More women in advanced pregnancy seem to be coming to the hospital.

- The team is tired, because last night they worked on a woman with postpartum hemorrhage.

You consent the last patient for theater through an interpreter. This takes some time as all the family are present and the army commander accompanying the patient has grave reservations about whether debridement of the leg could result in amputation. You explain that urgent debridement is necessary to avoid possible amputation if infection continues. Amputation is dreaded by the patients. You spend some time repeating your explanation. The acceptance of the work of the surgical team in the field is dependent on cultural understanding and dialogue.

As you enter the operating theater, the team is preparing the first patient.

The day is coming to an end. In Africa this always happens fast. The operation list is over for the day and the postoperative patients have been checked. The woman with the postpartum hemorrhage is stable, but ought to have a blood transfusion. Only recently have rapid kits to check hemoglobin become available for the team. However, family members who are willing to donate blood have not been found.

After a long day in the hospital you are left to your thoughts.

Your background is upper gastrointestinal surgery, and, at home, the fractures are dealt with by the orthopedic surgeon.

Or your position back home is a trauma surgeon in a big trauma center, with all subspecialties available.

Or you are an experienced vascular surgeon, spending more and more time in interventional radiology.

Or you are a general surgeon, doing many laparoscopic cholecystectomies.

Whatever your background, at home the postpartem hemorrhage, the caesarian section, or the severe head injury would be dealt with by specialist colleagues and you are not within your comfort zone in Dorein. However, the patients presenting to you now in Dorein are a reality and they expect you to treat them.

Your decision to take on this mission was based on a slightly naive motivation to do some good. By now it has become very clear to you that it is easy to actually do harm under these circumstances.

This is Dorein. It could have been Bangui, Muzaffarabad, Gao, Maiduguri, Juba, or so many other places where there are urgent surgical needs due to armed conflict or disaster.

Surgery in Conflict Zones

The ICRC has delivered surgical care to war wounded in field hospitals across the world since the 1960s when conflict in Yemen and the Nigeria-Biafra wars heralded a new era of challenges in the delivery of international humanitarian assistance within the context of protracted civil wars, which saw the burden of suffering among

civilians escalate to the unacceptable levels associated with modern warfare[11] (Figure 16.3). Analysis of civilian deaths in the current Syrian conflict makes for dismal reading: shelling is responsible for most civilian fatalities; up to one-fifth of violent deaths are among children; and air bombardment, shelling, and chemical weapons are more likely to result in fatalities among women and children than among men[12]. According to the Syrian Center for Policy Research, the war has claimed 470 000 lives, and over 11% of the population of Syria have been killed or injured[13]. It is estimated there are ten injuries for every fatality. In addition to direct injuries from conflict, the surgical burden also includes emergencies that present as a result of the destruction of the country's health care infrastructure[14].

Table 16.1 summarizes the surgical activity of the ICRC in 2015. Surgical activity includes the support of hospitals by the ICRC with drugs, equipment, training, and/or staff.

The mandate of the ICRC is to ensure the delivery of quality hospital care to the wounded and sick. Since 1963, the ICRC has operated well over 100 field hospital missions across Africa, Asia, and the Middle East. The unique role of the ICRC in the neutral, independent, and impartial delivery of health care has meant that the ICRC has had access to some of the most isolated and vulnerable populations of the world affected by conflict, poverty, and the lack of development that results from years of political unrest. Established in 1863, the ICRC is at the origin of the Geneva conventions (GCs) and the International Red Cross and Red Crescent Movement. It directs and coordinates the international activities conducted by the movement in armed conflicts and other situations of violence. Working in collaboration with national Red Cross and Red Crescent Societies, the reach of the ICRC into local communities, the scale of operations made possible through engagement with the local workforce, and the longevity of missions, has afforded the ICRC a history of sustainable field hospital programs and a depth of experience in the delivery of surgical care in the most austere of environments.

The work of the ICRC in situations of complex emergency – situations where lives and livelihoods are threatened by conflict, civil and political unrest, disaster, and the displacement of populations – and in situations of longstanding poverty and a lack of infrastructure, mean that the ICRC undertakes much of its activities among populations suffering from famine and malnutrition, where infectious diseases present public health emergencies, where access to regular medication is

Table 16.1 Activities in hospitals supported by ICRC in 2015. Activities include support of hospitals by the ICRC with drugs, equipment, training, and/or staff *Source:* ICRC

Department/ specialty	Number of patients
Surgery	Weapon-wounded 43 680 Non-weapon-wounded 92 287 Mine injuries 2293 Operative 119 666 (on average 2.7 procedures per patient)
Medical	190 000
Obstetrics and Gynecology	145 000
Outpatient	Surgical 510 000 Medical 1 000 000 Obstetric 240 000

prohibitive of the management of chronic disease, and where access to clean water and basic public services present major challenges to most of the population [15,16]. Although data on the prevalence of trauma and surgical disease in conflict zones are limited[17], we know that obstetric emergencies, road traffic crashes, general surgical emergencies, and the complications of infectious disease (typhoid perforations, for example) significantly add to local burdens of surgical disease [18,19,20]. There is growing evidence that untreated surgical disease vastly outnumbers war injuries in terms of surgical morbidity[21]. These regions of the world also suffer from a dire shortage of trained surgeons and primary health-care providers. The ICRC has surgical missions in some of the poorest regions of the world, and addressing the burden of surgical disease in these regions is inherent in the mandate of the ICRC.

Regions of the world with previously well-resourced health-care systems that are plunged into conflict face the same scarcity in health provision as internal infrastructure and health-care services become decimated[22]. The flight of local medical personnel compounds medical needs. Those who remain may work in conditions of fear and insecurity. As the health assistance division of the ICRC responds to the casualties of war, coordinated programs of the ICRC sanitation and economic security divisions work to alleviate the effects of a lack of infrastructure, desperate living conditions, and the loss of health and human rights associated with violent conflict, in partnership with local and international organizations.

Preparations for a Surgical Hospital Project

Planning and preparation for a hospital project at the ICRC is dependent on a mandate to deliver quality hospital care to the wounded and sick, an assessment of the needs of the population, and deciding on the nature of deployment necessary to meet the most pressing health needs.

ICRC hospital activities are considered in the following conflict situations:

- new acute crisis with a sudden high mortality rate due to violence
- expected acute crisis
- established crisis with continuous high mortality rate or other epidemiologic indicators
- new forms of violence
- long-term impact of violence

Table 16.2 and Figure 16.3 illustrate the life cycle of the process for ICRC field hospital deployment

Inherent in planning surgical activity is the ability to access and operate effectively in areas of conflict and instability. Populations (often in flight or bereft of the most basic means for living) need to be able to access emergency care safely and benefit from quality hospital care in a facility with functional infrastructure and effective administration and management. The field hospitals need to be properly resourced in line with ICRC and international standards[23,24]. These standards rely on the capabilities of the ICRC to improve or build infrastructures including facilities

Table 16.2 Lifecycle of the field hospital

Stage in lifecycle	Process	Components
1	Assessment of needs	Evaluation of the situation and health needs to be covered
2	Design of project	Evaluation of the scope and limitations of the project
		Definition of the strategic objectives of the project
3	Planning the project	Consideration of the resources necessary for the project
		Drafting a timeline for implementation
4	Running the project	Deployment, monitoring, and reporting of activities through project management: negotiation, adapting the project in terms of human resources and supplies, etc. Formative and summative clinician evaluations of project to ensure the highest standards of clinical care and best outcomes for patients Coordination of acute surgical care with local physiotherapy, rehabilitation, and prosthetics services provided by the ICRC, local, and international partners
5	Closing the project	Handing over the activities to local authorities

Source: ICRC

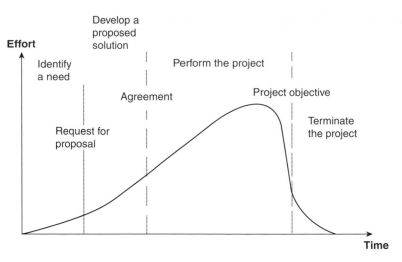

Figure 16.3 The process of the field-hospital project cycle
Source: ICRC

that protect patients from adverse weather, and facilities with potable water and sanitation arrangements, which promote hygiene in and around wards. Operating theaters need to be well lit, clean, and facilitate surgery in sterile fields. A reliable electricity supply and facilities for the sterilization of equipment are necessary. Drugs and medical supplies should be available and a system for safe waste disposal should be established. The ICRC has internal systems for the purchase, storage, and supply of equipment catalogued in accordance with ICRC protocols. Where possible, oxygen concentrators and pulse oximetry facilitate safe general anesthesia. Oxygen is not transported in pressurized cylinders. To avoid the waste of equipment or consumables, donations in the field are refused. There is a serious effort to harmonize the kits used by the different humanitarian actors. After a recent comprehensive review, WHO and the ICRC are now using the same emergency surgical kits.

Human resources include an operating-theater team, typically comprising a surgeon, anesthetist, operating theater nurse, and ward nurse. The ICRC adheres to international standards and a level of preparedness dependent on a pool of surgeons, anesthetists, and nurses with the skills to deal with war wounds, trauma, and general surgical emergencies. In addition, physiotherapists and biomedical technicians have key roles in the team. National Red Cross and Red Crescent Society staff and local personnel work with the ICRC team as operating theater assistants, nurses, porters, and physiotherapy assistants.

ICRC surgical facilities are supported by rehabilitation and prosthetic centers where patients continue their recovery and reintegration into society.

Hospitals vary in the level of support they provide according to what is necessary in terms of local provision. Where there is no means to provide health assistance locally, the ICRC substitutes health-care provision. Although each hospital project is unique to the context of deployment, all hospital activities involve:

- engineering of infrastructure and power supply
- management expertise in project, administration, and clinical services
- clinical services: surgical, medical, nursing care, and laboratory
- support services: biomedical, X-ray
- human resources: expertise and coordinated supply

The ICRC now recognizes five types of hospital programs (as proposed by the chief surgeon of the ICRC in 2015 – Figure 16.4). These may serve as a useful model:

- Type I: full substitution, where the hospital is staffed and managed by the ICRC. This applies to situations where virtually all local facilities have collapsed (often in the aftermath of disaster), or there are no other health facilities available for the population in need. Full substitution with continuous on-call cover for patient care requires at least two surgical teams. Examples include the ICRC hospital in Lokichokio, in Northern Kenya, from 1985 to 2006, a facility for the care of weapon-wounded patients from South Sudan, and the ICRC hospital in Muzaffarabad, Pakistan, in 2005 and 2006, in the aftermath of the earthquake.
- Type II: substitution within an existing facility. The ICRC takes over the responsibility of one department (for example, the surgical ward) and/or

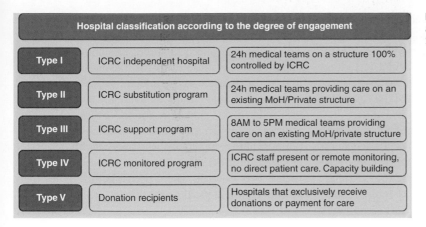

Figure 16.4 Hospital classification according to the degree of engagement Source: ICRC

Hospital classification according to the degree of engagement		
Type I	ICRC independent hospital	24h medical teams on a structure 100% controlled by ICRC
Type II	ICRC substitution program	24h medical teams providing care on an existing MoH/Private structure
Type III	ICRC support program	8AM to 5PM medical teams providing care on an existing MoH/private structure
Type IV	ICRC monitored program	ICRC staff present or remote monitoring, no direct patient care. Capacity building
Type V	Donation recipients	Hospitals that exclusively receive donations or payment for care

a group of patients (for example, weapon-wounded patients). This is currently the most common type of project. Examples include Goma in Congo, and Maiduguri in Nigeria.

- Type III: a support program, with staff present during the day (this may be a security restriction due to curfew). Examples include Bangui in the Central African Republic and Juba in South Sudan.
- Type IV: monitored programs, without direct responsibility for patient care. In some cases, these are "remote control" programs due to security constraints. In these programs, it is difficult to ensure the quality of care. Examples include Kandahar in Afghanistan and Laiza in Myanmar.
- Type V: donations of equipment and/or consumables without further clinical involvement. Currently more than 400 hospitals receive donations from the ICRC.

Surgical Standards

ICRC recruitment of surgeons is based on expertise in surgery in austere environments. Surgeons are expected to have broad skills in general surgery and orthopedics. Although most patients present with limb injuries, chest and abdominal injuries are common. Patients frequently present with infective complications and surgical decisions rest on the control of sepsis as a priority. War wounds are typically contaminated, contain devitalized tissue, affect more than one body compartment, involve multiple injuries in the same patient, and present late. Therefore, most of the casualties who reach treatment centers have limb injuries[25]. Over the last thirty years, the ICRC has published extensive surgical guidelines on the management of war wounds[24,25,26,27,28]. Detailing each of these is beyond the scope of this

chapter, but specific examples, such as the management of landmine injuries and the fashioning of amputation stumps that best fit a prosthesis and enable patients to mobilize and reintegrate into society, deserve special mention. An awareness of what happens to patients *after* surgery is crucial to maintaining quality in operative surgery. Surgical deployments on ICRC missions are generally longer than surgical field missions undertaken by NGOs and charities. Individual surgeons, therefore, have the opportunity to monitor outcomes at first hand and learn from more experienced colleagues; indeed, first-mission surgeons are accompanied by a senior surgeon and trainer.

There are multiple challenges to the delivery of quality surgical care and pitfalls that every surgical colleague and every organization engaging in clinical work abroad should be aware of. Today, most countries regulate medical care and licensing to assure the delivery of quality patient care. This may involve specific training, a minimum number of certain procedures performed every year for accreditation, continuous quality appraisal for medical licensing, the measurement of patient outcomes, or a register of complications. Surgeons working at home and overseas must meet these standards of competence. Host countries in conflict and disaster zones are likely to have similar rules for licensed practice and quality control. Field hospitals must comply with these rules.

Although it may be difficult to prepare for the wide variety of pathologies that surgeons may encounter in the field, in the absence of skilled specialist colleagues, surgeons should not undertake procedures they lack the skills to perform. At all times, the medical profession (and more so surgical colleagues) must be aware that one can do harm. The answer is perhaps to broaden surgical skills through supervised training at home and abroad. There are surgical courses tailored for surgeons embarking on missions and opportunities to learn from specialists at home. On mission, there are also opportunities to learn from colleagues, including local health personnel with considerable experience and wisdom. Every opportunity should be taken to work with local experts when they are available.

People in Aid, the Sphere project, and aid organizations themselves are increasingly advocating quality standards in the delivery of humanitarian aid. It is incumbent on surgical and medical programs to fulfill at least the minimum requirements of international standards for safe practice. The ICRC has agreed standards for practice and appraisal of staff. Host countries may have well-defined audit systems and requirements for local and visiting medical staff. Visiting medical staff must be appraised of local needs and be fit to practice in challenging field environments.

The ICRC quality standards cover patient, staff, and equipment needs in the field. Examples include the required amount of water per day per patient and the space specifications for hospital beds. In a hospital substitution project with 24-hour staff coverage, one surgical team does not suffice and a second team must be recruited and deployed as the project is planned. There should always be one physiotherapist per surgeon on mission as at least two-thirds of the surgical caseload include limb injuries. Regrettably, in reality, running programs compliant with these minimum requirements presents a challenge. Conflict environments are increasingly dangerous for both local and visiting health-care providers. Security threats prohibit the adequate staffing of hospitals to meet standards.

In the aftermath of the Haiti earthquake, concerns were raised in the media regarding the quality of the humanitarian assistance provided; specifically the rate and appropriateness of amputations performed received public attention. WHO and other organizations investigated and responded, formulating the foreign medical team (FMT) initiative, now renamed EMTs[19]. In 2013, the "blue book" was published, describing the requirements for teams to go to disaster zones[28]. The minimum standards regarding staff and equipment for mobile teams, field hospitals with limited surgical capacity, and full field hospitals were clearly defined. The next step, which is now ongoing, is the guidance for clinical practice in disasters and conflict, which differs from normal clinical practice. Experienced clinical staff must adapt their treatment

methods according to the different pathology and environments they encounter in the field.

One of the projects providing clear clinical guidance for the teams in the field is the "Management of limb injuries in disasters and conflicts" text[23]. An expert group with humanitarian, military, and academic input has updated the guidelines for the treatment of limb injuries in conflict and disaster zones. As sepsis compounds injuries in patients who present with delays, the emphasis in these guidelines is on damage control and radical debridement. These principles are increasingly accepted and practiced worldwide.

Summary

Surgical care for the weapon wounded and sick in conflict and disaster zones is clearly defined with internationally accepted guidelines for clinical care, the provision of resources, and infrastructure. There is an obligation to provide care that meets quality standards. Donors and host countries demand that surgical care is provided to the highest standard. As for the patients, they deserve the best.

Take-Home Messages

- Conflict and disaster present a burden of surgical need well beyond direct injury.
- Through experience spanning over forty years, the ICRC has accumulated expertise in the management of war wounded in austere and under-resourced environments.
- The ICRC's scheme for field hospital deployment, support, and substitution serves as a useful model for IOs as they plan their medical response to disasters and conflict.
- Preparation and organization are key to safe and effective practice in the field.
- Surgeons must work within their skill sets, but must seek to expand their skills, taking advantage of learning opportunities at home and in the field.

References

1. Shrime MG, Sleemi A, Thulasiraj RD. Charitable platforms in global surgery: a systematic review of their effectiveness, sustainability, and role in training. *World Journal of Surgery* 2015: **39**: 10–20.

2. Myles P, Haller G. Global distribution of access to surgical services. *The Lancet* 2010: **376** (9746): 1027–8.

3. Funk LM, Weiser TG, Berry WR, et al. Global operating theatre distribution and pulse oximetry

supply: an estimation from reported data. *The Lancet* 2010: **376**(9746): 1055–61.

4. Mock C, Cherian M, Juillard C, et al. Developing priorities for addressing surgical condition globally: furthering the link between surgery and public health policy. *World Journal of Surgery* 2010: **34**: 381–5.

5. Marck R, Huijing M, Vest D, et al. Early outcome of facial reconstructive surgery abroad: a comparative study. *European Journal of Plastic Surgery* 2010: **33**: 193–7.

6. Huijing MA, Marck KW, Combes J. Facial reconstruction in the developing world: a complicated matter. *British Journal of Oral and Maxillofacial Surgery* 2011: **49**: 292.

7. International Federation of the Red Cross and Red Crescent Societies. Emergency response units. Online article. http://www.ifrc.org/eru

8. The many victims of war: indirect conflict deaths. Global burden of armed violence (2008). Geneva Declaration Secretariat. Chapter 2. http://www.geneva declaration.org/fileadmin/docs/Global-Burden-of-Armed-Violence-full-report.pdf

9. Nott DM, Veen, H, Matthew P. Damage control in the austere environment. *The Bulletin of the Royal College of Surgeons of England* 2015: **96**(3): 82–3.

10. Hayward-Karlsson J, Jeffrey S, Kerr A, Schmidt H. Hospitals for war-wounded. Chapter 3.2, The admission sheet used in ICRC hospitals, and Chapter 4.2, The operating theatre. 2005: **46**: 113–16.

11. Coupland RM, Samnegaard HO. Effect of type and transfer of conventional weapons on civilian injuries: retrospective analysis of prospective data from Red Cross hospitals. *The British Medical Journal* 1999: **319**: 410–2.

12. Guha-Sapir D, Rodriguez-Llanes JM, Hicks MH, et al. Civilian deaths from weapons used in the Syrian conflict. *The British Medical Journal* 2015: **351**: h4736.

13. Black I (2016). The Guardian. Report on Syria conflict finds 11.5% of population killed or injured. Online article. https://www.theguardian.com/world/2016/feb/11/report-on-syria-conflict-finds-115-of-population-killed-or-injured

14. Trelles M, Dominguez L, Tayler-Smith K, et al. Providing surgery in a war-torn context: the Médecins Sans Frontières experience in Syria. *Conflict and Health* 2015.

15. Torno RR (2016). A legacy of 50 years of war: the failure of state development in South Sudan since independence. Theories of development. http://www.academia.edu/20373682/A_Legacy_of_50_Years_of_War_The_Failure_of_State_Development_in_South_Sudan_since_independence

16. Acerra JR, Iskyan K, Qureshi ZA, Sharma RK. Rebuilding the health care system in Afghanistan: an overview of primary care and emergency services. *International Journal of Emergency Medicine* 2009: **2**: 77–82.

17. Chu K, Trelles M, Ford N. Rethinking surgical care in conflict. *The Lancet* 2010: **375**: 262–3.

18. Sirwardhana C, Wickramage K. Conflict, forced displacement and health in Sri Lanka: a review of the research landscape. *Conflict and Health* 2014: **8**: 22.

19. Devakumar D, Birch M, Rubenstein LS, et al. Child health in Syria: recognising the lasting effects of warfare on health. *Conflict and Health* 2015: **9**: 34.

20. Chu KM, Ford NP, Trelles M. Providing surgical care in Somalia: a model of task shifting. *Conflict and Health* 2011: **5**: 12.

21. Ratnayake R, Degomme O, Roberts B, Spiegel P. Conflict and health: seven years of advancing science in humanitarian crises. *Conflict and Health* 2014: **8**(1): 1.

22. Burnham G, Hoe C, Hung YW, et al. Perceptions and utilization of primary health care services in Iraq: findings from a national household survey. *International Health and Human Rights* 2011: **11**:15.

23. ICRC. Management of limb injuries during disasters and conflicts. 2016.

24. The Sphere handbook (2018). http://www.spherehand book.org/

25. Mannion SJ, Chaloner E. Principles of war surgery. *The British Medical Journal* 2005: **330**: 1498–500.

26. Giannou C, Baldan M, Molde A. *War surgery*. Volume 2. ICRC; 2013.

27. Delauche MC, Blackwell N, Le Perff H, et al. A prospective study of the outcome of patients with limb trauma following the Haitian earthquake in 2010 at one- and two-year (the SuTra2 study). *PLOS Currents* 2013.

28. Norton I, von Schreeb J, Aitken P, Herard P, Lajolo C. *Classification and Minimum Standards for Foreign Medical Teams in Sudden Onset Disasters*. World Health Organization. 2013. Website. http://www.who.int/hac/global_health_cluster/fmt_guidelines_september2013.pdf

Wound Management in a Field Hospital Environment

Alan Kay

Introduction

Managing wounds will be the commonest surgical activity most field hospitals will need to deliver[1]. Even in situations where public health and medical care issues predominate, people will sustain wounds. It might be anticipated that the majority of these will be simple wounds that could be looked after by the patient or nonprofessional carers. Normal functions of society, however, are disrupted in situations where, for example, there is population displacement, conflict, disaster, or enduring civil unrest. Access to clean water with which to wash a simple wound and a straightforward dressing can no longer be guaranteed. There may also be considerable delay in the patient seeking care, creating an additional challenge of chronic wounds. So, the environments where we might be most likely to find field hospitals are where the ability to manage even simple wounds is compromised, generating a higher burden of difficult wound problems.

Wounds from weapons are often complex, requiring technically demanding methods of surgical reconstruction if the best outcomes are to be achieved. A field hospital may not be the best place to conduct such interventions. Sophisticated surgical technique may also require sophisticated supporting services, which may not be available.

This is the challenge of providing wound care in a field hospital: a complexity of wound problems not normally encountered having to be managed in sub-optimal facilities.

Delivering wound care in a field hospital requires a broad appreciation of the overall situation and context. Clinicians must avoid focusing solely on the immediate clinical problem of the individual patient in front of them: a more population-based approach is necessary. Similarly, the limits of the individual clinician's skill set must not be allowed to adversely influence the care delivered. There is a temptation to embark on treatments outside clinicians' normal expertise and practice on the basis that there may be no one else to provide the care. There is a very significant difference between "the best was done" and "I did my best." Inappropriate early care may remove options for later interventions.

Establishing the Context

The expertise underpinning field hospitals can deploy in a variety of ways, some examples being:

- a preexisting capability, which trains and rehearses together, may deploy as a formed unit in response to an acute situation
- the logistical support elements of a field hospital may be on standby and this is then populated by ad hoc clinical staff when required to deploy
- a long-term facility remains in place for many years with regular rotations of both logistical and clinical staff
- a small team of specialists may deploy to augment the capability of an existing facility

Whatever the situation, it is vital that a thoughtful assessment of all factors is made. This would seem obvious for command and logistical supporting elements, but is also essential for clinical staff when it comes to understanding what might be the best care to deliver. Delivering care in a situation of intense needs and compromised resources is not an excuse for lack of proper patient evaluation and planning of the optimal care possible under these circumstances. Proper evaluation and planning of how best to use what is limited will help mitigate against some of the constraints.

What is my stated mission?

This may define the type of patient that will be encountered and set limits on eligibility.

What is the underlying situation?

This could, for example, be a sudden-onset disaster (SOD), a war, or a collapse of an unstable state. It will help predict the nature of the injuries likely to be seen.

Where will I be?

This may provide information relevant to environmental control and risks to staff, as well as give an idea about likely travel times for patients.

What other facilities are in my vicinity and what capabilities do they have?

This should include existing indigenous capabilities, prehospital care arrangements, and nonprofessional care habits. This will help anticipate what might happen to the patients before they reach your facility.

What expertise, equipment, and logistical support does my facility have and how much of it?

This will set limits on aspects of your clinical capability and how much capacity you may have.

What preexisting indigenous or imported capability is there for specialist treatment and rehabilitation and where is it?

This may directly influence what clinical pathways you initiate.

This can be summarized as:

- Where are my patients and how will they get to me?
- Where am I and what can I do?
- Who is elsewhere and what can they do?

With this appreciation it is then possible to take the essential mental move from "This is what I can do" to "This is what I should do."

Clinicians must have the insight and humility to constrain their interventions to what is appropriate to the facility they are working in and to the population they serve. In military field hospitals, where the rapid onward movement of injured military personnel is planned and assured, a doctrinal approach to what should be done acts as a check on activity. In less rigidly disciplined philanthropic facilities, it can be more difficult to control the actions of individuals and often their patients will be living in that environment with the consequences of treatment for decades after the visiting medical team has gone home.

It is highly likely the answers to some of these questions will change as situations develop, further information is uncovered, and staff rotate. Clinicians must also be able to adapt their approach to respond to new circumstances.

General Measures in Wound Care

General Patient Wellbeing

Wound management is optimized if the patient's overall condition is as good as can be achieved. In acute wounding, adequate resuscitation is essential. Assessment of tissue viability and, therefore, debridement is compromised in a poorly perfusing patient. Compromised tissue will do less well with reduced oxygen delivery. The deleterious effects on wound healing of the systemic inflammatory response and metabolic response to trauma can be reduced in impact by good supportive care[2]. The nutritional state of the patient is important: the detrimental effects of chronic malnourishment need to be anticipated and managed. This includes consideration for reducing the patient's parasite load, although there is some debate about the efficacy of this. Prophylaxis against tetanus must be ensured. There is a complex interaction between pain, stress levels, and the metabolic response, and adequate pain management strategies need to be available[3,4,5].

The Clinical Environment

This is an area of considerable challenge. By the very nature of a field hospital, control of the clinical environment is more difficult. The climate within a facility is much more influenced by external factors. Maintaining patient normothermia is most easily achieved if the internal ambient temperature is middle-to-high-twenties degrees centigrade. If lower than this, the use of near patient warming devices such as fluid warmers, warm air over-blankets, and under-patient warming mattresses is of help. There is no evidence of harm from the ambient temperatures being in the high-thirties degrees centigrade, but it is uncomfortable for patients and staff alike. Even tented facilities can be equipped to improve environmental control, creating clinical white space through the use of liners and additional outer shading layers plus air conditioning units.

Simple hygiene is of importance. Outcomes in wound management are adversely affected by infections. The potential for significant cross-contamination via staff and equipment is high. There is no reason why basic infection prevention and control measure cannot be followed[6]. Handwashing with soap and water and/or use of antiseptic hand rubs after each individual patient contact should be mandated and policed: there is no excuse for failures in such practices by staff. In genuine mass-casualty situations, the bedding down of large numbers of patients, sometimes in the open, makes it difficult to keep such areas clean, but the clinical spaces used for interventions and procedures should have clear protocols to maintain minimum standards of cleanliness.

Patient confidentiality should be respected with invasive interventions and, ideally, examinations being screened from general view.

Paying attention to the maintenance of standards in the clinical environment brings a sense of professionalism and "protected space" that instils confidence and morale among patients, as well as improving outcomes.

Antibiotics

The continued rise of antimicrobial resistance has led to attempts to more tightly restrict the use of antibiotics in normal clinical practice[7]. With respect to wound care, while infections will be treated, there are more general trends away from prolonged antibiotic prophylaxis. In the field hospital environment, assumptions are made about degrees of possible wound contamination which make the use of prophylaxis more appropriate, but this must be tempered with a rational approach. Prolonged use of broad-spectrum antibiotics simply as a precaution will result in the emergence of complex resistant strains of microorganisms.

The mainstay of wound care remains physical interventions with surgery, but for ballistic, blast, and contaminated wounds, it is accepted that there must be concomitant administration of antibiotics as prophylaxis[8]. Antibiotics alone cannot replace the need for surgery.

Field hospitals should have a clear policy of antibiotic use, which is appropriate to the environment in which it is operating. Individual clinicians must not be allowed to override the policy with attitudes based on their nondeployed practice.

A basic approach to antibiotic use in wound care is:

- prophylaxis should be with broad-spectrum antibiotics, which cover those organisms known to cause early wound infections, predominantly *Staphylococcus*, *Streptococcus*, and *Clostridium* species
- the first dose should be administered as soon after wounding as possible
- a second dose is given at the time of debridement
- a third dose is given about six to eight hours after that

Indications for prolonging prophylaxis beyond three doses are:

- exposed bone
- penetrating eye injuries
- penetrating central nervous system injuries

- where there is retained contamination within anatomically difficult areas, such as joints

Consideration of antibiotic choice should include tissue penetration for eye and central nervous system wounds, and additional anaerobic organism cover for bowel injuries.

If the wound is clinically infected at presentation, then use the same antibiotics as for prophylaxis. If the infection fails to clear or develops after prophylaxis, change to an antibiotic based on a knowledge of likely resistance patterns within the local geographical area.

If the field hospital has a microbiological laboratory capability, a policy of using wound surveillance swabs will help build a picture of local pathogens and resistance.

Initial Wound Surgery

With full situational awareness and the patient's general condition attended to, wounds are ultimately a surgical condition. The core requirement for any surgical wound management is to ensure an adequate debridement.

An examination of the patient beyond a primary survey is required to identify all wounds and any functional deficit. Radiological imaging of all ballistic injuries should be mandated where the facilities allow [9]. Findings should be documented. All wounds require some attention. For small wounds that do not breach the deep fascia and with no clinical evidence of damage to functional structures, this may be achieved by simple washing of the wound and applying a dressing.

For significant wounds this is not simply a case of cleaning and removal of nonviable tissue. Wound debridement should be seen as much as a diagnosis as it is a treatment and may be better referred to as initial wound surgery (IWS).

Patients who have wounds and are physiologically unstable should have a damage control resuscitation approach initiated[10]. This may include damage control surgery if other measures do not stem massive ongoing hemorrhage. Once control of hemorrhage and other leakage, such as bowel contents, is achieved, a period of additional resuscitation might be required to normalize physiology before further surgical interventions are appropriate. Full surgical attention to all patients may also not be possible in the case of overwhelming workload in a mass-casualty incident. The principles of damage control relate to the deranged physiology of an individual patient. When it is resource issues that direct truncating interventions, this is better referred to as abbreviated surgery.

In both situations, the process of formally debriding wounds might be delayed. As a minimal wound intervention, rapid lavage to reduce surface contamination can be performed quickly. There can be a tendency for the superficial components of wounds to be neglected, particularly in penetrating torso injuries; after complex correction of life-threatening damage to intracavity organs, it is easy to forget that the injuring object will have had to enter the body, and sometimes leave it, resulting in surface wounds. It must be made clear in the surgical notes following damage control or abbreviated surgery if there are wounds that require later debridement.

At some point every significant wound must undergo formal IWS and this should be performed as early as possible after the wound is sustained[11,12]. There is no clear evidence as to how long is too long to wait to perform a debridement. Perceived wisdom is that this should ideally be performed on wounds within six hours. There is, however, growing support for the approach that it is less harmful to wait for surgery to be done well by appropriately experienced clinicians rather than try and meet nonevidence-based timelines by utilizing inexpert generalists[13].

Very simple wounds can be managed by nonsurgeons at the bedside on wards or in emergency departments. It is essential that adequate analgesia is administered and the inability to control pain during the procedure is an indication in itself for referral to surgical care. A key requirement for the nonspecialist is to ensure all injured structures are identified, either by examination of function or by direct observation through the existing defect. Again, if this is not achievable, referral is indicated, and it is inappropriate for nonsurgeons to extend wounds for exploration. Bleeding that cannot be controlled with simple pressure and elevation is another indication for referral. The wound must have nonviable tissue and contamination removed, and this may require sharp excision. Doctors and other appropriately trained health-care professionals can perform this, but nonprofessional staff should not be permitted to go beyond irrigation.

For wounds where exploration is required, the IWS should be performed in an operating theater under adequate local, regional, or general anesthesia. The aim is to identify all injured structures, generate a surgical plan, perform any essential interventions

including removal of nonviable tissue and contamination and then apply a dressing. A structured approach to this is as follows.

Wound Hygiene

The patient as a whole should be viewed as being dirty. Clothing should be removed, but kept to give back to the patient later. A very wide area of uninjured skin around the wound should be cleaned using a soapy solution in warm water and then dried. This is not a formal surgical preparation, but a basic hygiene clean known as a social wash. Ideally, the whole patient should be cleaned, but this may not be practicable preoperatively.

Nonsurgical Control of Hemorrhage

General oozing from the wound can be controlled with a pressure dressing and/or elevation.

There are several types of topical hemostatic agents available[14]. These are primarily designed for prehospital use to mitigate for a lack of surgical capability where tourniquets and pressure dressings prove inadequate, such as in junctional areas. Their use within hospital should be limited to extreme situations only; for example, an overwhelming number of casualties. Once within a field hospital, where surgeons and operating theaters are available, the approach to continuously bleeding wounds should be formal surgical control.

If the patient has a tourniquet in place, either from prehospital or applied on arrival during the primary survey, this should be evaluated before the wound is addressed. If the initial tourniquet has been on for significantly more than two hours, discussions about managing the patient's general condition, overall distal viability, and potential need for fasciotomies should be had before it is released. If the tourniquet is a simple windlass type, as is common for prehospital use, this should be replaced by a pneumatic one as soon as is practicable. This can be placed proximal to the windlass, but not inflated initially. It should also not be applied too tightly such that it constricts venous flow when not inflated. The existing tourniquet can then be released and the wound observed. If there is no significant hemorrhage, then the pneumatic tourniquet does not need to be inflated immediately but should remain in place as a precaution or for use during debridement. This then allows an assessment of distal vascularity.

If, on releasing the tourniquet, there is significant bleeding, inflate the pneumatic tourniquet, and formal surgical vascular control should be obtained. Having an inflated pneumatic tourniquet in place makes the patient a priority for surgery.

Opinions on whether to debride a tourniquet-controlled exsanguinated limb or not vary and there is no hard evidence to support either view. Some feel that an injured limb is already undergoing a degree of vascular insufficiency and further periods of nonperfusion are potentially detrimental to the tissues. Others state that proper evaluation is not possible in a bloody field and the ongoing additional bleeding is not good for the patient and may increase demands on limited blood product stocks. Having an agreed approach in advance is preferable to having to make ad hoc decisions in the heat of the moment.

Nonpneumatic tourniquets designed for the pre-hospital environment are not appropriate for per-operative use. If a tourniquet is used during surgery, it should be released prior to any dressings to allow final assessment of tissue viability and control of any residual bleeding. It should be noted that on letting down a tourniquet, there is always a hyperemic surge with associated increase in bleeding and a sudden release of anaerobic metabolic products into the general circulation, which may have physiological sequelae in a shocked patient. It is important to communicate with the rest of the team that the tourniquet is about to be let down so any patient optimization can be performed. It is advisable to wrap the limb in gauze swabs and temporarily elevate it as the tourniquet is released to reduce the impact of the hyperemia.

General Wound Inspection

Much can be gleaned by observation with the patient under anesthesia in a controlled, well-lit environment, dressings off, bleeding controlled, and dirt and clothes removed. New wounds may have been uncovered during the social wash. Patterns in wounding can be assessed; for example, if there are several wounds, are they linked? Are there obvious signs of abnormal position suggesting fractures, dislocations, or tendon division? At this stage it is worth reviewing any radiological imaging and establish if all required views have been obtained. Any findings should be documented accurately; in particular, the size and position of wounds. There is always a possibility that these peroperative findings will form part of the evidence base for future legal considerations. With that in mind, it is important to avoid speculating as to the origin of wounds such as bullet versus fragment or

entry versus exit. Your responsibility is to describe what you find as a professional description of fact, not to extrapolate that into opinion as to causation. The legal jurisdiction under which the field hospital functions should not unduly influence clinical practice, but clinicians must be aware of what their responsibilities are in terms of how information and material that may become evidence should be handled.

Having fully observed the location of all wounds and made an assessment of likely damage to anatomical structures, the patient can be formally prepped and draped for surgery with the exposed operative field based on an appreciation of likely procedures. For example, a high groin wound that may have caused a vascular injury should be prepared to permit proximal control to be obtained at the level of the iliac vessels, a vein graft to be harvested from the uninjured leg, and fasciotomies to be performed.

Information about the planned procedure should be shared with the full surgical team in the form of a safe surgery brief such as the World Health Organization (WHO) checklist[15]. This can be performed very rapidly in emergency situations and being in field conditions is not an excuse for missing out this vital patient safety step[16].

The process of performing the various surgical stages listed below has been broken down to aid explanation. In reality, for practicality and efficiency, the steps will be overlapping.

Wound Edge Excision

The rim of skin around any wound will have a degree of contamination and contusion. Skin has a good blood supply and is relatively resilient, so any excision can be minimal. Even heavily contused, degloved or abraded skin may survive and if it does progress to necrosis the risk to the patient of leaving small amounts of dead superficial tissue is very low. It is prudent to remove a 1 mm rim of skin from around a wound and only remove more if it is obviously nonviable. Over-exuberant excision risks converting a wound that is suitable for delayed direct closure into one that requires a more complex reconstruction.

Wound Extension

It is rare to be able to visualize the full extent of a wound through the skin defect. Wounds should be extended surgically to properly explore and this must include deep fascia. Also, a wound will become edematous and the rise in tissue tension restricts perfusion. Any deep contamination is more likely to cause suppuration if trapped. The process of opening a wound by extension "unbridles" the tissues, allowing free drainage of exudate and swelling without pressure increase. This is the origin of the term debridement.

Wound-extension incisions should be along normal lines of election in the limbs; that is, longitudinal with a horizontal component across flexion creases and in a way that allows fasciotomies and access to neurovascular bundles to be performed if necessary. In the torso and head and neck, extensions should be planned to anticipate underlying injuries and/or along natural skin creases. The extensions should only be so long as to decompress fully the zone of injury and allow what further procedures are required.

Wound Exploration

A thorough exploration of the wound is made to establish what structures have been injured and to assess viability of tissue and the degree of contamination. Some low energy projectiles can separate tissue planes without causing much visible disruption; it is important to spot subtle signs such as air or hematoma. Preoperative imaging can play a very useful part in predicting wound tracks. The anatomical position of the patient on the operating table is unlikely to be the same as when they were injured, and wound tracks will not necessarily be in straight lines. The exploration may well involve extending the wound further; in particular through deeper structures. It is not necessary to lay open every wound fully if it is clear that no significant deeper structures are damaged, and contamination and cavitation are likely to be minimal. This requires a degree of surgical judgment.

Great care must be taken not to increase the risk of vascular compromise to tissues as wound extensions and explorations are performed. It should also be performed in a way that does not remove potential reconstructive options. Limbs should be explored by raising the skin in the subfascial plane and preserving perforating vessels where possible.

Establishing a Surgical Plan

Wound extension and exploration essentially provide a wound diagnosis. Decisions now must be made about what needs to be done during this surgical procedure and what is better to be left. Devitalized tissue and contamination should be excised. In the majority of field hospital situations, the basic principle will be that

of delayed repair. Immediate repair of damaged structures and closure of wounds that are caused by ballistic or blast mechanisms, sustained in a heavily contaminated environment, and where optimal care is not guaranteed is a highly risky approach. There are, however, some situations where immediate repair is necessary, and this should be performed as part of the IWS. There are also injuries where temporizing measures can be used. These decisions must be made with a full appreciation of the overall situation and context as outlined above.

Essential Surgical Interventions

Damage-control procedures to save life are, of course, essential. The main indication for repair at the time of initial wound surgery is restoration of vascularity. If larger vessels are damaged, a decision is needed as to the impact that will have on the viability of remaining tissues[17,18]. If repair will confer no benefit in terms of more distal viability, it is appropriate to ligate a damaged vessel. If by restoring flow there will be better functional recovery, then primary repair is indicated, even if this requires a patch repair or interposition graft. In contaminated wounds, autologous graft should be used in preference to artificial materials. If the surgical capability to perform a repair is not available or it is not appropriate because a damage control or abbreviated surgery approach is indicated, shunting of vessels can be performed[19]. This can also be done as a temporizing measure to allow a patient to be moved to a facility with greater capability in terms of vascular repair. If it is planned for a field hospital to receive patients with significant wounds, but it possesses no vascular surgery skills beyond ligation, questions need to be asked about the suitability of the facility to be allocated that role.

Ongoing contamination, such as leaking bowel, must be controlled.

The presence of compartment syndrome or a risk of it developing is an indication for fasciotomies as part of initial wound surgery. Similarly, retrobulbar hematomas should be released by lateral canthotomy.

Excision of Devitalized Tissue and Contamination

Removal of all visible contamination is a goal that is not always easy to achieve. Large pieces loose in a wound can be picked out individually. Finer material will often be firmly adherent to tissue and cannot be wiped off or irrigated out. Efforts to sharply excise all such material may remove otherwise healthy tissue. Material impregnated by a blast or ballistic mechanism will often follow tissue planes and it is possible to remove this by delicate excision of adventitial layers leaving functional structures intact. It has been shown that small metallic objects such as bullets and fragments which are deeply embedded in viable tissue can be safely left[20]. Any foreign body encountered during wound excision should be removed, but it may not be necessary to go hunting for every fragment seen on imaging. Fragments that are intraocular, in a synovial joint, or where they may cause impingement with the potential for erosion should be removed, although specialist surgical expertise may be required. More caution needs to be used with embedded environmental nonmetallic materials, and experience has shown that, if left, these will rapidly lead to local pus formation.

Decisions about how much tissue to excise are not solely related to assessment of viability at the time of debridement. Differing tissues have differing resilience and there are differing consequences of the way dubiously viable tissue is managed.

There are general factors to consider:

- Is the patient's physiological state contributing to apparent nonviability and will this improve?
- Is there any risk that a change in the patient's condition may go unnoticed, such as poor staff levels on the ward or the patient being moved to another facility?
- Will future workload make it difficult to reassess the wound in the operating theater at an appropriate time?

It may be appropriate to leave some dubiously viable tissue if there is a degree of confidence in the control there will be over the patient's postoperative care. If there is any doubt over what might happen to the patient in the next few days, it is more appropriate to be more radical in how much tissue is excised.

Then there are tissue specific factors to consider:

- As described above, skin is reasonably resilient and well vascularized and should be preserved as much as possible to aid later wound closure.
- Fat is poorly vascularized and has little functional benefit, so can be excised fairly radically. Caution should be taken in over-thinning the fat layer immediately beneath the skin as this can compromise the dermal blood supply.
- Deep fascia, tendons, and ligaments are also poorly vascularized, but have a very low metabolic demand and are difficult to assess viability. There is also little harm in leaving them at IWS as long as gross contamination is removed. These are structurally resilient and useful tissues and worth preserving initially so simple trimming of ragged edges is all that is required. If nonviable, they tend to lose structural integrity over time and can be excised later.

- Muscle is very sensitive to trauma and, even with its good vascularity, is liable to undergo necrosis. It is also liable to become infected once dead, and retained nonviable muscle presents a risk to the patient. It is therefore usual not to preserve dubiously viable muscle. Surface contamination of muscle can be removed by excision of the epimysial layer while preserving function.
- Neurovascular bundles should be preserved at IWS and function not compromised by over-exuberant excision of contamination. Heavy contamination can be removed by careful excision of the loose adventitial tissue. Care should be taken to avoid unnecessarily dividing small side branches as this can lead to further devascularization and denervation of surrounding muscles. There is no indication to tag the ends of divided structures, particularly nerves. Tagging in itself causes a degree of further damage and, at later surgery, any reconstructive surgeon will know how to find the structures with the normal approach being to first identify healthy tissues outside of the zone of injury.
- Bone fragments, no matter how comminuted, should be retained if there remain attachments to soft tissues and, therefore, a blood supply. Completely loose fragments should be removed.

There are no reliable, near patient, intraoperative investigations that are appropriate for the field-hospital environment that can give useful information about tissue viability. Assessment relies on the visual inspection by the surgeon. It would seem intuitive that the experience of the surgeon is the most sensitive measure, but this has not always been found to stand up to scientific scrutiny[21]. Small-vessel bleeding from tissue may confirm vascularity, but gives no indication about potential tissue survivability at the cellular level. Lack of bleeding in itself does not mean tissue will not survive as tissues may reperfuse as the patient's general condition improves. Contractility of muscle does demonstrate that the muscle is currently functioning and, therefore, alive, but progressive necrosis over the next few days is well recognized. Gross distortion of normal macroscopic architecture usually results in nonviable tissue.

As bleeding is encountered it should be addressed. Continuing to work in a bleeding field is a poor surgical method as it further insults the patient's physiology and makes assessment of tissues more difficult. Electrocautery, preferably bipolar, is useful for individual vessels but should not be used to scorch raw bleeding areas. This leaves a necrotic layer and makes assessment at later surgery more difficult.

The tissues of the hands and face are highly specialized and with little redundancy. Loss of form and function in these areas has a huge impact on the patient's ability to perform in society. Every effort must be made to preserve tissue so as to maximize the reconstructive options. IWS should be as minimalistic as possible with the focus being on removal of gross contamination and preservation of blood supply. Involvement of specialists in hand and facial surgery should be sought as early as is realistically possible.

Amputation at IWS

Primary amputation to a defined level at IWS is not advocated. There are several factors that might influence the final level of an amputation, including patient preferences, and it is unlikely all the information will be available immediately.

Cases will present where there has been complete or near complete traumatic amputation by the mechanism of injury. It may also be obvious that even if the limb is still attached there will be no effective reconstructive options once all nonviable tissue is removed. In these cases, the process of removing nonviable tissue remains the same and this may result in what would be recognized as an amputation. What should not be done is excision of any viable tissue in anticipation of a predicted final amputation level. This includes bone, which, if viable, can be left longer than the soft tissues. This has been found to be useful in splinting the tissues and handling during procedures.

This approach means at IWS a significant limb wound is debrided, not amputated, even if the result of debridement is a shortened limb.

Wound Irrigation

With essential surgical procedures and excision of nonviable tissue complete, the final part of removal of contamination is wound irrigation. This will aid in washing out loose debris. More importantly, it will also reduce the total bacterial load in the wound and lower the chance of the residual microscopic contamination progressing to invasive infection.

Large volumes of low-pressure warm isotonic solutions are preferable[22]. Using fingers to gently agitate the tissues helps loosen material and ensures deeper recesses are reached. Evidence suggests that high-pressure irrigation systems can drive contamination deeper into tissues and potentially increase the risk of infection[23]. There is little clinical evidence to give guidance on how much fluid to use, but common practice is for about 3 L for each limb that has simple wounds, increasing to about 9 L for heavily contaminated open fractures. This places a significant resupply burden on a busy field hospital. A practical alternative is to use water that is clean enough to drink as the initial irrigating fluid and use sterile crystalloid for the last liter. Irrigating with common antiseptic solutions such as iodine, hydrogen peroxide, and chlorhexidine has not been shown to improve clinical outcomes[24,25].

A final check is made of the wound as irrigation can reveal new areas of contamination and restart some bleeding. If any deep pockets with narrow openings leave significant dead space, simple soft plastic ribbon drains can be used.

Any temptation to loosely close the tissues to restore anatomical alignment with sutures must be resisted. If vital structures need acute coverage, then this should be a formal surgical procedure.

Dressings

The vast majority of wounds will not undergo direct closure at IWS. The open wound requires a dressing. Many dressings are designed to help achieve wound healing, but in this context the aim is to prevent further wound deterioration until the next trip to theater.

A key element in managing a field hospital is to preserve resources and this includes the resilience of the staff. Having appropriate dressing regimens helps control workload by keeping unnecessary interventions to a minimum.

Factors influencing the choice of dressing include the following:

- patient comfort
- ease of application
- resilience to movement and interference
- allowing free drainage of exudate from the depths of the wound, but also preventing strike-through of the dressing

- it should not require frequent dressing changes nor laborious nursing care
- it should comply with prescribing legislation
- it should be familiar to staff in their normal practice

There is no clear evidence based on trials of clinical practice that show better outcomes if dressings with antiseptic properties are used[26].

IWS is aimed at converting a contaminated traumatic wound into a safe surgical wound that can be left until a planned delayed primary closure, normally in the operating theater at about five days later. The dressing should be designed to not require changing during this time. Following this principle, collective experience led to the development of a standard approach to wound dressings, which was advocated by the International Committee of the Red Cross (ICRC) and used extensively over several decades[27].

Standard ICRC Dressing

The basis is a large volume of bulky absorbent material, usually made from fluffed-up simple gauze, which is loosely laid on the wound, not packed into it. It can have additional cotton wool applied on top if necessary. This is held in place using crepe bandages or sticky tape if on the torso. There is no requirement for a wound/gauze interface layer such as Vaseline gauze. The dressing must not be tight, but the bulkiness has been found to effectively splint wounds, which reduces pain levels. It is usual for dark blood-colored fluid to stain the outer crepe and this has a characteristic, slightly metallic, odor to it. At about day five, the dressing is removed under appropriate anesthesia in the operating theater with the expectation of seeing healthy tissue, no wound tension, no evidence of pus or infection, and condition right for closure.

Topical Negative Pressure Dressings

Efforts have been made to develop mechanical devices that alter the wound biology such that healing is facilitated to potentially remove the need for surgical closure. One such method is to apply negative pressure, which essentially sucks on the wound. Initially termed vacuum-assisted closure (VAC), a trademarked commercial name, it was later more generically described as negative-pressure wound therapy. The sealed nature of such dressing with exudate collected in a container was attractive for use in field hospital settings, but the more complex practicality of applying the dressing,

need for an electrical pump, and the cost made it inappropriate for most situations, particularly in humanitarian missions. Some ad hoc adaptations using low-technology materials were developed, but these were more individual surgeon based rather than organizational capabilities[28].

Experience within military evacuation chains involving intercontinental transfers found the strike-through of exudate in simple gauze dressing was unsatisfactory. Access to negative pressure dressings was easier within this robust pathway and, despite no proven efficacy, the principle was explored. As the intent was only to provide an appropriate dressing to keep a wound from deteriorating rather than trying to stimulate healing, the words "therapy" or "closure" became inappropriate and the term "topical negative pressure (TNP) dressing" became common.

Collective anecdotal experience soon demonstrated the significant benefits of TNP in terms of basic hygiene, patient comfort, and ease of nursing care [29]. Exceptionally complex blast injuries appeared to do very well with the patients remaining unexpectedly stable. The USA utilized a foam-based system, while the UK preferred gauze. The gauze used was a loose open-weave pattern, which by coincidence happened to be impregnated with a bactericidal agent. There is no evidence this agent influenced the efficacy of the dressing. The TNP was also used extensively in the receiving firm base hospitals, and wound practices evolved as experience was gained. No formal trials have been performed in the field hospital environment, but TNP has become a preferred method of dressing in many organizations.

A method of utilizing TNP is as follows. The gauze is loosely placed along every tissue plane that has been opened. If the wound has deeper tracts, drainage tubes can be placed to follow the gauze and several drains can be placed in each wound. Looser amounts of gauze are then added to fill the wound, but not tightly packed. Proprietary adhesive film sheets are then used to seal the wound. When using gauze, it is possible to link wounds across normal skin with a bridge of gauze and the adhesive film can circumferentially wrap a limb as long as it is laid on without tension rather than stretched across. Using the appropriate connections via the drainage tubes, the sealed dressing is linked to a suction pump, which is set to run continuously at negative 80 mmHg. As the negative pressure is applied, the dressing shrinks down and becomes firm. This effect has been used to splint limbs. It is also possible to incorporate other tubes in the dressing such as urinary catheters and chest drains. This method can also be used for dressing laparotomy wounds, which, because of damage control principles, are not going to be closed immediately although an interface layer, such as a plastic sheet, should protect the bowel.

Gauze alone should not be placed over neurovascular bundles that have been denuded of their adventitial covering or where there has been a vascular repair. In this situation, a nonadherent interface layer is required. Several materials have been tried and there is no conclusive best product. It seems as if plastic type material is better and a perforated silicone dressing is commonly used.

TNP on the face has not been frequently used with efficacy, and safety has not been fully established.

If using foam, it is important to use only open-cell material. In some situations, when using ad hoc TNP, foam from packaging has been used and this can be of a closed-cell pattern. This does not transmit the negative pressure to the wound and exudate is trapped. Foam also seems to do less well if placed on intact skin, so linking wounds with foam bridges is not used as often.

Immediate Tissue Cover at Initial Wound Surgery

There are significant risks to primarily closing wounds that are caused by ballistic and blast mechanisms, heavily contaminated and where ongoing care cannot be guaranteed. It remains a mantra that these wounds must never be closed at IWS; "must," "always," and "never" rarely apply in medical practice and there are a small number of situations where at least a degree of immediate wound closure is advantageous for the patient. The term "closure" does not necessarily imply skin closure and what is required is cover of certain structures with viable tissue. The principle of this needing to be tension free remains and it is important to factor in the likelihood of further wound swelling. It is essential that any wound considered for immediate cover has undergone debridement. Covering dead or contaminated tissue will lead to a poorer outcome.

Some specific tissues do not do well if left exposed and should be covered: the central nervous system and meninges, the globe of the eye, synovium and cartilage of joints, and intraabdominal and intrathoracic organs. Bone devoid of periosteum does better if covered but, if not possible, will tolerate a simple dressing as long as it is kept moist.

Some tissues, because of good blood supply and the importance of retaining function through anatomical alignment, benefit from closure as early as possible: the face, hands, and genitals. Intraoral mucosa should be primarily closed to cover exposed facial skeleton or through-and-through wounds, but not if it risks further necrosis by excessive mobilization or tension.

Vascular repairs and skeletonized neurovascular bundles should be covered with viable tissue if possible.

Coverage by skin closure should only be performed at IWS if this can be achieved by returning the skin to its normal position or where there has been minimal loss. The raising of large local or distant flaps may well alter skin perfusion and should be performed with caution on acutely injured tissues. Transposing muscle is an alternative, but this requires knowledge of specific muscle blood supply, and care should be taken not to damage small feeding vessels. Extreme caution must be exercised if considering closing any wound caused by blast.

Ongoing Care

Beyond standard postanesthetic care, specific wound care delivered on the wards is essential if best outcomes are to be achieved. Regular observations of the patient's general condition should be performed and documented to look for changes that may indicate hemorrhage, ischemia, and infection. Pain levels should be monitored and appropriate analgesia administered.

Part of the success of the approach of IWS followed by delayed primary closure is permitting wound perfusion by allowing swelling without a rise in tissue pressure. Removing tension by surgical incisions is then aided by reducing further edema by resting the wound and elevation. If the bulky dressing is not supportive enough, it can be augmented by a plaster backslab. The lack of swelling under tension also reduces pain levels.

Movement of the tissues involved in the wound should be minimized and this may involve a degree of immobilization. This needs to be balanced against a need to maintaining as near a normal range of motion as possible in other parts of the body. Avoidance of chest-related complications is essential and where possible the patient should sit up when not asleep and be supervised in respiratory therapy.

Attention needs to be paid to providing the correct nutritional requirements and this may include correcting preinjury deficiencies.

The correct approach to managing psychological problems related to injury is not straightforward. Complex multifactorial issues may be involved in the patient's psychological state, and field-hospital staff may have differing cultural norms. Distinguishing between normal adjustment behavior following injury and true mental health pathology is difficult, and inappropriate interventions can be counterproductive. The field hospital should have an expertly informed approach to psychological wellbeing, and care must include providing a supportive environment.

Planning the Next Surgical Intervention

The intent of IWS is to have a wound that remains stable in its dressing after an adequate debridement. If the surgical plan is that the next intervention is delayed primary closure, then there should be no need to change the dressing. Routinely taking dressings down on the ward simply to satisfy curiosity is additional workload, adds to patient discomfort, and increases infection risks for no benefit. The plan should be for the patient to be taken to the operating theater and, under appropriate anesthesia, have the dressing removed and an assessment made on the suitability for delayed primary closure (DPC).

ICRC experience has been that this is best performed about five days after the IWS. DPC still aims to achieve healing by primary intention. Leaving it for too long means the wound will progress to heal by secondary intention with more fibrosis and a poorer result. How long is too long is variable, but DPC should be planned for within the first week. Contemporary military experience has provided anecdotal evidence that DPC can be safely performed earlier in certain situations. In some recent conflicts, military field hospitals resourced to perform only IWS within an evacuation chain for military personnel were tasked with an additional responsibility to deliver definitive treatment for local nationals. The pressure on bed availability drove a demand to discharge these patients as quickly as was deemed safe. Having closed wounds was a requirement, so reducing the time to DPC was advantageous. It was found that ballistic wounds caused by bullets or metallic fragments could be safely closed two days after IWS. Wounds with a significant blast element or heavy environmental contamination were treated more cautiously and left for the traditional five days and often required further debridement prior to DPC. It should be noted that this approach was being taken in field hospitals that had a degree of semipermanent buildings with good environmental control and supervised by surgeons who were experts in complex wound management. It is unknown if this will be a safe approach in more austere environments.

Having DPC as the next planned step is appropriate if the surgeon is entirely confident that the debridement performed at IWS was adequate and complete. If there are doubts about tissue viability or debridement was abbreviated, the next intervention should be planned for around 48 hours. This has traditionally been referred to as a "second look", but should more accurately be described as a further debridement with the emphasis on the principle that something is going to be done, rather than just an observation being made.

If damage control surgery only has been performed, the next stage should occur as soon as the patient is physiologically stable. This second intervention is essentially the formal IWS.

If at any point the patient's general condition deteriorates, there is unexpected further hemorrhage, there are clinical indications of wound infection, or distal ischemia develops, consideration should be given to formally inspecting the wounds in the operating theater under anesthesia. It should be remembered that the signs of systemic inflammatory response and infection can be very similar, and clinical judgement is required. It is not appropriate to perform wound inspections on the ward.

At some point during the period between IWS and DPC, a thorough reexamination of the patient needs to be performed. This is to identify any missed injuries or functional deficits and is often termed the "tertiary survey[30]."

DPC

Wound healing through primary intention is preferable to secondary intention. This is because the latter takes longer to achieve and results in a greater degree of fibrosis with poorer function. The cellular responses that lead to healing by fibrosis start immediately and primary closure minimizes the volume of tissue undergoing secondary intention healing rather than fundamentally altering wound biology. Delays in closure much beyond a week result in a sufficient degree of tissue changes such that pliability is reduced and closure becomes more difficult.

As has been described, closing the wounds most likely to be encountered in a field hospital too early is risky and the balance between reducing this risk and not getting too much fibrosis is to close wounds from about day two to day eight.

Primary intention healing is achieved by reducing the raw surface area and getting skin to skin closure. This removes the stimulus for wound contracture and the need for reepithelialization.

For safe and reliable DPC, the same conditions apply as at the end of IWS; there should be no residual nonviable or contaminated tissue, no undue tissue tension, and all damaged structures known about. At the planned next surgical intervention after IWS, a degree of wound exploration is required to ensure there are no areas of doubtful viability, but if the tissues look healthy it is unnecessary to completely reopen up every element of the wound. In blast injuries, even where IWS was very thorough and all obvious nonviable tissue had been excised, it is not unusual to see areas of further necrosis. This is not evidence of earlier poor decision-making; it is the natural wound evolution and is most commonly seen in muscle. Although the tissue architecture and small-vessel perfusion appeared intact at the first look, there was sufficient damage at a cellular level to cause progressive necrosis. If this is only apparent on a few small patches, this can be excised and DPC started. If there are larger areas, these should also be excised but DPC postponed until a further return to the operating theater after about 48 hours.

Similarly, there should be no evidence of infection; either cellulitis or frank pus. Some very small pockets of pus with no surrounding tissue inflammation can just represent the response to retained contamination. These can be irrigated and DPC performed. Any evidence of invasive infection requires systemic antibiotic treatment and a postponement of DPC.

The presence of injured deeper structures does not preclude DPC. If, for example, it is known a main nerve in a limb is divided, but repair is being delayed, possibly for weeks until the correct resources are available, it is sensible to perform DPC over the nerve injury rather than leave the wound open. It is essential that the requirement for further reparative interventions is recorded and the patient informed.

The wound should be reirrigated with warm isotonic crystalloid before closure. If it is obvious that closing superficial layers will create deeper cavities, soft plastic ribbon drains can be used to provide a route for exudate to escape. This will only be effective for small cavities that will naturally collapse in

a dressing. Larger areas should not be closed using deep sutures if it creates tension in the tissues; they should be left open to allow free drainage. This has been a situation where TNP dressings have proved useful and gradual elimination of such cavities has been achieved by sequential use of reducing volumes of gauze.

Closure of skin by direct suture should only be performed if the edges appose without tension. This will not be possible if there has been significant skin loss. Mobilizing skin by undermining through subcutaneous fat must not be attempted. If repositioning of skin to avoid tension is required, then formal flaps should be fashioned. This is why it is important that wound extensions during IWS are made in the subfascial plane with regard to future flap design. An alternative is to close the wound using a skin graft. It is not unusual in complex wounds for there to be a combination of these methods used to achieve closure.

Ideally monofilament nonabsorbable sutures should be used for direct skin closure and removed before crosshatch markings develop. Absorbable sutures remain as a foreign body long after they have lost any function in wound support and are a potential nidus for small abscess formation. Similarly, braided sutures can cause further damage to already injured tissues and allow wicking of surface contaminants. While these present only a very small risk in most routine surgical work, wounds that are having DPC in field hospitals are by their very nature at greater risk of developing complications and all surgical technique should be optimal. Metal skin staples may not give the most accurate of skin apposition in difficult contoured wounds, but are a good way of rapidly closing skin when there is pressure on time.

It is acceptable to partly close wounds and then return for further closure after another couple of days. This can be facilitated by the combined use of TNP and elasticated sloops, which gradually draw tissue in. This has been frowned on historically, but proved useful when dealing with massive tissue loss following improvised explosive device blast wounds. In normal practice, wounds of such extent that are not caused by blast would be closed using sophisticated surgical techniques such as free tissue transfer. The systemic response to these devastating blast injuries, however, is a relative contraindication to the more complex flap repairs, which are also not appropriate in most field-hospital conditions. Even when extensive experience of using sloops had been gained, their use in the primary dressing following IWS was not entertained; their place is as an aid once DPC has started. Combining sloops and TNP should not be viewed as the primary modality of wound care, but is a pragmatic solution in some complex situations.

Once skin has been sutured and the wound is essentially closed, a dressing is still applied. This will help absorb any seepage of exudate and, by providing a degree of splintage, reduce pain. A thin strip of gauze held in place by adhesive tape is often all that is required. As experience with TNP dressings developed it was noted that when used in partially closed wounds the TNP seemed to be beneficial to the sutured segment as well as the open part. TNP dressing were therefore used in the more complex closed wounds for the first couple of days after DPC. This again is anecdotal, but the sutured wounds seemed to be less painful, edema settled quicker, the patients mobilized more readily, and overall there were fewer wound complications.

If after DPC the sutured wound becomes clinically infected, there should be a very low threshold for reopening the wound so that viability of tissues can be reevaluated, tissue tension relieved, and any pus allowed to freely drain.

Skin Grafting as DPC

When it is not possible to close a wound by directly suturing skin to skin, an alternative is to use skin grafting as a method of DPC. In general, this will be autologous split thickness.

As harvesting a graft results in a wound elsewhere on the body (the donor site), the primary wound defect must be of a size that justifies the procedure. The donor site of a split-thickness skin graft will normally take about two weeks to reepithelialize so any wound that is anticipated to heal in less than this time should not be considered for grafting. It is generally accepted that wounds less than about 3 cm diameter do not need grafting apart from specialized areas such as face and hands.

For a skin graft to take, the recipient wound must have a sufficiently vascular base. This is not the same as a granulating wound bed: granulation tissue is a sign of a chronic wound and it will not have appeared during the time frame for DPC, even when TNP is used. If the wound bed looks viable, it will usually support a skin graft. This includes tissues that are traditionally viewed as not being particularly

vascular such as fat and fascia: these will normally accept a graft. Very poorly vascularized tissues such as bone devoid of periosteum and cartilage should not be grafted. Tendons do poorly when grafted, both in terms of graft take and the later functional problems with adhesions. The central nervous system, peripheral nerves, and skeletonized vessels will readily accept a graft, but there is a risk to later function and flap coverage is preferable.

As a skin graft is essentially avascular for a day or so until it takes, it is particularly prone to infection. A cellulitic wound or the presence of pus is a relative contraindication to skin grafting.

In the vast majority of cases, split skin grafts should be meshed. This helps prevent exudate lifting the graft from the bed and therefore increases take rates and also facilitates the contouring of the graft into the more complicated three-dimensional defects. Meshing can be achieved by simply making multiple small (about 0.5 cm) incisions in the graft. If a degree of "expansion" of the graft is required; that is, increasing the surface area it will cover by meshing, this can only be achieved if formal meshing machines are used. It should be noted that the standard meshing ratio of 1.5:1 is applicable for most situations. The ratio 3:1 can be used where there is a significant shortage of available graft. Ratios above this are extremely difficult to handle and should only be used by those with experience.

Hand knives to harvest skin are acceptable but, if at all possible, it is better to use an electric or compressed gas driven dermatome. Donor-site bleeding should be minimized by liberally infiltrating either subdermally or intradermally with weak epinephrine solution (1:1 000 000) about five minutes before harvesting. An alternative is to place gauze soaked in the epinephrine solution on the raw donor site after harvesting for at least five minutes before applying the dressing. The addition of a long-acting local anesthetic agent to the solution is efficacious for postoperative pain relief. There are numerous dressings advocated for donor sites and the choice will be predominantly dictated by availability[31]. It should be noted that Vaseline gauze is not a nonadherent dressing: at body temperature the Vaseline becomes liquid and is quickly absorbed leaving the remaining gauze to become very firmly stuck to raw surfaces. It is better to leave a donor-site dressing in place until it is shed as the wound heals rather than remove it as a planned dressing change.

There are similarly numerous ways to secure a skin graft and it is likely that the most success will be achieved by using the method that the surgeon is most familiar with. For situations where the treating team is not very familiar with skin grafting, suturing a graft in place with a few interrupted tacking sutures is often the safest. Evidence for very early mobilization following skin grafting originates from specialized plastic surgery units and may not extrapolate to field-hospital conditions[32]. It is probably safer to use a bulky dressing with or without a plaster backslab, keeping the area rested and, if possible, elevated until the first change of dressing at about day five. The use of TNP as a dressing to secure a skin graft has gained popularity and is now the method of choice in many organizations[33]. It is worth reemphasizing that, in the contexts mentioned above, TNP is advocated because of the practical aspects of managing the dressing and patient comfort; not as a wound therapy aimed at achieving healing.

Nonacute Wounds

It must be anticipated that some patients will present with wounds that are not acute and may have either not received any treatment or have been mismanaged. There are many reasons why this might happen, examples being:

- a SOD such as an earthquake disrupts all normal means of accessing health services
- an enduring conflict prevents free movement for individuals
- the patient's priorities are not their wound and they only present when the wound prevents them from performing what they consider to be more important activities
- wounds have been primarily closed and without proper debridement by inexperienced health-care workers

The wound biology will have progressed toward healing by secondary intention and achieving direct closure is unlikely. It is unusual for such patients to be in need of urgent interventions and it is worth spending time on optimizing the patient and carefully considering all factors before committing to a specific clinical pathway. An appropriate approach is to:

- remove the factors preventing the wound from healing such as necrotic tissue, contamination, infection, malnourishment
- confirm the wound has entered a healing phase by witnessing the formation of granulation tissue
- only then decide on the method of wound closure

If there is clear evidence of invasive tissue infection, systemic antibiotics should be administered. Wounds that have been primarily closed and with any signs of wound tension or infection should have the sutures removed. If the facilities are available, samples should be cultured for microbiological assessment.

These wounds may benefit from a less radical surgical approach. Obviously necrotic tissue and contamination does need to be removed surgically and tissue tension released along the same lines as IWS. Cellulitic tissue may resolve with antibiotics. Some structures with key functions such as certain tendons and nerves, even if directly involved in a suppurating wound, may not need excision. Bone infection is particularly complex and requires a highly specialized approach.

Unlike managing acute wounds, having a regimen of daily irrigation and change of dressings can be advantageous, but hygiene habits to control cross infection must be meticulous. Physically abrading the wound during the dressing change can help to disrupt biofilm[34]. There is no unequivocal clinical trial evidence of benefit in using antiseptic solutions for irrigating chronic wounds. Similarly, there is no conclusive evidence to support superiority of one particular type of dressing. If definitive care of chronic wounds is to be achieved in a field hospital environment, the aim is the generation of a viable bed, as normally demonstrated by the presence of granulating tissue, which allows closure by skin grafting or, in some cases, a flap.

Reconstruction

A field hospital is not a good environment to undertake definitive reconstructive surgery. The time, environmental control, surgical skill set, equipment, consumable resources, rehabilitation services, and so on are rarely all present. There are, however, occasions when it may be best for the patient and should be done. Before embarking on any reconstructive surgery, it is essential that a full assessment of the situation and context is made and understood by the clinicians. Examples of various scenarios include the following:

- In most military field hospitals, the military patients are being moved along a controlled evacuation chain and the aim is to do only what is necessary to preserve life and prevent deterioration such that definitive care delivered at the end of the chain can achieve maximal outcome. If IWS (including essential immediate cover and vascular interventions) has been performed correctly and there is no delay in onward movement, there is no requirement to embark on reconstructive procedures.

- Where a field hospital has been deployed in response to a SOD it may be many weeks before the normal health system has recovered, but it is anticipated there will be a return to a well-developed service. In such a scenario it is appropriate to get wounds healed as early as is safe by using simple reconstructive measures that can be revised by more sophisticated techniques later and done in such a way as to not remove options for that later reconstruction.

- In the enduring instability of a failed state, a field hospital might be the most sophisticated medical facility available for many years and any wound-closure techniques should be aimed at getting the best functional outcomes possible within the resources available using reconstructive options appropriate to the setting. If such surgery is a frequent requirement for the facility, it would be inappropriate to deploy surgeons who do not have the skill set to perform the types of reconstruction likely to be required.

The optimal reconstructive pathway for any given wound is influenced by many factors. Compared to working in a more sophisticated environment, those factors related to resources and context in a field hospital are more likely to have a greater impact on decision-making than the patient's individual requirement. That said, if the reconstructive technique used is not appropriate for the patient, it is unlikely to result in a satisfactory outcome.

Having to redo or revise surgical procedures due to poor technique or decision-making is not only bad for the patient but also an unnecessary additional burden on resources. Salvaging a poor result will often increase the complexity of the techniques required and make what was originally a manageable situation into one that is beyond the capability of the facility.

There is a balance between a more prolonged course of using repeated simple but very reliable measures and a single more complex procedure that carries a greater risk of failure but achieves the goal in a shorter period of time.

Clinicians need to make decisions that fit within the resources made available to them. In terms of maximizing the effectiveness of a field hospital, surgeons have a responsibility to take an approach that aims to "get it right first time." This requires choosing techniques that:

- work reliably in their hands
- work for the wound
- work for the patient
- work in the situational environment

Surgeons may be presented with nonacute cases where there is a request to improve appearance or function. Common conditions are congenital deformities and scar contractures. The emotional impact on decision-making can be high particularly when children are involved and there is often an expectation that just doing something will make things better. The temptation to embark on elective reconstruction that is beyond the normal experience and skill set of the surgeon must be resisted.

Timing of Reconstruction

Open wounds are detrimental to the patient's general condition, stimulating an ongoing catabolic state and increasing the risk of infection. The aim is to close a wound as soon as is safe. The principle of DPC is to provide a safety buffer of time in situations where there is risk in earlier closure such as in blast and ballistic injury and in compromised clinical environments such as a field hospital. Reconstruction is simply a form of wound closure that focuses on restoring maximal form and function and should also be performed as early as is safe.

Reconstruction can be performed immediately as part of IWS where vital structures require covering. This normally involves use of flap closure as skin grafting does not provide robust viable immediate cover. This type of reconstruction does not necessarily have to be the definitive option. Flaps can be raised as a temporizing maneuver and then revised or replaced at a later time.

More commonly, early reconstruction occurs as part of DPC. Beyond direct suture, split skin grafting is frequently the most appropriate option. It is a technique that is still within the capability of most surgical generalists, it gets wounds healed relatively safely and quickly, and it does not generally remove options for later revision reconstruction. In certain anatomical areas, a full thickness graft may give a better result. If the wound does not have a healthy bed that will allow a graft to take, flap closure will be required.

In well-resourced specialist centers, it is normal practice to try and cover wounds, particularly with open fractures, with flaps within five days[35]. The evidence that flap closure performed after this time is more likely to have complications is not conclusive and almost certainly does not relate to the techniques likely to be used in field hospitals. Ensuring the patient's general condition is satisfactory and the wound is clear of nonviable tissue and contamination is more important than striving to meet target timelines.

Wounds that have been closed with a planned temporizing method or have not had a good result from simple techniques can be revised by more complex procedures at any time in the future and there is no definite time limit. It is accepted that, the earlier revision surgery is carried out, the more likely there is to be a beneficial improvement particularly in limbs, where joint mobility is essential for function. There is, however, some degree of spontaneous improvement in terms of scar tissue maturation, particularly if active scar management techniques are used. Scars will not fully mature for up to a year or two and this should be a factor in making decisions on revision.

Methods of Reconstruction

The greater the surgeon's breadth of reconstructive skills, the more likely they will be able to find a solution that fits with the other requirements. It is unrealistic, however, for every surgeon to have undertaken full plastic-surgery training. Having a limited number of specific techniques will help a generalist offer some capability for definitive reconstruction.

Plastic surgeons have traditionally described a "reconstructive ladder" where techniques are stratified by complexity. This can lead to the misconception that the simple measures are tried first and the ladder is ascended as each previous rung fails. In reality, the most suitable option should be chosen first irrespective of its place on the ladder. Listed below is a range of techniques and individuals can gauge what they see as the limit of their own skill set.

In terms of definitions:

- A graft is a volume of tissue that is moved from one part of the body to another, having been completely detached, and then reacquires its blood supply from the recipient wound bed.
- A flap is a volume of tissue that is moved from one part of the body to another while retaining its own integral blood supply. Flap nomenclature is descriptive and combines terms used to indicate the tissues in the flap, its shape, its type of blood

supply, and how it is moved. There is a lot of overlap in terms and this can cause confusion.

All techniques will only be successful if there has been adequate IWS and are more likely to succeed with the patient's general condition optimized.

Healing by Secondary Intention

The mainstay of this approach is dressings. In small wounds, particularly when multiple, direct closure may be of questionable benefit and it is an appropriate alternative to simply dress the wounds. For larger wounds, the prolonged time taken for healing and the poorer quality of the result make healing by secondary attention a less attractive option. Wounds of more than 3 cm diameter will almost certainly do better if managed with a skin graft although the use of TNP dressings may extend this. The wounds still need to be actively managed. Any evolving necrosis should be debrided and a check kept for developing infection. Dressings will need to be changed with the frequency dependent on progress. There are numerous commercially available wound care products that claim to increase healing speeds. Each organization should have a procurement policy for such products rather than leaving the selection down to an individual surgeon's idiosyncratic beliefs. Secondary intention healing results in fibrosis; scar management should not be neglected.

Healing by Primary Intention

This can be achieved with either primary or DPC, most commonly through direct suture.

Split Skin Grafts

This relies on harvesting a skin graft of partial thickness so that some dermal elements and epidermal appendages remain at the donor site to allow it to heal by simple reepithelialization without stimulating contracture. Once reepithelialized, the donor site can be reharvested for a limited number of times as long as some dermis remains. In theory, the whole of the body's skin can be harvested, but in practical terms, even with meshing, it is difficult to get enough skin graft to cover more than about 40% of the total body surface area. The practicalities of skin grafting are covered above. Split skin grafted areas will often develop hypertrophic scarring and contracture. This is particularly seen when using meshed graft as the holes of the mesh are effectively healing by secondary intention. Scar management is essential.

Full Thickness Skin Grafts

The lack of the full thickness of dermis in a split skin graft reduces elements of skin function and generates a scar. A graft of full thickness of the skin should yield near scarless results and give a better color match if a site matched donor site is chosen. The donor site needs to be small enough to be directly closed, thus limiting the available amounts of full thickness skin for grafting. Because of the additional distance from the wound bed, and hence blood supply, the reliability of take for a full thickness graft is diminished. It does, however, provide a pliable reconstruction that retains the qualities of the donor site. This includes hair bearing, which can be used in specialized areas. Common recipient sites that do much better with full thickness grafts are on the face and hands.

Composite Grafts

These have the same characteristics as full thickness skin grafts, but contain more than one tissue type. The most common use is where some structural support is required so cartilage is included or specialized lining such as mucosa. An example is the reconstruction of full thickness eyelid loss.

Allografts and Xenografts

Although widely utilized in normal practice, nonautologous grafts are rarely available in field hospitals and have virtually no role in wound care.

Biological Templates

These, particularly for dermis and bone, have a definite place in reconstruction, but remain expensive and require very exacting surgical conditions. Field hospitals are probably not a good environment for such techniques.

Tissue Expansion

The principles of tissue expansion are well established. If skin is stretched over a period of days or weeks, for example over a gradually inflating balloon, the epidermis will expand although the dermis thins. The use of balloons for tissue expansion is common but it must appreciated they are essentially an implant that requires a level of surgical sterility rarely found in field hospitals. External traction devices are readily available commercially and can be improvised, so are more easily used in more austere settings. The quality of the reconstruction is debated. Additional amounts of local tissue laxity can be achieved peroperatively by ad hoc use of catheter balloons, but this is not true tissue expansion.

Local Random Flaps

"Random" refers to there being no identifiable blood vessel conferring viability to the flap. Blood supply depends on cutaneous flow and limits the length to breadth ratio of the flap to about 1.5:1, but longer on the face. They are "local" because they need to be immediately adjacent to the defect to be advanced, rotated, or transposed as required. There are numerous designs and all are based on geometric principles that move tissue from an area of surplus to a defect. They are often of a small size. Some local random flaps of muscle can be used to cover deeper structures. A few common local flaps will be of use in field hospitals and learning the basic geometry of design is relatively easy.

Local Axial Flaps

In certain anatomical locations, the design of a local flap can incorporate a known vessel, conferring more reliable vascularity and thereby increasing its length to breadth ratio and robustness. They are called axial because the vessels run along the axis of the flap. An example is the scalp flap.

Distant Flaps

Certain axial flaps have such a robust blood supply that they can be raised with a very long length and be used to reach defects that are not immediately adjacent. These do not necessarily always include a paddle of skin, and muscle-only distant flaps are common. The tissue connection including the vessels is called the pedicle. An intact skin bridge can remain as part of the pedicle. Examples of this are the groin flap and deltopectoral flap. The flap can be "islanded" by disconnecting all tissue except the vessels and thereby increase the mobility. Examples are the radial forearm flap and latissimus dorsi flap. Some distant flaps do not rely on an axial vessel, but have skin raised along with the deep fascia to utilize the connecting perifascial vascular plexus fed by perforating vessels. An example is the medial fasciocutaneous flap of the lower leg. Distant flaps can also be composite to transfer a range of other tissues such as when a rib is incorporated with a pectoralis major flap. Distant flaps are the most likely method for complex reconstruction in field hospitals and the design of many can follow a planning template that does not require technically demanding dissection of small vessels.

Free Flaps

Where a flap has been islanded on its vessels, the next level of complexity is to divide the vessels to allow the flap to be moved to virtually any part of the body and then revascularize the flap by using microvascular anastomoses to vessels at the recipient site. This has become a standard technique in modern plastic surgery and gives the greatest flexibility in reconstructive options. It does require specific surgical skills, prolonged operating time with exacting physiological stability, and expert postoperative nursing care to ensure high success rates. Although there are examples of where free flaps have been used in field hospitals, it is not a technique that has a place in most scenarios[36].

Tendon Repairs

The most effective method of reconstructing tendon function is by early primary repair and allowing immediate gliding of the repair in a well vascularized soft tissue envelope[37]. This is challenging when the process of IWS and DPC is being followed and if there is no skilled physiotherapy support. Repairing tendons distal to the elbow requires a degree of familiarity with the anatomy and technique and, for those in the hand, significant expertise. There are numerous described methods of repair: the most straightforward being a two-strand core stitch augmented by a circumferential epitendinous suture.

The shortening of a muscle belly that is not held to length by an intact tendon insertion becomes relatively irreversible after about three weeks and the gap between the tendon ends becomes fibrotic. Primary tendon repair then becomes impossible. Reconstruction of this in the hand requires a tendon graft and usually a two-stage approach utilizing a spacer. Results will be disappointing without expert surgery and hand therapy. This is a situation that is probably best left for delayed reconstruction by a specialist team.

Nerve Repairs[38]

There is clear evidence that the result of repairing peripheral nerves is better the earlier it is performed.

Any advantage from immediate repair is probably lost, however, if the excision of damaged nerve ends and the general state of the wound bed are not optimal. In the presence of blast or crush, which will include ballistic injury, nerve repairs are better delayed until DPC. Repair should be by epineurial suture under magnification. Traditional teaching has been to avoid any tension in a nerve repair. There is a growing consensus that a degree of nerve mobilization and some tension is better than having to resort to a nerve graft. If, however, there is an appreciable nerve gap, then an autologous cable nerve graft will be required, and this can be safely performed at DPC. This requires expertise and it is probably better to not repair a nerve and leave it for late reconstruction rather than repair it badly.

Late nerve reconstruction, be it for missed injuries, planned delay, or revision because of poor outcome, is best left to a specialist team.

References

1. Wong EG, Dominguez L, Trelles M, et al. Operative trauma in low-resource settings: The experience of Médecins Sans Frontières in environments of conflict, postconflict, and disaster. *Surgery* 2015: **157**(5): 850–6.

2. Lord JM, Midwinter MJ, Chen YF, et al. The systemic immune response to trauma: an overview of pathophysiology and treatment. *The Lancet* 2014: **384**: 1455–65.

3. Wilmore DW. Metabolic response to severe surgical illness: overview. *World Journal of Surgery* 2000: **24**(6): 705–11.

4. Malchow RJ, Black IH. The evolution of pain management in the critically ill trauma patient: emerging concepts from the global war on terrorism. *Critical Care Medicine* 2008: **36**(7 Suppl): S346–57.

5. Demling RH. Nutrition, anabolism, and the wound healing process: an overview. *World Journal of Plastic Surgery* 2009: **9**: 65–94.

6. Hospenthal DR, Green AD, Crouch HK, et al. Infection prevention and control in deployed military medical treatment facilities. *The Journal of Trauma and Acute Care Surgery* 2011: **71**(2 Suppl 2): S290–8.

7. World Health Organization. Antimicrobial Resistance. Online article. https://www.who.int/antimicrobial-resistance/en

8. Penn-Barwell JG, Murray CK, Wenke JC. Early antibiotics and debridement independently reduce infection in an open fracture model. *The Journal of Bone and Joint Surgery* 2012: **94**(1): 107–12.

9. Dick EA, Ballard M, Alwan-Walker H, et al. Bomb blast imaging: bringing order to chaos. *Clinical Radiology* 2018: **73**(6): 509–16.

10. Hodgetts TJ, Mahoney PF, Kirkman E. Damage control resuscitation. *Journal of the Royal Army Medical Corps* 2007: **153**(4): 299–300.

11. Malhotra AK, Goldberg S, Graham J, et al. Open extremity fractures: impact of delay in operative debridement and irrigation. *The Journal of Trauma and Acute Care Surgery* 2014: **76**(5): 1201–7.

12. Enninghorst N, McDougall D, Hunt JJ, Balogh ZJ. Open tibia fractures: timely debridement leaves injury severity as the only determinant of poor outcome. *The Journal of Trauma and Acute Care Surgery* 2011: **70**(2): 352–6.

13. Prodromidis AD, Charalambous CP. The 6-hour rule for surgical debridement of open tibial fractures: a systematic review and meta-analysis of infection and nonunion rates. *Journal of Orthopaedic Trauma* 2016: **30**(7):397–402.

14. Boulton AJ, Lewis CT, Naumann DN, Midwinter MJ. Prehospital haemostatic dressings for trauma: a systematic review. *Emergency Medicine Journal* 2018: **35**(7): 449–57.

15. World Health Organization. Surgical Safety Checklist. Online article. https://www.who.int/patientsafety/safesurgery/checklist/en

16. Arul GS, Pugh HE, Mercer SJ, Midwinter MJ. Human factors in decision making in major trauma in Camp Bastion, Afghanistan. *Annals of the Royal College of Surgeons of England* 2015: **97**(4): 262–8.

17. Debakey ME, Simeone FA. Battle injuries of the arteries in World War II: an analysis of 2471 cases. *Annals of Surgery* 1946: **123**(4): 534–79.

18. Hughes CW. Arterial repair during the Korean war. *Annals of Surgery* 1958: **147**(7): 555–61.

19. Rasmussen TE, Clouse WD, Jenkins DH, et al. The use of temporary vascular shunts as a damage control adjunct in the management of wartime vascular injury. *The Journal of Trauma and Acute Care Surgery* 2006: **61**(1): 8–12.

20. Bowyer GW, Cooper GJ, Rice P. Small fragment wounds: biophysics and pathophysiology. *The Journal of Trauma and Acute Care Surgery* 1996: **40**(3 Suppl): S159–64.

21. Sassoon A, Riehl J, Rich A, et al. Muscle viability revisited: are we removing normal muscle? A critical evaluation of dogmatic debridement. *Journal of Orthopaedic Trauma* 2016: **30**(1): 17–21.

22. Bhandari, M, Jeray KJ, Petrisor BA, et al. A trial of wound irrigation in the initial management of open fracture wounds. *The New England Journal of Medicine* 2015: **373**(27): 2629–41.

23. Hassinger SM, Harding G, Wongworawat MD. High-pressure pulsatile lavage propagates bacteria into soft tissue. *Clinical Orthopaedics and Related Research* 2005: **439**: 27–31.

24. Crowley DJ, Kanakaris NK, Giannoudis PV. Irrigation of the wounds in open fractures. *The Journal of Bone and Joint Surgery* 2007: **89**(5): 580–5.

25. Penn-Barwell JG, Murray CK, Wenke JC. Comparison of the antimicrobial effect of chlorhexidine and saline for irrigating a contaminated open fracture model. *Journal of Orthopaedic Trauma* 2012: **26**(12): 728–32.

26. Fries CA, Ayalew Y, Penn-Barwell JG, et al. Prospective randomised controlled trial of nanocrystalline silver dressing versus plain gauze as the initial post-debridement management of military wounds on wound microbiology and healing. *Injury* 2014: **45**(7): 1111–6.

27. Giannou C, Baldan M, Molde A. *War surgery*: volume II. 2013. ICRC.

28. Mansoor J, Ellahi I, Junaid Z, Habib A, Ilyas U. Clinical evaluation of improvised gauze-based negative pressure wound therapy in military wounds. *International Wound Journal* 2015: **12**(5): 559–63.

29. Penn-Barwell JG, Fries CA, Street L, Jeffery S. Use of topical negative pressure in British servicemen with combat wounds. *Eplasty* 2011: **11**: e35.

30. Hajibandeh S, Hajibandeh S, Idehen N. Meta-analysis of the effect of tertiary survey on missed injury rate in trauma patients. *Injury* 2015: **46**(12): 2474–82.

31. Serebrakian AT, Pickrell BB, Varon DE, et al. Meta-analysis and systematic review of skin graft donor-site dressings with future guidelines. *Plastic and Reconstructive Surgery – Global Open* 2018: **6**(9): e1928.

32. Wallenberg L. Effect of early mobilisation after skin grafting to lower limbs. *Scandinavian Journal of Plastic and Reconstructive Surgery and Hand Surgery* 1999: **33**(4): 411–3.

33. Yin Y, Zhang R, Li S, Guo J, Hou Z, Zhang Y. Negative-pressure therapy versus conventional therapy on split-thickness skin graft: a systematic review and meta-analysis. *International Journal of Surgery* 2018: **50**: 43–48.

34. Hurlow J, Bowler PG. Clinical experience with wound biofilm and management: a case series. *Ostomy Wound Management* 2009: **55**(4): 38–49.

35. D'Alleyrand JC, Manson TT, Dancy L, et al. Is time to flap coverage of open tibial fractures an independent predictor of flap-related complications? *Journal of Orthopaedic Trauma* 2014: **28**(5): 288–93.

36. Klem C, Sniezek JC, Moore B, et al. Microvascular reconstructive surgery in Operations Iraqi and Enduring Freedom: the US military experience

performing free flaps in a combat zone. *The Journal of Trauma and Acute Care Surgery* 2013: **75**(2 Suppl 2): S228–32.

37. Khor WS, Langer MF, Wong R, et al. Improving outcomes in tendon repair: a critical look at the evidence for flexor tendon repair and rehabilitation. *Plastic and Reconstructive Surgery* 2016: **138**(6): 1045e–58e.

38. Trehan SK, Model Z, Lee SK. Nerve repair and nerve grafting. *Hand Clinics* 2016: **32**(2): 119–25.

Chapter 18

Orthopedics in a Field Hospital

Elhanan Bar-On and Patrick Herard

Introduction

Field hospitals will invariably be deployed in situations in which the medical needs far exceed the surge capacity of the local medical facilities. Most deployments will be either following major natural disasters such as earthquakes, storms and floods, human-made disasters – armed conflicts or industrial accidents – widespread epidemic outbreaks and large-scale refugee migrations[1–5]. Deployments may be short or long term, and the field hospital will treat large numbers of patients with pathologies resulting from the event as well as routine medical problems in the local population – serving as a supplement or substitute to the local medical system[6]. Most deployments will be in low- and middle-income countries in which the baseline of medical services is suboptimal during routine times and is further challenged by the calamity.

As a result of this situation, the prime factor in the operational scenario of a field hospital, when compared to a permanent hospital operating in routine conditions, is an extreme imbalance between the medical requirements and the ability to deliver adequate care to as many patients as possible. The need to diminish this imbalance will dictate the operational principles at all service levels.

While the above "principle of imbalance" is pertinent in all fields of medicine within the field hospital, its relevance is increased tenfold in the field of orthopedics. This is true because of increased needs as well as diminished ability to deliver care.

The orthopedic needs vary widely depending on the operational scenario. However, the two most common situations in which field hospitals are deployed – following major earthquakes and during armed conflicts – produce large numbers of complex injuries requiring a long series of surgeries with subsequent rehabilitation. On the other side of the imbalance scale is the ability to deliver care. Whereas many of the medical and surgical specialties require only basic diagnostic and therapeutic equipment, enabling the caregiver to deliver an adequate standard of care under austere conditions or in a prehospital facility, the situation in orthopedics is very different. At the diagnostic level, the minimal requirement is an X-ray machine producing basic radiographs. X-ray capability, although required by the World Health Organization (WHO) standards in all field hospitals[7], may sometimes be unavailable. Moreover, in some areas of the body, three-dimensional imaging (CT or MRI) is essential to make an accurate diagnosis and these modalities are currently unavailable in the field-hospital setting. This limited diagnostic capability will directly influence the type and level of care that can be delivered in a field hospital. At the therapeutic level, there are two major problems preventing delivery of a standard of treatment that parallels that given in a full-service permanent hospital:

1. Modern orthopedic treatment utilizes an amount and diversity of equipment unparalleled in any other surgical field. This is true of surgical instruments, but more so of hardware and implants utilized for fracture fixation and limb reconstruction, while unsalvageable joints are currently treated by partial or total joint replacement; requiring a large armamentarium of implants. The logistic reality of a field hospital deployment will enable availability of only a very limited hardware stock.

2. The skeletal system's susceptibility to infection and the extreme difficulty in treating these infections, once established, dictate the need to perform orthopedic surgical procedures under severe aseptic conditions. These conditions are unattainable in most field hospitals.

Both these factors dictate an extreme change in the paradigm of orthopedic treatment in a field hospital when compared to that practiced in a regular hospital in a high resource country.

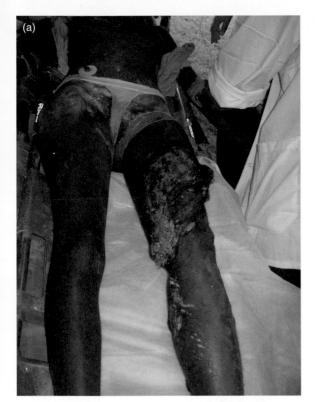

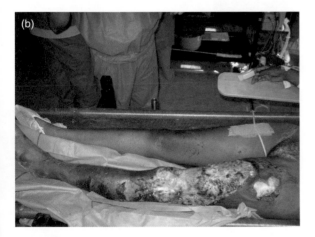

Figure 18.1a Crush injury of left lower limb in patient extracted after six days under rubble

Figure 18.1b Same patient following initial debridement

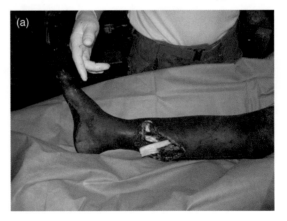

Figure 18.2a Open fracture with devitalized tibia

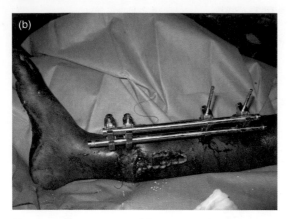

Figure 18.2b Same patient following several debridements, 4 cm shortening, soft tissue coverage, and external fixation

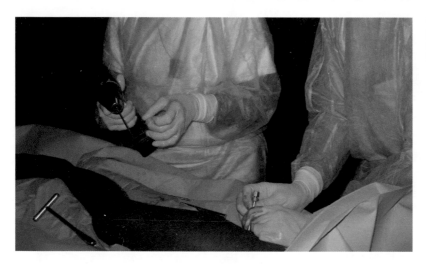

Figure 18.3 External fixation without fluoroscopy, using a nonsterilizable home drill, maintaining sterility at pin–patient interface

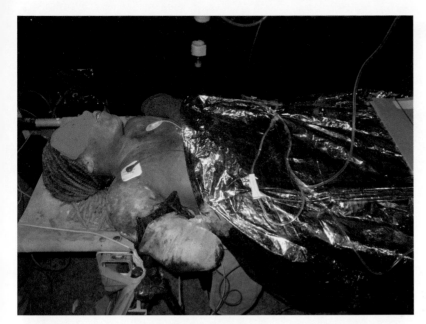

Figure 18.4 Patient after field amputation of the upper limb to enable extraction from under the rubble

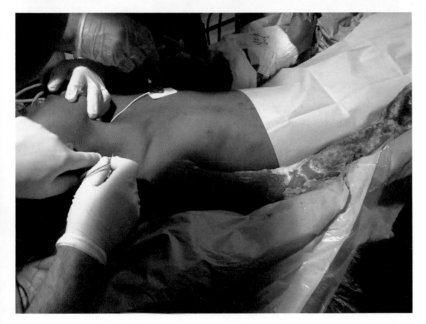

Figure 23.1 Wound debridement under interscalene block in the aftermath of the 2010 Haitian earthquake

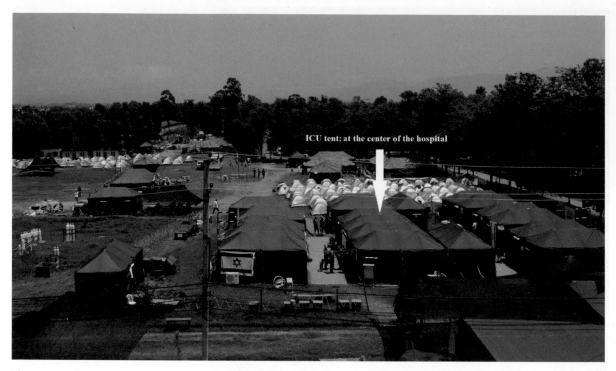

Figure 24.1 The ICU tent positioned in the center of the field hospital, in proximity to the different units it serves

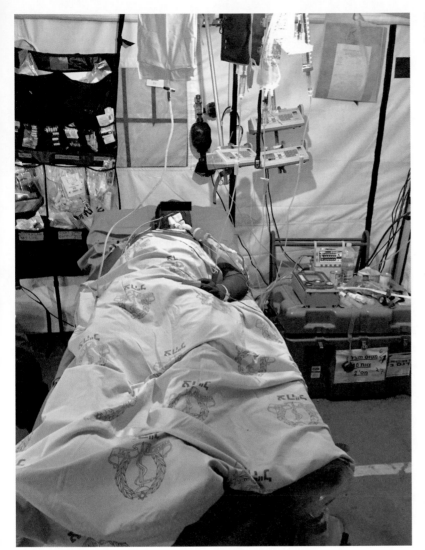

Figure 24.2 A critically injured casualty in the ICU station; equipment is smaller for efficiency and space saving

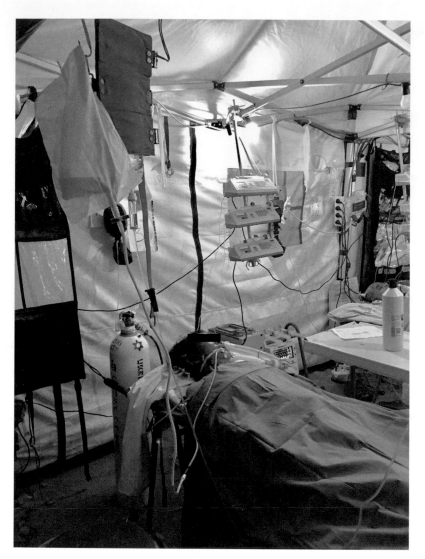

Figure 24.3 Proximity between patient beds

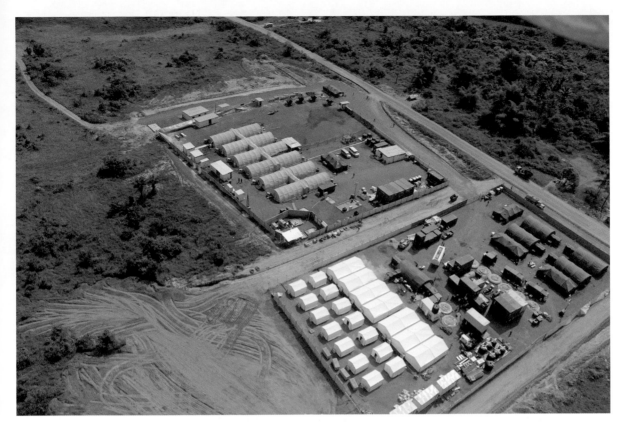

Figure 25.1 Aerial view of the US public-health service Monrovia Medical Unit, 2015

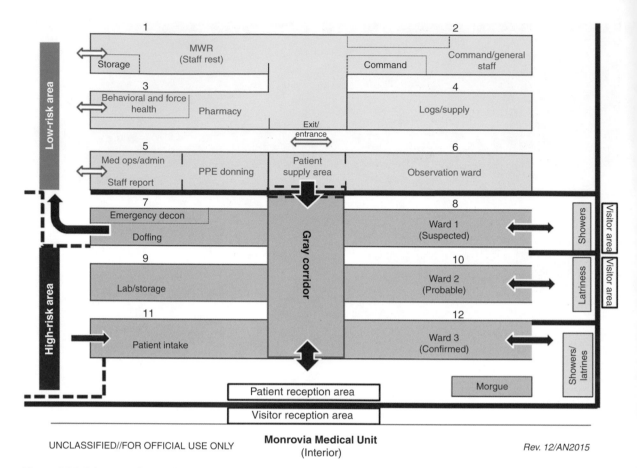

Monrovia Medical Unit
(Interior)

Rev. 12/AN2015

Figure 25.2 Schematic of US public-health service Monrovia Medical Unit Layout, 2015

Deployment Scenarios

The factors governing the orthopedic needs during field hospital deployment include the following:

1. The type of event prompting deployment. Scenarios prompting field hospital deployment include natural disasters and human-made calamities. Among natural disasters, earthquakes cause the highest number of musculoskeletal injuries requiring orthopedic treatment[8–10]. The reason lies in the nature of the disaster. The energy released during an earthquake is unequalled in any other event. Most of the energy released is mechanical energy, causing collapse of buildings, and most injuries are caused by falling debris resulting in fractures, soft tissue wounds, and crush injuries. The number and type of injuries will therefore depend on the magnitude of the earthquake, the level of urbanization, the type and quality of building, and the time of day of the occurrence. Additional causes of musculoskeletal injuries during earthquakes include falling or jumping from heights, falls during escape, and burns due to fires erupting during the earthquake. In natural disasters such as tsunamis, storms, and floods, despite a high number of people killed in the disaster, the number and severity of injuries will be much lower than in an earthquake[1,11–13]. However, common to all disaster scenarios, musculoskeletal injuries will predominate as the leading cause of morbidity.

   In armed conflicts, the types of injuries encountered will depend on the nature of the conflict and the types of weaponry used. These range from traditional weapons such as machetes and small arms, to antipersonnel or antitank landmines, and heavy weaponry such as artillery and air bombardment[14–19].

2. The phase of the deployment in the timeline following the event. Field hospitals will typically not start operating before day four following the event. Therefore, patients sustaining life-threatening internal or multiorgan injuries will either have perished or will have been treated in local facilities. Field hospitals deployed in the first weeks following the disaster will encounter acute injuries, followed by early complications; mainly infections and the consequences of crush injuries. Subsequent deployments will encounter late complications: chronic infections, nonunion, malunion, and rehabilitation problems[1,20].

3. The capabilities of local medical facilities and adjacent emergency medical teams (EMTs) in the disaster zone, as well as the capabilities of medical facilities outside the disaster zone, and the evacuation capabilities to these facilities. These factors, together with the level of coordination in the EMTCC and health cluster managing the disaster, will directly affect the caseload encountered in the field hospital. The caseload will also be affected by the baseline capabilities of the local medical system and the health status of the population prior to the disaster[3,21–24].

Injury Epidemiology

The epidemiology of injuries encountered in field hospitals will vary according to the deployment circumstances. However, in all cases it will be very different from that found in everyday practice. The musculoskeletal injuries encountered following earthquakes and armed conflicts will be mostly high energy injuries. In earthquake deployments, 60% of patients treated due to trauma will suffer limb injuries. Nineteen percent of all patients treated and 54% of those admitted will have fractures, and 31% of these fractures will be open. Lower limb fractures predominate (62%), followed by upper limbs (23%) and axial skeleton injuries (14%)[3,9,20,25–39].

2%–5% of those injured and 12%–25% of hospitalized patients will develop crush syndrome[40,41].

In armed conflict zone deployments, 50%–75% of injuries encountered will be limb injuries; 60%–80% of them to the lower limbs. Thirty-nine percent will have fractures; 50% of them open[14–19]. The injury patterns will depend on the nature of the conflict, the populations involved (military vs civilian), and the type of weaponry used. Assault rifles utilized in close combat will cause single or multiple localized injuries. Shelling and bombing will inflict multiple superficial or deep complex wounds caused by fragments. Antipersonnel mines will inflict blast injuries and traumatic amputations of the lower limbs. Traditional cold weapons such as machetes and pangas, used in intersocietal strife, will result in slash wounds – more commonly to the upper body. The combat scenario will also induce secondary injuries caused by conventional mechanisms: falls while running, high-speed motor vehicle accidents, and injuries caused by collapsing bombed buildings. Burns may be caused by erupting fires or due to cooking in unsafe conditions in temporary habitations.

Surgical and Medical Needs

The abovementioned injury patterns dictate a wide array of surgical and medical needs. These will range from the need to treat a large number of superficial soft tissue injuries requiring basic outpatient surgical capabilities to complex limb injuries requiring major surgical procedures: fracture fixation, complex soft injury treatment and coverage, and amputations at various levels. Multisystem injuries will also require interventions and collaboration with other surgical and medical specialists. Due to the timetable of setup of field hospitals and the poor sanitary conditions prior to admission, many of the wounds encountered will be infected, requiring extensive surgical debridement and antibiotic coverage. In long-term deployments, the sequelae of the acute injuries and the rehabilitation needs will have to be addressed. In addition, patients with routine orthopedic problems will seek treatment even in the early phase following the disaster and these needs will predominate in field hospitals deployed in nondisaster scenarios[3,6,24].

Treatment Capabilities

The treatment capabilities in a field hospital will, by definition, be lower than those in a permanent medical facility. They will vary widely between the teams deployed by various governmental and nongovernmental agencies. WHO has outlined minimal standards for treatment capabilities of EMTs[7].

A type 1 EMT is not defined as a field hospital. It is a mobile or stationary team performing casualty collection and limited triage. It is capable of providing care for minor injuries and illnesses, and stabilization of more seriously injured casualties, preparing them for evacuation to a facility with higher capabilities. Orthopedic treatment capabilities will include basic wound treatment and fracture stabilization by plaster casts or splints.

Type 2 and 3 EMTs are classified as field hospitals. A type 2 facility has basic and emergency surgical capabilities and postoperative support. A type 3 EMT is an advanced field hospital with specialized multidisciplinary surgical and intensive-care capabilities. The orthopedic treatment capabilities will vary among different field hospitals, but should include musculoskeletal imaging capabilities, extended wound care, surgical fracture fixation, and amputation of unsalvageable limbs. Postoperative care,

intensive medical and nursing care, and early rehabilitation should be available[8].

Facility

A field hospital should have several loci in which orthopedic care can be delivered. Initial assessment and care will be given in the triage and emergency department. The orthopedic department should be housed in a specific designated area. Wound care, closed reduction, and casting of fractures will be performed in this area. Local anesthesia can be administered, and regional blocks or conscious sedation may be available in some facilities. Outpatient care and follow-up of patients will be performed in this department[28,43].

All field hospitals will have at least one operating theater with one surgical table in type 2 and two tables in type 3 facilities. Regional and general anesthesia and appropriate monitoring will be available.

Patients requiring hospitalization will be treated in the inpatient departments. When possible, surgical patients should be in separate departments enabling specialized nursing, wound care, and pain control. Children should preferably be hospitalized in a separate pediatric ward[44,45].

Personnel

Orthopedic surgeons will be found in type 3 and possibly in type 2 EMTs. In lower-level facilities, orthopedic care will be provided by general surgeons or other health-care personnel. The number of orthopedic surgeons required will depend on the type of the disaster and the resultant caseload, and the number of orthopedists available will depend on the size of the facility and the dispatching organization. Ideally, there should be adequate orthopedic personnel to staff both the orthopedic department and the operating theater simultaneously. The orthopedic workforce can be augmented by task shifting with nonorthopedic surgeons or physicians working under the supervision of orthopedic specialists[3,8].

Nursing and paramedical staff would ideally include personnel specifically trained in caring for orthopedic patients. Practically, such personnel are scarce and will not be readily available, but onsite training is possible including wound, pin, and plaster-cast care. An orthopedic nurse should head the team in the orthopedic department, maintaining order and adequate stock management of the casting and bandaging supplies. The surgical nurses or technician team should include at least one team leader familiar with orthopedic equipment. Physiotherapists should be included in all deployments in high trauma volume scenarios to provide early rehabilitation and predischarge instruction. Due to the unique characteristics of deployment in a field hospital, especially in a postdisaster setting, all staff should undergo predeployment preparation. If there is only one orthopedic surgeon on the staff, he or she should have significant previous field experience in disasters and austere environments.

Larger teams should include personnel with previous experience as well as those exposed to the scenario for the first time to enlarge the pool of experienced personnel available for future deployments. Local health professionals and additional foreign volunteers can be incorporated into the staff, but their credentials should be scrutinized in order to ensure adequate professional standards[27,46,47].

Equipment

Surgical equipment availability, as well as the level of asepsis, will be main limiting factors in the orthopedic treatment capabilities of a field hospital. The minimal equipment set should include the following:

Orthopedic department and emergency department
1. Surgical instruments for basic wound care and suture
2. Bone cutter for digit amputations
3. Bandaging and elastic bandages
4. Splints for temporary splintage and Thomas splints
5. Plaster of Paris and cast padding
6. Cast cutting instruments and/or saw
7. Skeletal traction kit
8. A Spica table (can be constructed on site)
9. Crutches

Operating theater
1. Basic soft tissue instruments
2. Basic bone instruments: bone cutters and Gigli and hand saw
3. External fixation set, preferably with self-drilling Schanz pins; tapered thread pins should be avoided
4. Hand drill

Power instruments (drill and saw) may be available in some field hospitals. These should be with rechargeable batteries rather than electric cable or air powered. Low-priced hardware store drills can be used, but surgical techniques will have to be modified as these are not sterilizable.

Most field hospitals will not include internal fixation in their armamentarium due to inadequate aseptic conditions in the surgical theater, as well as cost and payload considerations. Recently, some nongovernmental organizations (NGOs) have reported limited use of internal fixation in facilities in which adequate aseptic conditions have been attained[27,47–49].

C-arm fluoroscopy will rarely be included in the armamentarium of a field hospital due to price, payload, and maintenance considerations.

Treatment Principles

Treatment principles will be dictated by the deployment scenario and the capabilities of the specific field hospital. Due to all the abovementioned factors, the paradigm governing orthopedic treatment in a field hospital is completely different from that governing routine orthopedic care in a permanent hospital and will be administered according to the principles of damage control medicine, usually deferring definitive and reconstructive surgery to a permanent hospital outside the disaster or conflict area or postponing it until recovery of the local permanent facilities[50].

The first priority will be the treatment of secondary life-threatening or limb-threatening injuries. These will be usually due to massive penetrating trauma, vascular compromise, blast injuries, crush injuries, open fractures with extensive soft tissue damage, or severe infections. Although the governing principle will be "life over limb[25,51]," this principle has sometimes been misinterpreted and has led to unnecessary amputations[46]. The basic principles of a thorough assessment of the patient coupled with a recognition of the available treatment modalities and their appropriate application can lead to an optimal outcome in these suboptimal conditions.

Crush Syndrome

Crush injuries will be encountered mostly in earthquake scenarios due to injuries to the limbs caused by falling debris, with the most severe injuries being caused by prolonged entrapment under the rubble (Figure 18.1a). Besides the severe local injury to the

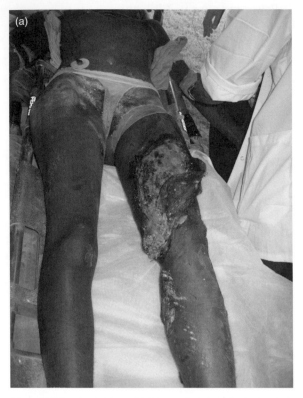

Figure 18.1a Crush injury of left lower limb in patient extracted after six days under rubble (A black and white version of this figure will appear in some formats. For the color version, please refer to the plate section.)

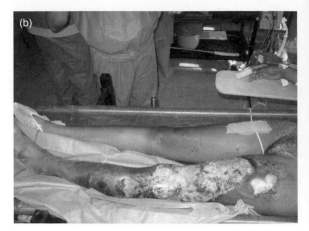

Figure 18.1b Same patient following initial debridement (A black and white version of this figure will appear in some formats. For the color version, please refer to the plate section.)

limb with extensive soft tissue damage and possible fractures, patients may develop crush syndrome, which is a multiorgan injury with potentially life-threatening consequences. Local hemorrhage and fluid shifting will cause hypovolemic shock, hyperkalemia, and hypocalcemia, together with cytotoxin and endotoxin release, which may cause cardiac dysfunction and decreased renal blood flow; myoglobinuria and hormonal changes may lead to renal failure. Systemic treatment of crush syndrome will require intensive care and possible peritoneal or hemodialysis and therefore these patients should be treated in a type 3 EMT or in a hospital outside the disaster zone. Treatment of the local injury includes debridement of all nonviable tissues. Assessment of tissue viability will be by gross appearance, bleeding, and muscle response to diathermy[40,41,52,53] (Figure 18.1b).

Compartment Syndrome

Compartment syndrome is a limb-threatening condition with the potential to become life threatening. The most common locus is the leg, but it can appear in other segments including the thigh, foot, or forearm. Compartment syndrome may occur minutes to hours following the injury and, when diagnosed acutely, it must be treated as a surgical emergency. In a field hospital, devices for measurement of compartment pressures or tissue oxygenation are generally unavailable and impractical, and diagnosis will be based on clinical examination, with progressive pain unresponsive to analgesia being the cardinal sign raising suspicion of acute compartment syndrome. Other signs such as paresthesia, pallor, and paralysis are less specific and waiting for them to appear may delay diagnosis and treatment. Acute compartment syndrome is treated by an emergency fasciotomy of all involved compartments as irreversible tissue damage starts occurring six hours after onset. This, however, holds true only for those compartment syndromes diagnosed up to 24–36 hours from onset. When the diagnosis is delayed beyond that time frame, fasciotomy should not be performed as the tissue damage is irreversible and fasciotomy may cause severe infections, which may become limb or life threatening. Late diagnosed compartment syndrome will therefore be treated by supportive medical measures. Amputation will be reserved for unsalvageable and/or life-threatening limbs[53,54].

Infections

Infected wounds are among the leading causes of morbidity and mortality in the field-hospital setting. Several factors are responsible for this high rate and severe nature of these infections:

1. The severe nature of injuries often caused by high-energy mechanisms causing open fractures and extensive soft-tissue damage. These will be encountered following earthquakes and armed conflicts with blast and mine injuries.
2. Multiple soft-tissue injuries of varying severity encountered following fragment injuries.
3. The delay in deployment of field hospitals and the prolonged time lapse from the time of injury to initiation of care, often in a contaminated environment with poor sanitary conditions and lack of access to prehospital care.
4. Inadequate preliminary debridement, and unindicated primary wound closure.

The primary orthopedic treatment of infected wounds is surgical debridement. A wide exposure of the injury site is required. All nonviable tissues should be removed including soft tissues and devitalized bone fragments. The first dressing change should be performed two to five days after the primary procedure and subsequently at 48-hour intervals as needed until the local infection is controlled. Copious drainage or systemic symptoms may dictate earlier wound inspection. These second-look procedures should include secondary surgical care as needed. Large deep debridements should be performed in the operating theater while smaller and superficial ones can be managed in the orthopedic clinic or as a bedside procedure. However, adequate pain control must be provided in all cases.

The flora encountered in cultures from the infected wounds varies in different types of disaster settings but commonly is predominated by multiple drug-resistant bacteria[55–58].

The use of antibiotics is somewhat controversial in this setting. Most protocols will administer antibiotics as an adjunct treatment to surgery, especially if systemic signs of infection are present, but some protocols do not administer antibiotics before cultures are obtained, to avoid development of drug-resistant bacteria. In all protocols antibiotics are considered adjunct treatment and the importance of surgical debridement as the mainstay of treatment cannot be overemphasized, with closure always delayed until infection control is obtained[17,59–64].

Laboratory capabilities, available in all type 3 and some type 2 facilities, should include blood counts, ESR, CRP, and cultures. When available these will assist in surgical decision-making[7].

Fractures

The prerequisite for modern open surgical treatment of fractures is a clean surgical environment. Although this has been achieved in some field hospitals, in most of the deployed field hospitals the absence of sterile surgical milieu, internal fixation hardware, and C-arm fluoroscopy will dictate a completely different treatment approach to fracture care. However, the basic goals of treatment remain similar: fracture reduction to an acceptable position, provision of optimal conditions for union, early mobilization when possible, and preventing complications such as infection and joint stiffness.

Closed Fractures

Closed limb fractures will almost always be treated by closed reduction and cast immobilization. As radiography is a meager resource and a bottleneck in the field-hospital setting, the quality of reduction should be assessed clinically, with postreduction X-rays reserved for selected cases. Cast wedging can be used to improve alignment. Due to the high risk of infection, minor malalignment, or incongruity of intra-articular fractures should be accepted, and surgeons should resist the urge to perform open reduction as it is better to have osteoarthritis than osteomyelitis. The exception to this rule is the treatment of femoral fractures in adults. Skeletal traction is a treatment option, but it requires prolonged bed rest with possible nursing problems. In addition, prolonged hospital bed occupancy will be at the expense of other patients requiring surgery and a hospital bed is a scarce commodity in this setting. Home traction may be an option, but, in an earthquake stricken area, many of the patients will not have a home. Therefore, in extreme disaster scenarios with no foreseeable option for safe internal fixation, external fixation of closed femoral fractures is an acceptable option enabling early mobilization and ambulation[25,66]. However, some NGOs consider external fixation contraindicated in closed femoral fractures due to the risk of primary or secondary infection and in light of the availability of safe secondary fixation in their facilities[27,65].

Pediatric femoral fractures should be treated by closed reduction and immobilisation in a spica cast with adequate analgesia or conscious sedation. Infants can be treated with a soft spica made from cast padding and an elastic bandage or with Pavlik harness if available[67].

Open Fractures

The priority in treatment of open fractures is the prevention and treatment of infection. Therefore, initial treatment will always be debridement of non-viable and infected tissues (see chapter 17). The viability of soft tissues will be assessed by color, consistency, bleeding, and contractility. Divided nerves and tendons have traditionally been trimmed and marked for later reconstruction, but this approach has been challenged due to the introduction of a foreign body with a potential for infection. Primary repair of nerves and tendons should not be attempted. An effort should be made to preserve viable periosteum as it will induce bone formation and fracture union. Infected and devitalized bone fragments and those with no periosteal attachment should be excised. The exception is large articular osteochondral fragments, which may be cleansed and replaced for possible incorporation. Medullary canals should be inspected and curetted for contamination. Foreign bodies should be excised if they are readily accessible or if their location is potentially damaging: adjacent to neurovascular structures, intra-articular, or in weight-bearing areas. All wounds should be left open following the initial debridement and repeat debridements as described above should be performed until the wound is clean and soft tissue coverage of the bones can be achieved.

Fractures should be realigned clinically at the first debridement. The method of fracture fixation will be determined by the state of the soft tissues and the fracture configuration. In relatively small wounds, a plaster slab may be used, allowing windowing or change of the

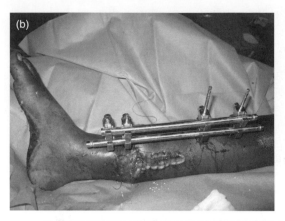

Figure 18.2b Same patient following several debridements, 4 cm shortening, soft tissue coverage, and external fixation (A black and white version of this figure will appear in some formats. For the color version, please refer to the plate section.)

dressings for wound care. This is especially appropriate for upper limb open fractures. In injuries with more extensive soft tissue damage, either skeletal traction or external fixation should be utilized. Skeletal traction is simpler, requires only one pin, thus reducing the chance of pin tract infection, and does not contaminate the involved bone. However, the patient is immobilized in bed, requires increased nursing care, and increases hospital-bed occupancy. External fixation, although more expensive, requiring expertise and carrying a somewhat greater risk of pin tract infection, gives improved fracture stability, enables wound access, and allows early limb and patient mobilization and discharge from the hospital. It therefore remains the method of choice for fixation of open long-bone fractures in a field-hospital setting (Figure 18.2a–b). External fixators can be placed without C-arm fluoroscopy, based on clinical examination or a previous radiograph of the fracture. Self-drilling Schanz pins are preferable, but not essential, and conical threaded pins should be avoided as they cannot be backed out if necessary. Sterility of the site of pin insertion site as well as of the drill and pins must be maintained. A sterilizable power drill is preferable, but a home hardware drill can be used, maintaining sterility of the parts of the drill and pins in contact with the limb (Figure 18.3). Some protocols/NGOs will avoid using power drills due to the potential for damage in inexperienced hands and insert all pins with a hand drill[66,68,69,70].

The external fixator can be replaced by a plaster cast once wound closure is achieved and the fracture is stable. Alternatively, patients requiring reconstructive surgery can be converted to a circular fixator or

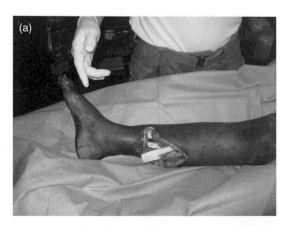

Figure 18.2a Open fracture with devitalized tibia (A black and white version of this figure will appear in some formats. For the color version, please refer to the plate section.)

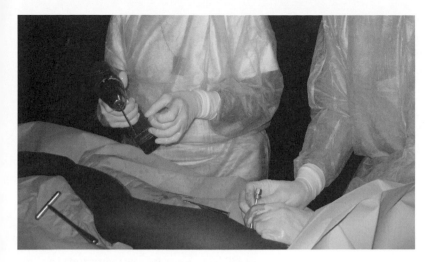

Figure 18.3 External fixation without fluoroscopy, using a nonsterilizable home drill, maintaining sterility at pin–patient interface (A black and white version of this figure will appear in some formats. For the color version, please refer to the plate section.)

internal fixation if required, providing adequate surgical conditions have become available[27,65,71,72]. However, when applying an external fixator, the surgeon must bear in mind that it may be the definitive treatment for the fracture in this setting. Conversion to internal fixation, although practiced in everyday settings, carries a high risk of infection and should therefore be avoided in a field hospital.

Internal fixation should never be used in an acute phase field hospital with inadequate surgical sterility. The only exception is Kirschner wires, which may be used for stabilizing fractures or dislocations in the hand or foot. Internal fixation for limited indications has been reported from field hospitals in which adequate surgical asepsis has been attained. This has mainly been intramedullary nailing of femoral fractures using the SIGN nail, which does not require fluoroscopy for insertion. Nailing of tibias is avoided due to a high infection rate[27,65].

Amputations

Although in some cases an amputation of a limb may be a lifesaving procedure, most amputations (except those of toes and some finger amputations) will cause significant long-term disability and dependency on prosthetic devices. The decision to amputate a limb will therefore be based on many factors including:

- the general condition of the patient
- the condition of the limb
- the surgical capabilities in the hospital
- the rehabilitation capabilities in the region
- social conditions and available welfare support
- cultural and religious attitudes to body image and mutilation in the local population

The considerations guiding the decision-making process, when compared to that in everyday practice in the high-resource countries, may be completely different in the setting of a field hospital operating in an underserved region following a major disaster or armed conflict. Several scoring systems have been devised to aid in this decision-making[73,74]. They attempt to prognosticate the chance of salvaging the limb according to various parameters relating to the injury mechanism, patient age and general health condition, and the status of the limb. They have also been used to try and forecast the probability of a patient returning to work following an amputation or limb reconstruction. These scores are based on surgical and rehabilitation capabilities in developed countries and may have to be modified for use in austere settings. However, scoring and recording the status of the limb before amputation is of ethical and medicolegal importance[75,76].

Absolute Indications

1. Uncontrollable sepsis. In these cases, an amputation will constitute a lifesaving procedure. However, amputation should almost never be performed as the primary procedure and the definition of a limb as a source of uncontrollable infection should be made only if systemic sepsis persists despite major debridement of all infected tissue and antibiotic coverage. One must also ensure that there is no other occult source of infection besides the limb.
2. Prolonged limb ischemia with irreparable vascular damage. This will depend on the time of ischemia, the degree of mutilation and the vascular reconstructive capabilities in the field hospital or the possibility of evacuating the patient to a facility with

more advanced capabilities. Irreversible ischemia is the one factor that constitutes an indication for amputation in all published limb trauma scores[73].

Field Amputations

There may be situations in which the only way to extricate an entrapped person from under the rubble will be to amputate a limb. These cases are rare and controversial, but if the procedure is deemed necessary, the ethical principles of informed consent should be maintained and the amputation should be performed by personnel with adequate surgical experience. Adequate fluid resuscitation should be administered, hemorrhage control should be attainable, and adequate analgesia should be given[77] (Figure 18.4).

Relative Indications

1. Severe crush injuries. These may also be life threatening as mentioned above, but these effects may already be irreversible at the time of surgery and the efficacy of amputation as a lifesaving procedure in these cases remains controversial [40,41,53,54,76].
2. Extensive tissue loss. This may be due to the injury itself or may be the result of debridement of infected or nonviable tissues. Although some limbs may appear unsalvageable on admission, tissue loss is usually not an indication for primary amputation.

Bone loss may be treated by acute shortening with planned future lengthening or intercalary bone grafts. Muscle loss and motor nerve damage can be treated by muscle transfers or arthrodesis and sensory loss at the time of injury may recover. Major skin loss can be treated with flaps or skin grafts. Unfortunately, in some past disasters, amputation has been performed too liberally by persons with inadequate experience, resulting in unnecessary physical and emotional damage, and multiple avoidable revision procedures. Although the surgical capabilities in a field hospital are inadequate for performing reconstructive procedures, they may become available in other facilities later on. Therefore, although some limb injuries will be so mutilative as to preclude any limb salvage, the decision to amputate these limbs should be taken by surgeons with experience in major limb trauma in austere settings.

3. Rehabilitation capabilities. An amputation through clean tissue proximal to the injured area with early closure and rehabilitation may result in an early return to the work circle and if the amputation is below the knee, the overall function may be comparable to that of a limb undergoing extensive reconstructive surgery, although longer-term follow-up studies have shown increased satisfaction in patients undergoing limb salvage. However,

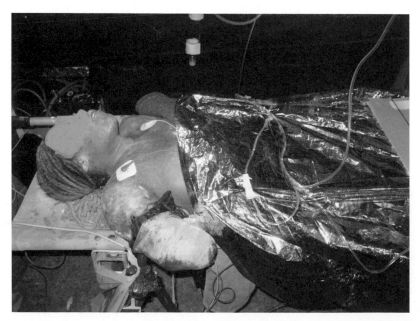

Figure 18.4 Patient after field amputation of the upper limb to enable extraction from under the rubble (A black and white version of this figure will appear in some formats. For the color version, please refer to the plate section.)

successful function following amputation depends on the availability of a rehabilitation system, which includes physiotherapy starting in the early postoperative stage with continued long-term treatment and capabilities of prosthetic manufacture and fitting. These capabilities must be sustainable in the long term as the prosthesis will need repair and replacement, and stumps may require future surgical care. Following the 2010 Haiti earthquake, 30% of amputees required revision surgery[78]. In addition, the amputee will require vocational training and psychologic and social support. Therefore, the availability of rehabilitative care is a prerequisite for effective amputation treatment. Lacking this care, an amputee will be severely disabled and will pose a heavy economic and emotional burden to his or her family[76].

4. Cultural and social considerations. The attitude to amputees varies greatly between cultures. In some, it carries a severe stigma and may add psychologic and social stress in a patient who may already be physically and emotionally challenged. Some religions sanctify the wholeness of the body and find mutilative procedures unacceptable. In addition, the economic burden of prolonged rehabilitation in an environment in which public welfare resources and support are scarce or unavailable may be devastating for the injured patients and their families. These factors may significantly affect the decision between amputation and attempts at limb preservation, sometimes at the expense of functional outcome. Therefore, the importance of informed consent following detailed explanation of the possibilities and potential outcome is essential before performing an amputation, for both ethical and medicolegal reasons. The explanation should be given not only to the patients but also to their families with the aid of an interpreter when necessary.

5. Surgical principles. A detailed description of the various amputation techniques is beyond the scope of this text, but the following principles should be adhered to in the field hospital setting: Initially, all viable tissues should be preserved to enable stump coverage. Stumps should be left open initially to be closed or covered as secondary procedures. Guillotine amputations should be avoided. Length should be preserved, especially in the upper limbs. Amputations through joints have the advantage of diminished bleeding.

Amputations requiring bone fusion should be avoided[17,75,76].

Axial Skeleton

Axial skeleton injuries will rarely be treated surgically in a field hospital. Unstable pelvic fractures should be stabilized with an external fixator to reduce internal hemorrhage. Stable fractures of the pelvis and spine are treated with pain control, bed rest, and mobilization as tolerated, and those requiring open surgery will be transferred to facilities with appropriate capabilities[80–82].

Pediatric Considerations

Children constitute a special population whose vulnerability is accentuated in disaster situations. Their dependence on adults will be even greater if their parents have been killed, injured, or separated, raising practical and ethical problems. Most field-hospital deployments will be in low- and middle-income countries in which children constitute a high percentage of the population. In contrast, many of the governmental, military, and NGOs dispatching these field hospital are not geared for treatment of children both from the personnel and the equipment standpoints. These factors must be taken into consideration at the preparation stage of the deployment and appropriate adjustments should be made, bearing in mind that personnel with specialized pediatric training are usually proficient in treating adults while the opposite may not hold true. In the operational stage, when possible, children should be hospitalized in a separate pediatric ward staffed by personnel experienced in treating children including pediatricians, pediatric nurses, and physiotherapists. Pediatric mental health workers can be included to start treatment of post-traumatic disorders at an early stage. Medical clowns have shown a growing participation in field hospital activity[44,45].

Orthopedic treatment in children is also significantly different to that in the adult population. Open growth plates have the potential to remodel residual deformities following fracture malunion, but if injured by the trauma or surgery, a damaged growth plate may cause significant limb deformity or shortening requiring late reconstructive surgery. In open fractures, some bone fragments, which would be discarded in adults, carry a potential for reincorporation and should be preserved. The child's periosteum has a powerful bone-regeneration capability and all attempts should be made to preserve it. Stump overgrowth can be a significant problem in growing children, causing skin breakdown. It can be prevented or treated secondarily by capping the end of the amputated bone with cartilage either from the amputated limb or from the iliac crest [83,84]. Special attention should be given to pain management in children and medications have to be dosed appropriately[26,67,85–87].

Routine Orthopedic Problems

Most field hospitals will be deployed in underserved regions where the local population has limited access to orderly care and carries high morbidity rates of chronic diseases. Even in severe disaster situations, by the second week of deployment, a high percentage of patients seeking care in the field hospital will be due to nondisaster-related problems. Although most of these patients will suffer from nonorthopedic problems, many will seek care due to chronic musculoskeletal diseases such as arthritis and back pain, as well as late sequelae of congenital deformities, trauma, and musculoskeletal infections. Some of these patients will have pathologies rarely seen in high-resource countries such as polio and tuberculosis. The availability of medical care provided by teams from high-resource countries, and the fact that care is delivered free of charge, further increase the patients' expectations and the caseload in the hospital. Orthopedic surgeons working in a field hospital may be tempted to undertake surgical treatment of these cases both from altruistic motives as well as due to the urge to perform elaborate surgery for these challenging cases. This temptation should be resisted bearing in mind the limited capabilities in the field hospital and the high potential for surgical complications, and the surgeon should adhere to the principle of "primum non nocere[3,4,6,94,95]."

Follow-Up Care and Rehabilitation

Most field hospitals will be deployed for short periods of several weeks during the acute phase of a disaster, delivering orthopedic damage-control treatment of the injuries. Therefore, most of the patients treated in the hospital will require follow-up treatment elsewhere, ranging from wound care and cast removal, through pin care and removal of external fixators, to treatment of complications and late reconstructive

surgery. Many of the patients will require short- or long-term rehabilitation. This treatment will be given either in field hospitals deploying for prolonged periods, in local facilities, which resume activity following the acute period, or in referral facilities outside the disaster zone. Despite the organizational chaos that follows major disasters and conflicts, there are certain measures that should be taken in a field hospital to ensure a continuum of care for the patients treated [21,89–93].

Medical Records

All patients should be discharged from the hospital with a written discharge letter detailing the injury, previous treatment, care given in the hospital, and orders and recommendations for follow-up treatment. If possible, copies of the relevant radiographs should be given to the patient. As the patients will often not be able to understand the language of the written letter, a detailed oral explanation should be given to the patients and families in their own language. Generic forms describing cast and wound care in the local language should be prepared in the field hospital to be distributed to the patients on discharge. If the patient requires periodic dressing changes, the date of the last change should be written on casts and dressings[96,97].

Collaborations

Information should be gathered at the earliest phase of deployment regarding existing services and facilities in the disaster zone and the possibility of evacuating patients to centers out of the area for continued treatment. Contact should be established with these facilities either directly, through liaison officers, or through a coordination center or health cluster. This will enable the patients to be referred on discharge directly to one of these centers, thus ensuring a continuum of care. Direct collaboration during the deployment between a field hospital and a functional fixed medical facility has been shown to be beneficial. It enables relieving the fixed facility of the large number of patients requiring orthopedic damage control surgery that is performed in the field hospital while patients requiring internal fixation are treated in the fixed facility. In addition, it enables continued care of patients treated in the field hospital once it terminates the deployment. Close collaboration with local medical teams will also help avoid discreditation of the local medical system, which was found in Haiti following the 2010 earthquake, bearing in mind that this system will have to continue providing care to the population long after the field hospitals and medical teams return to their home countries[7,24,46,98–103].

Future Trends

Increasing awareness of the need for orthopedic care in field hospitals and following disasters has spurred advances in available technology, as well as in organization of treatment, education, and accreditation of emergency medical teams (EMTs) and facilities. Some of these are described in different chapters of this book.

Orthopedic care can be greatly improved by the introduction of a clean surgical environment, which is already available in some field hospitals. The availability of lighter portable C-arm fluoroscopy will further enhance the capability to perform internal fixation. Hardware such as the SIGN nail specifically designed for use in austere and low-resource environments can aid in performing more definitive orthopedic surgery in the field hospital setting. However, these advances must be made cautiously, avoiding violation of surgical and sterility standards. Treatment requiring multiple consecutive surgical procedures should be avoided unless one is confident that the expertise to perform these procedures will be available locally once the field hospital has departed. Care must be taken not to overload the limited payload with large armamentariums of orthopedic hardware, and hardware should be limited to versatile sets which can be used in a wide array of injuries.

Major advances are being made in the diagnosis and treatment of chronic compartment and crush syndrome. New diagnostic tools are being developed[104] and improvements in hemodialysis systems and teams are being established to try to save more people following crush injuries sustained during earthquakes[40].

The growing awareness of the major differences in delivering orthopedic treatment in austere environments and following disasters from that delivered routinely in high-resource countries, as well as recognition of the potential for the necessity of this expertise in the case of a major disaster in these countries themselves, has prompted major organizations involved in orthopedic training worldwide such as the AO Foundation, AAOS, Royal College of Surgeons, and SICOT, in collaboration with large NGOs such as WHO, the International Committee of the Red Cross (ICRC), and Médecins Sans Frontières (MSF) to initiate publications, courses, and think tanks to define guidelines for orthopedic treatment in disaster settings[105]. This knowledge

should be disseminated among EMTs operating in disaster and conflict areas and will optimize the orthopedic treatment provided in field hospitals.

Summary Points

- a typical deployment scenario will be characterized by extreme imbalance between needs and capabilities
- highest incidence of musculoskeletal injuries is in earthquakes and conflicts
- treatment policies are dominated by damage control approach
- all open fractures are assumed to be infected
- first priority is treatment of life- or limb-threatening infections by wide debridement, repeated as necessary, with adjunct antibiotics
- external fixation is the mainstay of open fracture stabilization
- closed fractures are treated by closed reduction and cast immobilization
- no open reduction and internal fixation are performed in field hospital setting, but only in specialized facilities with adequate sterility
- no fasciotomies should be performed for chronic compartment syndrome
- crush syndrome should be treated by forced diuresis, urine alkalization, and dialysis if available
- amputation should be performed for nonviable limbs by experienced surgeons, following thorough explanation and written consent
- specific pediatric anatomy and needs should be considered when treating children
- early rehabilitation should be included in the field hospital capabilities
- collaboration with local caregivers will greatly enhance the treatment capabilities during deployment and will ensure continued care of the patients treated in the field hospital

References

1. von Schreeb J, Riddez L, Samnegård H, Rosling H. Foreign field hospitals in the recent sudden-onset disasters in Iran, Haiti, Indonesia, and Pakistan. *Prehospital and Disaster Medicine* 2008: **23**: 144–51.

2. Kirsch T, Sauer L, Guha-Sapir D. Analysis of the international and US response to the Haiti earthquake: recommendations for change. *Disaster Medicine and Public Health Preparedness* 2012: **6**: 200–8.

3. Bar-On E, Abargel A, Peleg K, Kreiss Y. Coping with the challenges of early disaster response: 24 years of field hospital experience after earthquakes. *Disaster Medicine and Public Health Preparedness* 2013: **7**: 491–8.

4. Amital H, Alkan ML, Adler J, Kriess I, Levi Y. Israeli Defense Forces Medical Corps humanitarian mission for Kosovo's refugees. *Prehospital and Disaster Medicine* 2003: **18**(4): 301–5.

5. Leaning J, Guha-Sapir D. Natural disasters, armed conflict, and public health. *The New England Journal of Medicine* 2013: **369**(19): 1836–42.

6. Bar-Dayan Y, Leiba A, Beard P, et al. A multidisciplinary field hospital as a substitute for medical hospital care in the aftermath of an earthquake: the experience of the Israeli Defense Forces Field Hospital in Duzce, Turkey, 1999. *Prehospital and Disaster Medicine* 2005: **20**(2): 103–6.

7. Norton I, von Schreeb J, Aitken P, Herard P, Lajolo C. *Classification and minimum standards for foreign medical teams in sudden onset disasters*. Geneva: World Health Organization; 2013.

8. Kreiss Y, Merin O, Peleg K, et al. Early disaster response in Haiti: the Israeli field hospital experience. *Annals of Internal Medicine* 2010: **153**(1): 45–8.

9. Clover AJ, Jemec B, Redmond AD. The extent of soft tissue and musculoskeletal injuries after earthquakes; describing a role for reconstructive surgeons in an emergency response. *World Journal of Surgery* 2014: **38**: 2543–50.

10. Doocy S, Daniels A, Packer C, Dick A, Kirsch TD. The human impact of earthquakes: a historical review of events 1980–2009 and systematic literature review. *PLOS Currents* 2013: **16**: 5.

11. Doocy S, Daniels A, Murray S, Kirsch TD. The human impact of floods: a historical review of events 1980–2009 and systematic literature review. *PLOS Currents* 2013: **16**: 5.

12. Doocy S, Daniels A, Dick A, Kirsch TD. The human impact of tsunamis: a historical review of events 1900–2009 and systematic literature review. *PLOS Currents* 2013: **16**: 5.

13. Doocy S, Dick A, Daniels A, Kirsch TD. The human impact of tropical cyclones: a historical review of events 1980–2009 and systematic literature review. *PLOS Currents* 2013: **16**: 5.

14. Murray CJ, King G, Lopez AD, Tomijima N, Krug EG. Armed conflict as a public health problem. *The BMJ* 2002:**324**(7333): 346–9.

15. Gosselin RA, War injuries, trauma and disaster relief. *Techniques in Orphopaedics* 2005: **120**: 97–108.

16. Ley PF, Hamdan TA, Baldan M, Gosselin RA. Orthopedics in conflicts and disasters, in Gosselin RA, Spiegel DA, Foltz M (eds.), *Global orthopedics, caring for musculoskeletal conditions and injuries in austere settings*. New York: Springer; 2014: 493–504.

17. Giannou C, Baldan M. *War surgery*. Volume 1 and Volume 2. Geneva: ICRC; 2009, 2012.

18. Schoenfeld AJ, Belmont PJ. Traumatic combat injuries, in Cameron KL, Owens BD (eds.), *Musculoskeletal injuries in the military*. New York: Springer; 2016.

19. DePalma RG, Burris DG, Champion HR, Hodgson MJ. Blast injuries. *The New England Journal of Medicine* 2005: **352**(13): 1335–42.

20. Teicher CL, Alberti K, Porten K, et al. Médecins Sans Frontières experience in orthopedic surgery in postearthquake Haiti in 2010. *Prehospital and Disaster Medicine* 2014: **29**(1): 21–6.

21. Hotz GA, Moyenda ZB, Bitar J, et al. Developing a trauma critical care and rehab hospital in Haiti: a year after the earthquake. *American Journal of Disaster Medicine*. 2012: **7**(4): 273–9.

22. Walk RM, Donahue TF, Stockinger Z, et al. Haitian earthquake relief: disaster response aboard the USNS comfort. *Disaster Medicine and Public Health Preparedness* 2012: **6**(4): 370–7.

23. Sechriest VF second, Wing V, Walker GJ, et al. Healthcare delivery aboard US Navy hospital ships following earthquake disasters: implications for future disaster relief missions. *American Journal of Disaster Medicine* 2012: **7**(4): 281–94.

24. Bar-On E, Blumberg N, Joshi A, et al. Orthopedic activity in field hospitals following earthquakes in Nepal and Haiti: variability in injuries encountered and collaboration with local available resources drive optimal response. *World Journal of Surgery* 2016: **40**(9): 2117–22.

25. Missair A, Pretto EA, Visan A, et al. A matter of life or limb? A review of traumatic injury patterns and anesthesia techniques for disaster relief after major earthquakes. *Anesthesia & Analgesia* 2013: **117**(4): 934–41.

26. Morelli I, Sabbadini MG, Bortolin M. Orthopedic injuries and their treatment in children during earthquakes: a systematic review. *Prehospital and Disaster Medicine* 2015: **30**(5): 478–85.

27. Herard P, Boillot F. Quality orthopaedic care in sudden-onset disasters: suggestions from Médecins Sans Frontières-France. *International Orthopaedics* 2016: **40**(3): 435–8.

28. Bar-On E, Lebel E, Kreiss Y, et al. Orthopaedic management in a mega mass casualty situation. The Israel Defence Forces Field Hospital in Haiti following the January 2010 earthquake. *Injury* 2011: **42**(10): 1053–9.

29. Blumberg N, Lebel E, Merin O, Levy G, Bar-On E. Skeletal injuries sustained during the Haiti earthquake of 2010: a radiographic analysis of the casualties

admitted to the Israel Defense Forces field hospital. *European Journal of Trauma and Emergency Surgery* 2013: **39**(2): 117–22.

30. Awais S, Saeed A. Study of the severity of musculoskeletal injuries and triage during the 2005 Pakistan earthquake. *International Orthopaedics* 2013: **37**(8): 1443–7.

31. Elmi A, Ganjpour Sales J, Tabrizi A, Soleimanpour J, Mohseni MA. Orthopedic injuries following the East Azerbaijan earthquake. *Trauma Monthly* 2013: **18**(1): 3–7.

32. Guha-Sapir D, Vos F. Earthquakes, an epidemiologic perspective on patterns and trends, in Spence R, So E, Scawthorn C (eds.), *Human casualties in earthquakes.* New York: Springer; 2011: 13–24.

33. Helminen M, Saarela E, Salmela J. Characterisation of patients treated at the Red Cross field hospital in Kashmir during the first three weeks of operation. *Emergency Medical Journal* 2006: **23**: 654–6.

34. Phalkey R, Reinhardt JD, Marx M. Injury epidemiology after the 2001 Gujarat earthquake in India: a retrospective analysis of injuries treated at a rural hospital in the Kutch district immediately after the disaster. *Global Health Action* 2011: **4**: 7196.

35. Kaim Khani GM, Baig A, Humail M, Memon M, Quarashi MA. Musculoskeletal injuries among victims of the Battagram, Pakistan earthquake in October 2005. *Prehospital and Disaster Medicine* 2012: **27**(5): 489–91.

36. Mulvey JM, Awan SU, Qadri AA, Maqsood MA. Profile of injuries arising from the 2005 Kashmir earthquake: the first 72h. *Injury* 2008: **39**: 554–60.

37. Ramirez M and Peek-Asa C. Epidemiology of traumatic injuries from earthquakes. *Epidemiologic Review* 2005: **27**: 47–55.

38. Roy N, Shah H, Patel V, Coughlin RR. The Gujarat earthquake (2001) experience in a seismically unprepared area: community hospital medical response. *Prehospital and Disaster Medicine* 2002: **17**: 186–95.

39. Sami F, Ali F, Zaidi SH, Rehman H, Ahmad T, Siddiqui MI. The October 2005 earthquake in Northern Pakistan: patterns of injuries in victims brought to the Emergency Relief Hospital, Doraha, Mansehra. *Prehospital and Disaster Medicine* 2009: **24**: 535–9.

40. Sever MS, Vanholder R. Management of crush victims in mass disasters: highlights from recently published recommendations. *Clinical Journal of the American Society of Nephrology* 2013: **8**(2): 328–35.

41. Bartal C, Zeller L, Miskin I, et al. Crush syndrome: saving more lives in disasters: lessons learned from the early-response phase in Haiti. *Archives of Internal Medicine* 2011: **171**(7): 694–6.

42. Matsuzawa G, Sano H, Ohnuma H, et al. Patient trends in orthopedic traumas and related disorders after

tsunami caused by the Great East Japan Earthquake: an experience in the primary referral medical center. *Journal of Orthopaedic Science* 2016: **21**(4): 507–11.

43. Lehavi A, Meroz Y, Maryanovsky M, et al. Role of regional anaesthesia in disaster medicine: field hospital experience after the 2015 Nepal Earthquake. *European Journal of Anaesthesiology* 2016: **33**(5): 312–3.

44. Farfel A, Assa A, Amir I, et al. Haiti earthquake 2010: a field hospital pediatric perspective. *European Journal of Pediatrics* 2011: **170**(4): 519–25.

45. Burnweit C, Stylianos S. Disaster response in a pediatric field hospital: lessons learned in Haiti. *Journal of Pediatric Surgery* 2011: **46**(6): 1131–9.

46. Jobe K. Disaster relief in post-earthquake Haiti: unintended consequences of humanitarian volunteerism. *Travel Medicine and Infectious Disease* 2011: **9**(1): 1–5.

47. Sonshine DB, Caldwell A, Gosselin RA, Born CT, Coughlin RR. Critically assessing the Haiti earthquake response and the barriers to quality orthopaedic care. *Clinical Orthopaedics and Related Research* 2012: **470**(10): 2895–904.

48. Dewo P, Magetsari R, Busscher HJ, van Horn JR, Verkerke GJ. Treating natural disaster victims is dealing with shortages: an orthopaedics perspective. *Technology and Health Care* 2008: **16**(4): 255–9.

49. Alvarado O, Trelles M, Tayler-Smith K, et al. Orthopaedic surgery in natural disaster and conflict settings: how can quality care be ensured? *International Orthopaedics* 2015: **39**(10): 1901–8.

50. Dhar SA, Bhat MI, Mustafa A, et al. Damage control orthopaedic in patients with delayed referral to a tertiary care center: experience from a place where Composite Trauma Centers do not exist. *Journal of Trauma Management & Outcomes* 2008: **29**(2) 2.

51. Bertol MJ, Van den Bergh R, Trelles Centurion M, et al. Saving life and limb: limb salvage using external fixation, a multi-centre review of orthopaedic surgical activities in Médecins Sans Frontières. *International Orthopaedics* 2014: **38**(8): 1555–61.

52. Li W, Qian J, Liu X, et al. Management of severe crush injury in a front-line tent ICU after 2008 Wenchuan earthquake in China: an experience with 32 cases. *Critical Care* 2009: **13**(6): R178.

53. Reis ND, Michaelson M. Crush injury to the lower limbs. Treatment of the local injury. *Journal of Bone and Joint Surgery (Am)* 1986: **68**: 414–8.

54. Gerdin M, Wladis A, von Schreeb J. Surgical management of closed crush injury-induced compartment syndrome after earthquakes in resource-scarce settings. *The Journal of Trauma and Acute Care Surgery* 2012: 14.

55. Murphy RA, Ronat JB, Fakhri RM, et al. Multidrug-resistant chronic osteomyelitis complicating war injury

in Iraqi civilians. *The Journal of Trauma and Acute Care Surgery* 2011: **71**(1): 252–4.

56. Teicher CL, Ronat JB, Fakhri RM, et al. Antimicrobial drug-resistant bacteria isolated from Syrian war-injured patients, August 2011-March 2013. *Emerging Infectious Diseases* 2014: **20**(11): 1949–51.

57. Gilbert DN, Sanford JP, Kutscher E, et al. Microbiologic study of wound infections in tornado casualties. *Archives of Environmental & Occupational Health* 1973: **26**(3): 125–30.

58. Marra AR, Valle Martino MD, Ribas MR, et al. Microbiological findings from the Haiti disaster. *Travel Medicine and Infectious Disease* 2012: **10**(3): 157–61.

59. Lichtenberger P, Miskin IN, Dickinson G, et al. Infection control in field hospitals after a natural disaster: lessons learned after the 2010 earthquake in Haiti. *Infection Control & Hospital Epidemiology* 2010: **31**(9): 951–7.

60. Miskin IN, Nir-Paz R, Block C, et al. Antimicrobial therapy for wound infections after catastrophic earthquakes. *The New England Journal of Medicine* 2010: **363**(26): 2571–3.

61. Yun HC, Murray CK, Nelson KJ, Bosse MJ. Infection after orthopaedic trauma: prevention and treatment. *Journal of Orthopaedic Trauma* 2016: **30**(Suppl 3) S21–6.

62. Wang Y, Lu B, Hao P, Yan MN, Dai KR. Comprehensive treatment for gas gangrene of the limbs in earthquakes. *Chinese Medical Journal (Engl)* 2013: **126**(20): 3833–9.

63. Leininger BE1, Rasmussen TE, Smith DL, Jenkins DH, Coppola CJ. Experience with wound VAC and delayed primary closure of contaminated soft tissue injuries in Iraq. *Trauma* 2006: **61**(5): 1207–11.

64. Edsander-Nord Å. Wound complications from the tsunami disaster: a reminder of indications for delayed closure. *European Journal of Trauma and Emergency Surgery* 2008: **34**(5): 457–64.

65. Phillips J, Zirkle LG, Gosselin RA. Achieving locked intramedullary fixation of long bone fractures: technology for the developing world. *International Orthopaedics* 2012: **36**(10): 2007–13.

66. Lebel E, Blumberg N, Gill A, et al. External fixator frames as interim damage control for limb injuries: experience in the 2010 Haiti earthquake. *The Journal of Trauma and Acute Care Surgery* 2011: **71**(6): E128–31.

67. Bar-On E, Lebel E, Blumberg N, Sagi R, Kreiss Y. Pediatric orthopedic injuries following an earthquake: experience in an acute-phase field hospital. *The Journal of Trauma and Acute Care Surgery* 2013: **74**(2): 617–21.

68. Boillot F, Herard P. External fixators and sudden-onset disasters: Médecins Sans Frontières experience. *International Orthopaedics* 2014: **38**(8): 1551–4.

69. Awais S, Saeed A, Asad Ch. Use of external fixators for damage-control orthopaedics in natural disasters like the 2005 Pakistan earthquake. *International Orthopaedics (SICOT)* 2014: **38**: 1563–8.

70. Clover AJ, Rannan-Eliya S, Saeed W, et al. Experience of an orthoplastic limb salvage team after the Haiti earthquake: analysis of caseload and early outcomes. *Plastic and Reconstructive Surgery* 2011: **127**(6): 2373–80.

71. Scalea TM, Boswell SA, Scott JD, et al. External fixation as a bridge to intramedullary nailing for patients with multiple injuries and with femur fractures: damage control. *Journal of Orthopaedic Trauma* 2000: **48**(4): 613–23.

72. Dhar SA, Mutt MF, Hussain A, et al. Management of lower limb fractures in polytrauma patients with delayed referral in a mass disaster. The role of the Ilizarov method in conversion osteosynthesis. *Injury* 2008: **39**: 947–51.

73. Bosse MJ, MacKenzie EJ, Kellam JF, et al. A prospective evaluation of the clinical utility of the lower-extremity injury-severity scores. *Journal of Bone and Joint Surgery* 2001: **83**(1): 3–14.

74. Teicher C, Foote NL, Al Ani AM, et al. The short musculoskeletal functional assessment (SMFA) score amongst surgical patients with reconstructive lower limb injuries in war wounded civilians. *Injury* 2014: **45**(12): 1996–2001.

75. Herard P, Boillot F. Amputation in emergency situations: indications, techniques and Médecins Sans Frontières France's experience in Haiti. *International Orthopaedics* 2012: **36**(10): 1979–81.

76. Knowlton LM, Gosney JE, Chackungal S, et al. Consensus statements regarding the multidisciplinary care of limb amputation patients in disasters or humanitarian emergencies: report of the 2011 Humanitarian Action Summit Surgical Working Group on amputations following disasters or conflict. *Prehospital and Disaster Medicine* 2011: **26**(6): 438–48.

77. Macintyre A, Kramer EB, Petinaux B, et al. Extreme measures: field amputation on the living and dismemberment of the deceased to extricate individuals entrapped in collapsed structures. *Disaster Medicine and Public Health Preparedness* 2012: **6**(4): 428–35.

78. Delauche MC, Blackwell N, Le Perff H, et al. A prospective study of the outcome of patients with limb trauma following the Haitian earthquake in 2010 at one- and two-year (the SuTra2 study). *PLOS Currents* 2013: **5**: 5.

79. Gosselin RA, Rmith DG. Amputations, in Gosselin RA, Spiegel DA, Foltz M (eds.), *Global orthopedics, caring for musculoskeletal conditions and injuries in austere settings.* New York: Springer; 2014: 481–92.

80. Dailey SK, Casstevens EC, Archdeacon MT, Mamczak CN, Burgess AR. Assessment of pelvic fractures resulting from the 2010 Haiti earthquake: opportunities for improved care. *The Journal of Trauma and Acute Care Surgery* 2014: **76**(3): 866–70.

81. Dong Z, Yang Z, Chen T, et al. Spinal injuries in the Sichuan earthquake. *The New England Journal of Medicine* 2009: **361**: 636–7.

82. Keshkar S, Kumar R, Bharti BB. Epidemiology and impact of early rehabilitation of spinal trauma after the 2005 earthquake in Kashmir, India. *International Orthopaedics* 2014: **38**(10): 2143–7.

83. O'Neal ML, Bahner R, Ganey T, Ogden JA. Limb deficiency osseous overgrowth after amputation in adolescents and children. *Journal of Pediatric Orthopaedics* 1996: **16**(1): 78–84.

84. Fedorak GT, Watts HG, Cuomo AV, et al. Osteocartilaginous transfer of the proximal part of the fibula for osseous overgrowth in children with congenital or acquired tibial amputation. *Journal of Bone and Joint Surgery* 2015: **97**: 574–81.

85. Trudeau MO, Baron E, Hérard P, et al. Surgical care of pediatric patients in the humanitarian setting: the Médecins Sans Frontières experience, 2012–2013. *JAMA Surgery* 2015: **150**(11): 1080–5.

86. Sabzehchian M, Abolghasemi H, Radfar MH, et al. Pediatric trauma at tertiary-level hospitals in the aftermath of the Bam, Iran earthquake. *Prehospital and Disaster Medicine.* 2006: **21**(5): 336–9.

87. Jacquet GA, Hansoti B, Vu A, Bayram JD. Earthquake-related injuries in the pediatric population: a systematic review. *PLOS Currents.* 2013: **27**: 5.

88. Khan F, Amatya B, Gosney J, Rathore FA, Burkle Jr FM. Medical rehabilitation in natural disasters: a review. *Archives of Physical Medicine and Rehabilitation* 2015: **96**(9): 1709–27.

89. Rathore FA, Gosney JE, Reinhardt JD, Haig AJ, Li J, DeLisa JA. Medical rehabilitation after natural disasters: why, when, and how? *Archives of Physical Medicine and Rehabilitation.* 2012: **93**(10): 1875–81.

90. Iezzoni L, Ronan LJ. Disability legacy of the Haitian earthquake. *Annals of Internal Medicine* 2010: **152**: 812–4.

91. Sheppard PS, Landry MD. Lessons from the 2015 earthquake(s) in Nepal: implication for rehabilitation. *Disability and Rehabilitation* 2016: **38**(9): 910–3.

92. Bartels SA, VanRooyen MJ. Medical complications associated with earthquakes. *The Lancet* 2012: **379**(9817): 748–57.

93. World Health Organization (2016). Emergency medical teams: minimum technical standards and recommendations for rehabilitation. Geneva: Licence: CC BY-NC-SA 3.0 IGO. Website. https://extranet .who.int/emt/guidelines-and-publications

94. Gosselin RA, Gialamas G, Atkin DM. Comparing the cost-effectiveness of short orthopedic missions in elective and relief situations in developing countries. *World Journal of Surgery* 2011: **35**(5): 951–5.

95. Lin G, Marom T, Dagan D, Merin O. Ethical and surgical dilemmas in patients with neglected surgical diseases visiting a field hospital in a zone of recent disaster. *World Journal of Surgery* 2016: **19** [Epub ahead of print].

96. Levy G, Blumberg N, Kreiss Y, Ash N, Merin O. Application of information technology within a field hospital deployment following the January 2010 Haiti earthquake disaster. *Journal of the American Medical Informatics Association: JAMIA* 2010: **17**(6): 626–30.

97. Jafar AJ, Norton I, Lecky F, Redmond AD. A literature review of medical record keeping by foreign medical teams in sudden onset disasters. *Prehospital and Disaster Medicine* 2015: **30**(2): 216.

98. Degennaro V Jr, Degennaro V Sr, Ginzburg E. Haiti's dilemma: how to incorporate foreign health professionals to assist in short-term recovery while capacity building for the future. *Journal of Public Health* 2011: **33**(3): 459–61.

99. Born CT, Cullison TR, Dean JA, et al. Partnered disaster preparedness: lessons learned from international events. *Journal of the American Academy of Orthopaedic Surgeons* 2011: **19**(Suppl 1): S44–8.

100. Peleg K, Kreiss Y, Ash N, Lipsky AM. Optimizing medical response to large-scale disasters: the ad hoc collaboration health care system. *Annals of Surgery* 2011: **253**(2): 421–3.

101. Abolghasemi H, Radfar MH, Khatami M, et al. International medical response to a natural disaster: lessons learned from the Bam earthquake experience. *Prehospital and Disaster Medicine* 2006: **21**(3): 141–7.

102. Gerdin M, Wladis A, von Schreeb J. Foreign field hospitals after the 2010 Haiti earthquake: how good were we? *Emergency Medicine Journal* 2013: **30**(1): e8.

103. Merin O, Kreiss Y, Lin G, Pras E, Dagan D. Collaboration in response to disaster: Typhoon Yolanda and an integrative model. *The New England Journal of Medicine* 2014: **370**(13): 1183–4.

104. Lee SH, Padilla M, Lynch JE, Hargens AR. Noninvasive measurements of pressure for detecting compartment syndromes. *Journal of Orthopaedic Rheumatology.* 2013: **1**(1): 5.

105. World Health Organization (2017). Management of limb injuries during disasters and conflicts. Online article. https://extranet.who.int/emt/guidelines-and-publications

Burn Care in a Field Hospital Environment

Alan Kay

Introduction

Field hospitals must expect to have to deal with burn injury[1]. An increased prevalence of injury from burns is a feature of situations where there is disruption to the functioning of society. In addition to the direct effects of burn injury as a result of weapon wounding, there is the enduring added risk of sustaining burns following alterations in behavior patterns, which remove normal safe working habits[2]. Children are disproportionally more likely to be injured[3].

Over several decades, the management of burn injury in developed health-care systems has improved significantly with survival and good quality of outcome being considered normal even following very large burns[4]. The improvement has been most marked where care is delivered by services incorporating:

- organized burn care networks
- highly resourced centers of excellence
- large multidisciplinary teams
- standardized care pathways
- use of very early aggressive surgery
- sophisticated critical care
- rigorous infection prevention and control measures
- long-term follow-up with specialized rehabilitation

Provision of this level of complex integrated care is beyond the scope of most field hospitals. That said, even when lacking ideal resources, individual burn care specialists can significantly improve outcomes by making sure basic principles of burn care are applied. Field hospitals may temporarily bring a level of expertise that exceeds the background capability of the indigenous health-care system to provide long-term support for burn survivors.

An implication of the complexity of burn care is the disproportionately high demand it places on resources. In a single field hospital during a short phase in a war fighting scenario, 3% of casualties had burn injuries, but these accounted for 27% of critical care bed usage[5].

This discrepancy between what is realistically deliverable in a field hospital and what would be considered normal outcomes by both the donor and host nations means a great deal of thought must go into understanding the situation in which the facility finds itself. Agreed approaches to clinical pathways for burns, including thresholds of care, are best made in advance. These must be consistent and integrated across the command area of responsibility rather than be idiosyncratic to individual facilities.

If there are several facilities under a unified organizational structure, rationalizing burn care resources should be considered. It would be prudent to ensure there is a degree of additional training to prepare individuals to deliver appropriate initial management. In a complex scenario, centralizing burns expertise to a single identified facility and transferring all burn casualties there is an option.

Pathophysiology

Burn injury has three potential elements:

- the cutaneous burn
- a systemic physiological response to the burn
- inhalation injury

Heat above about 43°C alters protein structure and causes damage to cellular function. A relationship between temperature, duration of exposure and the body's limited ability to self cool will dictate when tissue exposed to heat will undergo necrosis or sustain recoverable injury. Tissues damaged but not killed by heat will exhibit a marked inflammatory response. For smaller burns this will be limited to the local tissues around the area of burn necrosis, but above a certain threshold a more generalized inflammatory response is initiated. The volume of tissue directly injured by heat can be equated to the area of skin burned, normally expressed as a percentage of the total body surface area (% TBSA).

The inflamed tissues will exhibit marked capillary leakage and fluid will be lost from the intravascular space. Above a certain size of burn, compensatory mechanisms for this fluid loss can be exceeded, leading to physiologically significant hypovolemia, and the clinical manifestations are called burn shock. Burns over about 30% TBSA can trigger a systemic inflammatory response syndrome. The fluid loss occurs over several hours after the injury, and burn shock may not be seen immediately. As the fluid loss is predictable it can be corrected in part by the prophylactic administration of intravenous fluids and the effects of burn shock reduced[6]. It is established practice to use a cut-off of 15% TBSA burn (10% in children), above which additional intravenous fluids should be administered. There is no clear evidence that supports this value. There is growing acceptance that it is safe to give additional fluids orally in burns up to 20% TBSA and this is helpful when resources are scarce[7].

The depth of burn has little impact on the management of burn shock, but alters burn wound treatment. Superficial partial thickness burns should heal spontaneously if managed correctly. Deeper burns will normally require surgical excision and healing by skin grafting.

Inhalation injury is a combination of factors[8]. True heat damage to the upper airways causes a burn injury and airway obstruction secondary to swelling is the concern. Damage to the lower airways is rarely a heat phenomenon; it is normally a chemical injury caused by the inhaled noxious products of combustion. The deleterious effects on pulmonary function of this chemical injury can be delayed and the clinical manifestations may not be evident for hours. Systemic intoxication can occur if these chemicals are absorbed into the circulation.

Initial Management

No assumptions should be made about the adequacy of prehospital interventions. It is important to be certain that the burning process has been stopped and the burn wound has been cooled by using water for about 30 minutes[9]. The water does not have to be sterile. All clothing and jewelry should be removed. Burns are painful and distressing; adequate analgesia should be given as soon as possible. Nonsteroidal

antiinflammatory agents should be avoided in the first 48 hours due to the potential renal sequelae.

It is essential that patients with burns undergo a full trauma assessment as for any other type of trauma, and that standard procedures are followed until other injuries are treated or excluded. The systemic effects of a burn may take a while to become apparent and it is important to have a high level of suspicion for other injuries in patients who have signs of hypovolemia or reduced levels of consciousness soon after sustaining a burn. This is particularly important following combat-related burn injury. If there is early hypovolemic shock, this should be treated according to normal measures for hemorrhagic shock irrespective of the burn size.

Burn-injured patients are particularly susceptible to becoming hypothermic. Every effort should be made to keep the patient warm.

An assessment must be made as to the likelihood of inhalation injury by ascertaining the following:

- there is a history of:
    - being in an enclosed space with smoke or flame
    - reduced level of consciousness at any stage
- there are symptoms of:
    - coughing
    - difficulty in breathing
- There are signs of:
    - peri- or intraoral burns with soot in the mouth or sputum
    - stridor

If performed soon after injury, blood gas analysis and chest X-ray can initially be normal even in the presence of significant inhalation injury. If available, carboxyhemoglobin levels can be measured.

Venous access should be secured peripherally or, if necessary, centrally or via an interosseous needle. While it is preferable to avoid cannulating through burned skin, it is acceptable to do so if there is no other option. Blood samples should be analyzed for a full blood count and urea and electrolytes.

A rapid assessment of the size of the burn should be made. This can be done using either the Wallace rule of nines (Figure 19.1) or serial halving[10].

It is difficult to establish an accurate assessment prior to a thorough wash of the burn and it must be accepted that this will be a rough estimate. Initially, therefore, precise calculation of a fluid regimen is

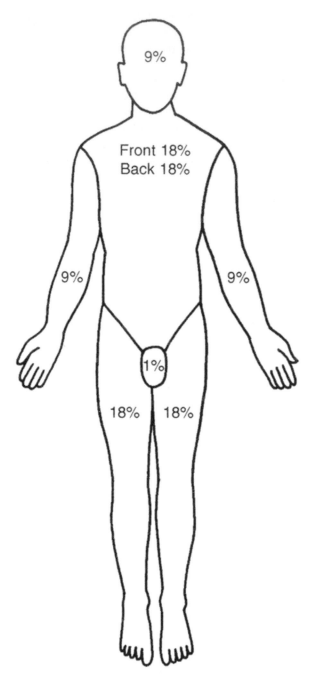

Figure 19.1 Rule of nines

unnecessary. Using the "rule of tens"[11]: 10 ml of crystalloid per hour for every estimated % burned (e.g., 40% TBSA = 400 ml per hour) is an acceptable initial administration rate until a more formal assessment is made. If it is not feasible to even make a rough estimate of burn size 500 ml of

crystalloid an hour will be safe for a short period. These amounts should be adjusted for small children.

For burns likely to be over 20% TBSA, a urinary catheter and a nasogastric tube should be passed.

It is not normal practice to give prophylactic antibiotics in civilian burn injuries, but combat burn injuries should be assumed to be contaminated. The normal antibiotic prophylaxis for combat casualties should be given for burns sustained in the combat environment. Appropriate measures should be taken to ensure the patient has tetanus immunity.

Further Care

Having assessed for other injuries, the likelihood of inhalation injury, and an estimate of the size of the burn, it is important to decide what further interventions are appropriate. Examples of differing situations that may influence decision-making are:

- the patient is part of an overseas military force and needs to be stabilized in preparation for long-haul aeromedical evacuation to receive definitive care in their home country
- the patient has a large burn and can be transferred without delay to a burn center a couple of hours away
- the patient is a local police officer with an inhalation injury in a country where there is no accessible critical care capability and your facility is only resourced for damage control surgery
- the patient is a child who has presented late with a large unhealed burn that exceeds the upper limit acceptable to the host nation's burn service

The likely clinical pathway and impact on resources over the following hours and days needs to be thought through before committing to a given treatment plan. Decisions may not be solely clinical and command elements should be involved.

Ongoing care, if deemed appropriate, requires multidisciplinary input and involves various aspects of the following.

Inhalation Injury

The initial concern is upper airway swelling, which is more likely to get worse in the first 24 hours. If any degree of upper airway obstruction is present, endotracheal intubation should be performed. Remember, the swelling is likely to be increasing. The majority of patients will be conscious and intubation will be impossible without first anesthetizing the patient. There is a significant impact from having a surgical airway and in difficult cases it should be considered an intervention of last resort.

In cases where there is a high suspicion of inhalation injury, but without evidence of upper airway obstruction, judgment is required to assess if it is considered safe to observe a casualty with a possible inhalation injury unintubated. If so, they should be nursed sitting up in an area where very regular observations can be made.

The pulmonary manifestations of burn injuries rarely occur early. If the airway is clear, the only likely effect of a burn that will cause compromise of respiration in the first few hours is a restriction of chest excursion by a deep circumferential torso burn. This is an indication for emergency chest escharotomy, described below.

Accurate Assessment of the Burn Wound Size

This requires total exposure of the whole body and a thorough wash. This is best performed in a warm, clean, and well-lit operating theater under general anesthesia. This also allows for any necessary surgical interventions to be performed and subsequent dressings. The process of induction of anesthesia can unmask burn-related hypovolemia and appropriate measures should be taken to avoid precipitous hypotension.

Warm antiseptic solution should be used, in large volumes if possible, with vigorous rubbing to remove dirt, carbonaceous residue, residual burned clothing, loose skin, and blisters. Some of the contamination found after explosions and in the battlefield environment contains oily-based products, and a soapy solution should be used. There is no role for delicate dabbing in a misguided attempt to be gentle on the wounds: this process requires aggressive cleaning. Leaving behind dead tissue and contamination will be more harmful.

With the burn fully exposed and cleaned, it is now possible to calculate its size and describe it in terms of % TBSA. Skin which has simple erythema alone is not considered burned. The best aid to this is the Lund and Browder chart (Figure 19.2), although some electronic mapping tools are becoming more available[12].

Calculation of Likely Fluid Requirements

With the % TBSA known, a more accurate assessment of intravenous fluid requirements can now be made.

For isolated burn injury, this relies on the use of mathematical formulas, of which there are many. The majority used by military medical services are crystalloid based, which should ideally be Ringer's lactate solution or Hartmann's solution. Normal saline has a tendency to cause more biochemical disturbances, in particular hyperchloremic acidosis. If the patient is receiving blood products for other injuries, the fluid requirements are dictated by the correction of the hemorrhagic hypovolemia and the burn crystalloid formula is ignored at this time.

The simple "rule of tens" described above works well for most average-size adults, but not for extremes of age or weight. It is an adequate starting point, but a more appropriate formula once a full assessment has been made is to use $2 \times$ % TBSA burned $\times$ body weight (kg)[13]. This gives a figure that is the volume of crystalloid in ml expected to be needed in the first 24 hours since injury. Half is given in the first eight hours and the second half given over the following 16 hours. (For example, 40% burn in a 20 kg child = $2 \times 40 \times 20$ = 1600 ml in 24 hours = 100 ml per hour for the first 8 hours, then 50 ml per hour for the subsequent 16 hours.)

To establish adult body weight, either ask the patient (if they are conscious) or make a guess by comparing body size to another person. For children, use weighing scales if at all possible. The use of normative data, such as the Broselow system, can have inaccuracies if applied to non-Western populations. Anecdotal experience in Afghanistan when treating local civilian children led clinical teams to downsize predicted values by one Broselow zone.

The volume of calculated additional fluid is based on a premise of losses from the time of injury. If there has been a delay in arrival, there may be a difference between the predicted requirement and the amount of fluid already given. Any volumes of "catch-up" should be spread over a few hours rather than administered as a rapid bolus, to avoid excessive edema formation. The calculated volumes are a guide only and act as a starting point. The rate of fluid administered should be dictated by the patient's physiological response. Should the patient exhibit classical signs of profound hypovolemia, treatment should resort to standard shock protocols irrespective of the burn.

Further Assessment of the Burn Wound

With the patient still in the operating theater, assessment of the burn and any other injuries continues.

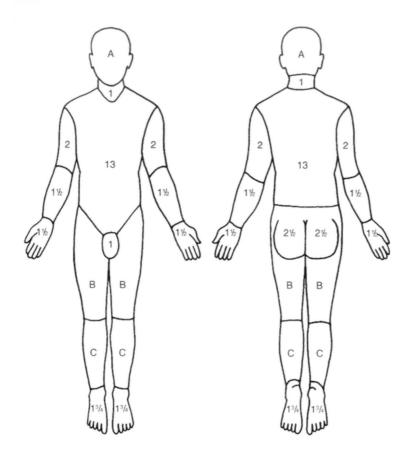

Relative percentage of areas affected by growth

Age in years	0	1	5	10	15	Adult
A – ½ of head	9½	8½	6½	5½	4½	3½
B – ½ of one thigh	2¾	3¼	4	4¼	4½	4¾
C – ½ of one leg	2½	2½	2¾	3	3¼	3½

Figure 19.2 The Lund and Browder chart

Any nonburn wounds need to undergo initial wound surgery. The depth of the burn wound requires evaluation. Accurate delineation of depth, however, requires experience and, at this level of care, is not going to dictate immediate ongoing wound management apart from identifying the need for escharotomies. It is not necessary, therefore, to spend a great deal of time and effort on this matter.

The simplest approach is to distinguish between superficial partial thickness burns, which have the potential to heal with only dressings, and deep burns, which usually require surgical excision and healing by use of skin grafts. Superficial partial thickness burns have a very thin layer of necrosis with underlying dermal inflammation causing hyperemia and capillary leakage. They therefore appear blistered, wet, and erythematous with an intact capillary refill. The necrosis in deeper burns damages the dermal blood vessels, ceasing flow and causing extravasation of red pigments. They appear dry, and can be a white color with areas of nonblanching red: so-called "fixed staining."

Circumferential deeper burn wounds are prone to a constricting effect since the layer of necrotic skin (eschar) shrinks as its water content reduces. This effect is further aggravated by ongoing capillary leakage in the deeper inflamed tissues, which causes more edema to accumulate under the unyielding eschar. This process leads to increased tissue pressure, reduced microvascular perfusion, and ischemia. This manifests itself clinically on the torso as restricted respiratory excursion or, in the limbs, a cold, very firm extremity with loss of distal capillary refill. The loss of distal pulses is a very late sign. This needs to be checked for during the initial assessment in the operating theater. In these cases, escharotomies are performed by dividing the eschar down into unburned tissue with the incision extending the whole length of the eschar. Where deep torso burns are compromising respiration, urgent chest escharotomies should be performed very rapidly and must incorporate a horizontal release below the costal margin that allows diaphragmatic descent. In extremis this can be done with a scalpel at the bedside, but is ideally performed as a formal surgical procedure in the operating theater with electrocautery to ensure hemostasis. To achieve full release, incisions must enter unburned skin and escharotomies will be painful: appropriate analgesia, preferably a general anesthetic, is essential. Limb escharotomies are not such an urgent priority and can wait for an hour or so. As such it should always be possible to perform them in an operating theater. Limb incisions should made down both the medial and lateral aspects. Significant structures at risk of damage during escharotomies are the ulnar nerve at the elbow and the common peroneal nerve just below the fibular head. Once completed, peripheral perfusion is reassessed to verify the effectiveness of the procedure.

With the exceptions of high-voltage electrical injury, fractures deep to the burn wound, or a concomitant vascular injury, fasciotomies of burned extremities are rarely required. In cases where a pulse or Doppler signal does not return after escharotomies are performed, fasciotomies should be considered. It should be appreciated that burn shock and the resultant high peripheral vascular resistance may make finding even a Doppler signal or palpable pulse difficult; further resuscitation may be needed.

Escharotomy is often performed about the same time as the positive effects of fluid administration and the rewarming of the patient are beginning to show physiological improvement in perfusion. Post-release limb hyperemia is, therefore, common and the escharotomy wounds can bleed profusely. Hemostasis must be meticulous.

Dressings

In normal hospital definitive care centers, further burn wound management is complex and may involve immediate burn wound excision and a variety of dressing regimes dictated by burn depth. In field-hospital environments, resources for such approaches are not available and no guarantee can be made about the accuracy of burn depth assessment. The approach should be to dress the burn wound at this stage. There is no universally agreed dressing regime and policy should be dictated by the following principles:

- no burn wound excision will have taken place
- it must be applicable for all burn depths
- it should have antiseptic properties
- it should minimize the drive of the systemic inflammatory response
- it should be easy to apply
- it should be comfortable for the patient
- it should not require frequent dressing changes or laborious nursing care
- it should comply with prescribing legislation
- it should be familiar to staff in their normal practice

There are no current dressing regimens that fully deliver this "ideal" and, as would be expected, there are a variety of practices in use. It must be emphasized that all burn wounds must be thoroughly scrubbed before applying any dressing. Common examples are:

- Gauze is soaked in 5% mafenide acetate solution (Sulfamylon) and applied directly to the burn wound and held in place with some form of bandage. This should be kept moist (but not saturated) with further wetting with the solution about every eight hours. The mafenide is known to cause wound pain and so this can be replaced at night with silver sulfadiazine – so-called "alternating agent" regimen.
- Cerium nitrate in silver sulfadiazine cream (Flammacerium) is applied thickly to the burn wound and then covered in Gamgee, which is held in place either with a bandage or adhesive sheet dressings. Ideally, this dressing should be changed daily, but it can be left in place for a few days.
- Silver nylon sheet dressing (e.g., Silverlon, Acticoat) is applied directly to the burn wound and held in place with some form of bandage. The manufacturers recommend keeping the dressing moistened with water, but the burn wound exudate is often enough to prevent desiccation. This dressing can be left undisturbed for up to five days.

All dressings should be inspected (not necessarily changed) at least daily to check for slippage, comfort, and excessive strikethrough. The patient's general condition should be taken into account and evidence of sepsis should prompt a consideration for a change of dressings.

The use of bags to dress hand burns is not used frequently now. Unconscious or heavily sedated patients should have hands fully dressed as above and splinted in the position of safe immobilization. Elevation of hand burns is very important. The advantage of hand bag dressings was the awake patient could assist in their own nursing care, particularly in mass-casualty situations or long evacuation journeys when the availability of professional staff may be limited.

Facial burns should be scrubbed as described above and a petroleum-based ointment applied regularly to prevent desiccation. There is no evidence that an antiseptic preparation is superior to plain Vaseline for the face. Ears should be covered with an antiseptic agent to prevent chondritis. It is difficult to assess scalp burns unless the hair is shaved off and this also makes dressing the head more hygienic.

The blink reflex is normally effective in protecting the eyes from heat injury, but it is important to properly examine the eyes for corneal damage, particularly in electrical arc injuries. The presence of foreign bodies and globe damage must be excluded if there has been a blast mechanism. In very deep facial burns, orbital compartment syndrome has been observed, particularly following high volumes of intravenous crystalloid administration. It may be necessary to perform a lateral canthotomy.

Ongoing Critical Care

The generalized physiological derangement following a significant burn injury is profound. Even following good surgical first aid and appropriate intravenous fluid administration as outlined above, the patient with a burn over about 30% TBSA may exhibit a marked systemic inflammatory response with progressive worsening of their condition. This deterioration should be anticipated and it is appropriate to care for these patients in a critical care environment. Burn injury produces changes in normal physiology, which does not resolve even with adequate management. These include a tachycardia, pyrexia of up to 38.5°C, and a leukocytosis, and can persist for several weeks even in uncomplicated burns. This complicates identification of infection.

Nasogastric feeding should be started as early as possible[14]. This helps maintain gut function and integrity. Peptic ulceration is not infrequent unless some form of prophylaxis is used; nasogastric feeding alone may not suffice and administration of gastric acid suppression drugs according to local protocols should be used as well.

Burn injury is a high risk for venous thromboembolism and standard prophylaxis regimens should be started unless there are other contraindications.

The formulas described above to calculate predicted intravenous fluid requirements provide a starting point and should not be viewed as a fixed regimen. With inconsistencies in the estimation of burn size and body weight, and the natural variation in inflammatory response, the calculated volumes are, at best, an initial guide. The amount of fluid administered must be directed by the patient's response. The effects of too much fluid, predominantly excessive tissue edema and pulmonary consequences, can be as detrimental as too little. The aim should be that fluid input should be no more than is necessary to ensure essential organ perfusion. Urine output is a good indicator of adequate circulatory status. A target is 0.5 ml of urine production per kg per hour for adults, with an upper limit of 1 ml per kg per hour. This should be doubled for infants. Children will also require maintenance fluids and a standard regimen should be used. Fluid input should be reduced if urine output exceeds these parameters.

Larger deep burns can lead to loss of circulating red cells. Blood product transfusion may be necessary, but care should be taken to ensure a low measured hemoglobin concentration is not simply dilutional.

Close monitoring of the patient is essential. Accurate measuring and recording of hourly fluid input and output must be performed along with pulse rate and blood pressure. The results must be acted on and fluid administration rates adjusted each hour according to the previous hour's figures. Where possible, blood samples should be taken at least every 6 hours in the first 24 hours, or more frequently if indicated, to measure hemoglobin, hematocrit, electrolyte, and blood gas values.

Even with large volumes of fluid administered, some patients will not maintain adequate essential organ perfusion. It has been a general finding that inexperienced clinicians respond to this by increasing fluid input, with the damaging consequences of excessive generalized edema[15]. The required level of sophisticated critical care interventions to give a realistic chance of survival from complex burn injury may well exceed both the clinician's skills set and the equipment available. In these situations, it is pragmatic to delay further surgery for at least 48 hours and, using the capability available, establish if the patient will survive the physiological insult.

Several decades of experience with returning severely burn-injured USA service personnel to continental USA for definitive care has shown that burn-injured casualties tolerate long-distance aeromedical transfer satisfactorily if carried out within the first week[16].

Further Surgical Interventions

Ideally, the role of a field hospital should be to stabilize patients sufficiently so they can be transferred on for definitive care. There are circumstances where the only source of definitive care is at the field hospital. For burn injury, this will entail healing the burn wound.

The standard approach by most expert burn services in developed health systems is to make an accurate diagnosis of burn depth. Burns that are considered likely to heal in less than two weeks are treated with a dressing regimen. Burns that are deeper will be excised within the first 24–48 hours and appropriate reconstructive methods employed[17]. In the absence of experience and resources sufficient to follow this approach, an alternative is to use dressings for two weeks and then to embark on surgical excision and skin grafting of what has not healed in that time.

To further minimize the impact on resources and the patient's physiology, surgery should performed in short controlled sessions rather than trying to deal with a large burn wound in a single operation. Excising and grafting an area no larger than 10% TBSA at a time is widely accepted as optimal for nonexpert teams. A further limit is the availability of autologous skin. Meshed autologous split skin graft will cover approximately 40% TBSA. To achieve cover of burns larger than this requires skills such as being able to reharvest donor sites and widely (> 3:1) meshing the skin.

Once a skin graft has taken, it is highly desirable for there to be ongoing scar management to reduce the chances of later scar contractures. If definitive burn surgery it to be undertaken, access to appropriate rehabilitation services should be ensured.

References

1. Wong EG, Trelles M, Dominguez L, et al. Surgical skills needed for humanitarian missions in resource-limited settings: common operative procedures performed at Médecins Sans Frontières facilities. *Surgery* 2014: **156**(3): 642–9.

2. Stewart BT, Trelles M, Dominguez L, et al. Surgical burn care by Médecins Sans Frontières-Operations Center Brussels: 2008 to 2014. *Journal of Burn Care & Research* 2016: **37**(6): e516–e24.

3. Spinella PC, Borgman MA, Azarow KS. Pediatric trauma in an austere combat environment. *Critical Care Medicine* 2008: **36**(7 Suppl): S293–6.

4. Gomez M, Cartotto R, Knighton J, Smith K, Fish JS. Improved survival following thermal injury in adult patients treated at a regional burn center. *Journal of Burn Care & Research* 2008: **29**(1): 130–7.

5. Roberts MJ, Fox MA, Hamilton-Davies C, Dowson S. The experience of the intensive care unit in a British Army field hospital during the 2003 Gulf conflict. *Journal of the Royal Army Medical Corps* 2003: **149**(4): 284–90.

6. Alvarado R, Chung KK, Cancio LC, Wolf SE. Burn resuscitation. *Burns* 2009: **35**: 4–14.

7. Peck M, Jeng J, Moghazy A. Burn resuscitation in the austere environment. *Critical Care Clinics* 2016: **32**(4): 561–5.

8. Walker PF, Buehner MF, Wood LA, et al. Diagnosis and management of inhalation injury: an updated review. *Critical Care* 2015: **19**: 351.

9. Wood FM, Phillips M, Jovic T, et al. Water first aid is beneficial in humans post-burn: evidence from a bi-national cohort study. *PLOS One* 2016: **11**(1): e0147259.

10. Smith JJ, Scerri GV, Malyon AD, Burge TS. Comparison of serial halving and rule of nines as a pre-hospital assessment tool. *Emergency Medicine Journal* 2002: **19** (Suppl): A66.

11. Bacomo FK, Chung KK. A primer on burn resuscitation. *Journal of Emergencies, Trauma, and Shock* 2011: **4**(1): 109–13.

12. Barnes J, Duffy A, Hamnett N, et al. The Mersey burns app: evolving a model of validation. *Emergency Medicine Journal* 2015: **32**(8): 637–41.

13. Chung KK, Wolf SE, Cancio LC, et al. Resuscitation of severely burned military casualties: fluid begets more fluid. *The Journal of Trauma and Acute Care Surgery* 2009: **67**: 231–7.

14. Raff T, Hartmann B, Germann G. Early intragastric feeding of seriously burned and long-term ventilated patients: a review of 55 patients. *Burns* 1997: **23**(1): 19–25.

15. Cartotto R, Zhou A. Fluid creep: the pendulum hasn't swung back yet! *Journal of Burn Care & Research* 2010: **31**(4): 551–8.

16. Renz EM, Cancio LC, Barillo DJ, et al. Long range transport of war-related burn casualties. *The Journal of Trauma and Acute Care Surgery* 2008: **64**(2 Suppl): S136–44.

17. Ong YS, Samuel M, Song C. Meta-analysis of early excision of burns. *Burns* 2006: **32**: 145–50.

Obstetrics and Gynecology in a Field Hospital

Avi Abargel and Shir Dar

Introduction

A field hospital can be deployed in many different scenarios. The needs are different in different scenarios and the field-hospital design should be modular, flexible, and "tailored" to meet the specific needs of the current mission.

Nevertheless, the inclusion of an obstetrics and gynecology team in a humanitarian mission will serve a crucial role in saving lives, bringing new lives to the disaster area, giving some comfort and hope for a better future to the affected population, and as a source of comfort to the field hospital staff.

Several studies have shown that males and females are affected differently by natural disasters due to biologic, social, cultural, and reproductive health differences. The average female:male death ratio is 3:1 in natural disaster areas[1]; 75% of most refugee populations are women and children including 30% adolescents. Out of the female population, 25% are in the reproductive stage of their lives (age 15–45) and 20% of them are pregnant[2,3]. While as many as 10% of natural-disaster victims seeking medical assistance may need an obstetrician or gynecologist[4], these needs are not usually given high selection priority [5], whereupon rescue teams are likely to lack those essential specialists.

In developing countries, it is customary for women with uncomplicated pregnancies not to seek medical support and to deliver without the aid of formal medical facilities; in Haiti, for example, only 25% of the deliveries are performed in medical institutions or under some other formal medical care. It is therefore not surprising that a field hospital with a gynecological team quickly becomes a referral center for other medical teams in the affected area, and approximately 50% of the cases the Israel Defense Forces (IDF) hospital gynecological team encountered in Haiti were complicated deliveries[6]. All these facts strengthen the need for experienced obstetrics and gynecology personnel to be included in international rescue team efforts and the need to ensure that they are provided with the necessary supplies to perform both routine and difficult deliveries.

The Effect of Earthquakes on Pregnancy Outcomes

An increase in miscarriages, premature deliveries, intrauterine growth restriction, and low birth weight infants has been reported following natural disasters[7]. Furthermore, increased seismic activity may increase delivery rate and preterm births up to 48 hours following an earthquake. A significantly higher rate of premature births was reported over a seven-month period in the wake of the 2007 earthquake in Japan[8].

Tan and colleagues compared 6638 pre-earthquake and 6365 post-earthquake newborns after a major earthquake in Wenchuan, China, in 2008. Those authors reported lower birth weights and low Apgar scores in the post-earthquake group. The ratio of preterm birth post-earthquake (7.41%) to pre-earthquake (5.63%) was statistically significant[9]. It is therefore not surprising that 5 of 16 (31.25%) deliveries at the IDF hospital in Haiti were preterm, compared to the much lower reported preterm delivery rate of 14.1% (WHO report)[10]. Tocolytic treatment, steroids (for lung maturity), specific antibiotics, and neonatal intensive care units (NICUs) should be included as part of the disaster rescue team's equipment to treat preterm deliveries.

Psychological Aspects of Earthquakes on Pregnant Women

Depression and post-traumatic stress disorder (PTSD) have been reported[11,12]. These could be related to the psychological burden imposed by the natural disaster forced displacement. In their systematic review, Harville and colleagues concluded that disasters of various types could impact maternal mental health, and that these mental-health issues need to be addressed either by psychologists if present or otherwise by the obstetrics and gynecology team[13].

The Obstetrics and Gynecology Team

Personnel

The composition of the team should be determined by the nature of the expected work at the disaster site.

Most of the surgeries performed in a field hospital, which is usually operational at the disaster area 80–120 hours after the earthquake, are orthopedic, and usually are semielective in nature and will occupy most of the operating room time. Conversely, the majority of cesarean sections in a disaster area will be urgent (the indications for cesarean sections will be discussed later in this chapter), resulting in the need to perform them independently. Therefore, our recommendation is to include at least two well-trained gynecologists,

but preferably three, along with one midwife and three nurses.

The Facility (figs. 20.1, 20.2, 20.3)

The Ob/Gyn domain should include a triage area, a hospitalization area, and a labor and delivery room; usually in three connected tents or rooms with an offered total dimension of 5–6 × 12 m (60–72 m²).

The triage and an examination tent/area (5–6 m × 3 m) should be equipped with a reception desk and a computer, a gynecological examination chair, and portable ultrasound.

The short-stay area should have room for 6–8 beds and cribs for postpartum/postsurgery patients (5–6 m over 6 m).

The labor and delivery tent/room (5–6 m over 3 m) should be equipped with a gynecological chair and a cardiotocograph (a fetal heartrate monitor and uterine contractions monitor), a newborn warmer, and all the equipment needed for the anesthesiologist to perform an epidural or spinal analgesia for vaginal delivery or cesarean sections. One should bear in mind that a cesarean section could be performed in this room if an emergency surgery is indicated and the operating room (OR) is occupied.

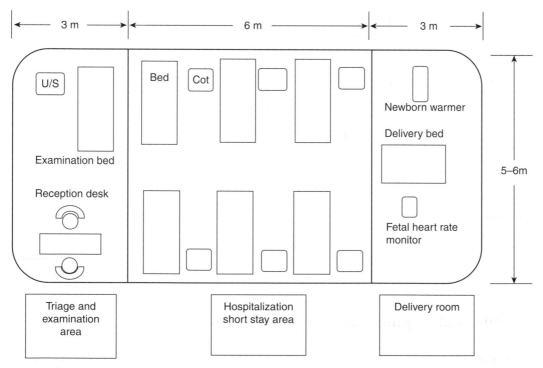

Figure 20.1 Obstetric ward layout

206

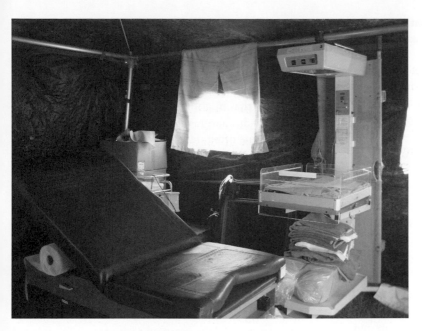

Figure 20.2 Labor and delivery tent

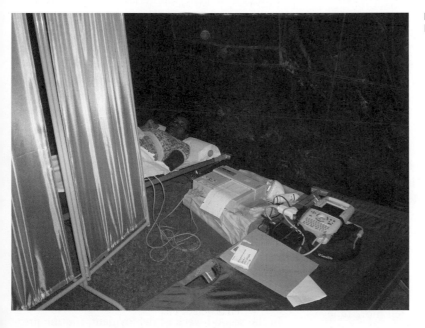

Figure 20.3 Monitoring active labor in hospitalization tent

Emergency Medical Team (EMT) Type 2: Inpatient Surgical Emergency Care

These teams have staff to provide inpatient acute care, and to perform general and obstetric surgery for trauma and other major conditions.

The team can perform a cesarean section, but the surgery is often performed by a general surgeon and not by Ob/Gyn specialists.

The nurses are ICU nurses and midwives are lacking. To allow at least some basic obstetrical care abilities, a type 2 EMT should include a surgeon who can perform a cesarean section and dilatation and curettage (D&C), and a nurse that can manage a vaginal delivery (preferably a midwife).

Those teams should have sets of surgical instruments for at least one cesarean section and one D&C.

Moreover, since these teams lack the ability to treat premature neonates, pregnant women with suspected preterm labor when the fetal estimated birth weight is less than 2000 g should not be treated in a type 2 EMT and should be transferred to a local hospital or to EMTs that have NICU capabilities.

Predeployment Planning

There are several major differences in patient management between a field hospital and a conventional facility:

1. Scarce resources limit the access to the OR and monitors
2. Lack of adequate hygienic environment may increase risk of infection
3. Limited number of hospitalization beds (shortens the stay after labor and surgery)
4. Many patients have no home to go back to, and forced to stay out on the street to recover
5. Lack of continuous medical follow-up

Cesarean section indications and considerations will differ from the typical paradigm and force the team to perform a cesarean section only when it is absolutely necessary.

1. Breech presentation: fetuses with expected birth weight 3700 g or less are to be delivered vaginally (provided there is a trained physician)
2. Intermittent fetal heart rate (FHR) monitoring: with only one FHR monitor, monitoring has to be carried out intermittently, with a higher tolerance to variable deceleration leading to a cesarean section
3. Managing the delivery according to the wellbeing of the woman and fetus and not strictly according to Freidman's curve, allowing women more time to deliver to avoid an unnecessary cesarean section as long as the FHR is normal
4. Ability to perform a cesarean section in the delivery room due to fact that all the cesarean sections are urgent and the OR may be unavailable due to the severe overload of trauma patients
5. Women after cesarean section should stay in the field hospital for three days

Predeployment Planning: Normal Vaginal Delivery

1. Managing the labor up to full dilation in the short-stay tent, preserving the delivery room for urgent cases that might appear without any notice
2. Early discharge: due to lack of sufficient beds, patients often need to be discharged prematurely; women after normal vaginal delivery should stay in the field hospital 6–8 hours or overnight
3. Intermittent FHR monitoring

The IDF Experience in the Field Hospital in Haiti

A total of 24 pregnant women sought medical care; none of whom had received routine prenatal care. There were 16 deliveries: 13 were vaginal births (including two twin deliveries) and three were cesarean sections. All the cesarean sections were performed in the delivery tent since the OR tent was occupied with other emergency surgeries. All three caesarian sections were urgent.

The first case was a case of premature rapture of membranes with umbilical cord prolapse. The second was a case of eclampsia and late decelerations on fetal monitoring, which necessitated an emergency cesarean section. The third case was a case of dying fetus with severe bradycardia and an estimated fetal weight of 980 g. He suffered severe fetal distress and died 15 minutes after birth.

Of the 16 delivered women, 8 (50%) had pre-eclampsia. There were 5 (31.25%) preterm deliveries at 30–32 weeks' gestation, and the newborns weighed between 980 g and 1700 g. There were two manual removals of the placenta.

The team also provided routine prenatal and gynecological care; the latter included two urgent gynecological procedures, vaginal-wall repair after pelvic fracture, D&C for severe perimenopausal bleeding, and 2 D&Cs for missed abortion.

In the second week of deployment, routine pregnancy follow-up care was provided, and minor gynecological problems were treated.

The IDF Experience in Japan Following the 2011 Tsunami

The large hospitals outside the disaster area continued to work and serve as a medical backup for the victims and, as a result, all the complicated patients and all the deliveries were treated there. The IDF team was asked to reach out to the pregnant survivors in the neighborhoods. A team consisted of an obstetrician with a portable ultrasound, an IDF midwife, and a local midwife. They visited the pregnant women and reassured them by offering examinations and ultrasound scans.

There were 20 pregnant women who were treated; 18 of whom received home care. All 20 underwent physical exams and ultrasound examinations, and two were found to require hospitalization (one with chronic hypertension and moyamoya disease and the other with suspected intrauterine growth restriction).

The IDF Experience in Nepal Following the 2015 Earthquake

In Nepal, the field hospital was adjacent to the military hospital in Kathmandu.

Since the ORs in the hospital were totally devoted to trauma patients, gynecologic procedures were performed in the field hospital, but part of the triage was done at the other facilities.

Medications and Medical Equipment

In organizing and deploying a concerted foreign medical-aid rescue effort, there is an inevitable cost–benefit conflict between the need to supply as much equipment as possible to maximize potential aid and the need to minimize both the expenditure and the bulk of shipment to be transported to the destination. While participating in the IDF hospital relief efforts in Haiti and Japan, it was the chapter authors' experience that there is little hope of obtaining additional supplies once the rescue team arrives at the devastated area. Without proper supplies and equipment, foreign-aid rescue teams are forced to improvise and contend with the lack of certain medications. It is thus vital to make every effort to anticipate as thoroughly as possible what will be the most essential medical needs of the specific population and to plan accordingly. In addition, packaging and storage must be thought out carefully for maximum exploitation of minimal transport space. The following are some examples of the challenges faced by the IDF field hospital's Ob/Gyn teams deployed in Haiti and Japan, arising from the lack of proper or sufficient medication:

- $MgSO^4$. Before the departure of the Haiti deployment, it was anticipated that the local population would have a high incidence of gestational hypertension and preeclampsia, but the extent to which these conditions were prevalent was highly underestimated. The supply of $MgSO^4$ was thus depleted after the first week.
- Oxytocin. On arriving in Port-au-Prince, it emerged that oxytocin had not been included among the supplies and it could not be found among the other medical teams in the area. Oxytocin was eventually discovered in a nearby Italian monastery (where the nuns presumably used it to assist women in childbirth).
- Vitamin K. This is not part of a regular medication arsenal and so it was not included. A three-day-old Haitian newborn was found to have massive rectal bleeding and was diagnosed as most likely suffering from hemorrhagic disease. Due to the absence of vitamin K, the newborn received a lifesaving blood transfusion from one of the IDF hospital physicians whose blood type was O negative.
- Steroids (for lung maturation in premature neonates). Given that preterm deliveries may occur more often due to natural disasters, betamethasone or dexamethasone should be included in the list of medications.

A list of recommended essential equipment and medications for Ob/Gyn relief teams, based on the chapter authors' experience in Haiti and Japan, is provided in Tables 20.1–3.

Ethical Issues

When operating in a disaster area, foreign-aid relief teams will inevitably confront unique ethical dilemmas; often arising from insufficient medical resources[13]. For example, prematurity became a major challenge with respect to resource utilization. It is clear that, with such limited resources, not every victim in need would be able to receive the necessary treatment. The quandary of whether to impose a minimum weight threshold for preterm infants to receive treatment is an ethical issue which Ob/Gyn teams operating in natural-disaster conditions should be prepared to deal with[14].

The survival rates of low birth weight infants delivered in a natural disaster area are dramatically diminished. Keeping in mind that the resources are extremely limited, Ob/Gyn teams operating in such areas are challenged to make difficult decisions in light of these shortcomings.

Table 20.1 Recommended essential equipment for Ob/Gyn relief teams

Item	Quantity
Ultrasound with vaginal and abdominal probe	1
Ultrasound printer	1
Fetal Doppler	1
FHR/contractions monitor	1
Manual vacuum extractor ("KIWI")	1+5
Delivery sets	50
Sponge holder	10
Portable IV pump/automatic syringe	2
Metal bivalve specula; different sizes	30
Tenacula	4
D&C set	1
Thermometers	5
Blood-pressure monitors	2
Gynecological chair	2
Gynecological lamp	2
Cesarean section sets	2
Episiotomy sets	2
Epidural sets	30
Curtains	6
Paper cover for bed	10
Cribs	5
Baby heater	1
Infant clothes	10
Baby blankets	6

In the IDF field hospital in Haiti, ad hoc ethical committees were established to resolve these complex ethical dilemmas (see Chapter 32) [13].

The Minimum Initial Services Package (MISP)[15]

The MISP for reproductive health is a coordinated set of priority activities designed to prevent and manage the consequences of sexual violence, reduce HIV transmission, prevent excess maternal and neonatal mortality and morbidity, and plan for comprehensive reproductive-health services in the early days and weeks of an emergency.

It is mandatory to report suspected cases of sexual violence to the local authorities or EMTCC/health cluster.

Summary

It is impractical to craft a single design for any and all international medical-aid disaster-relief team efforts. Each relief plan will be formed by a myriad of factors, including the magnitude of the natural disaster, its geographic location, the predisaster infrastructure, the phase of the relief operation (i.e., how many days after the disaster the team arrives), and what other teams and facilities are operational. Notwithstanding, the following are some identifiable lessons learned by the IDF hospital's Ob/Gyn relief teams deployed in Haiti and Japan.

Table 20.2 Recommended medications for Ob/Gyn relief teams

Medication	Quantity	Medication	Quantity
Oxytocin ampoules 10 U/ml	50	Amoxicillin/clavulanate tabs	200
Methylergonovine maleate ampoules 0.2 mg	30	Amoxicillin/clavulanate IV	60
Meperidine hydrochloride 10% ampoules	20	Doxycycline tabs 100 mg	100
Promethazine ampoules 25 mg	100	Ciprofloxacin tablets	200
Glycerin suppositories 2 g	400	Ciprofloxacin IV ampoules	200
Magnesium sulfate 10 mg ampoules	10	Metronidazole 500 mg tablets	100
Clotrimazole cream 1%	20	Contraceptive pills (21 pills)	50
Clotrimazole vaginal suppository 0.5 g	60	Naproxen 500 mg tablets	1800
Diflucan 150 mg tablets	20	Acyclovir cream 5% tube	10
Metronidazole gel 0.75%	20	Rho(D) immune globulin 300 µg	10
Estrogen 100 mg tabs	210	Ampicillin IV/IM 1 g	30
Medroxyprogesterone 5 mg	200	Nifedipine 20 mg tablets	80
Indomethacin suppository 100 mg	40		

Table 20.3 Recommended disposables for Ob/Gyn relief teams

Item	Quantity
Ultrasound gel tubes	10
Covers for vaginal probes	100
Large disposable specula	50
Medium disposable specula	50
Small disposable specula	20
Sterile and nonsterile surgical gloves	100
Urinary pregnancy kits	100
Umbilical clamps	20
Nitrazine swabs	20
Amniotic hooks	2
Single-use catheters	20
Urinometers	5
Infusion kit	30
Catheter kit	10

Table 20.4 MISP objectives and activities

1. Identify an organization(s) and individual(s) to facilitate the coordination and implementation of the MISP by:
   - ensuring the overall reproductive health coordinator is in place and functioning under the health coordination team
   - ensuring reproductive health focal points in camps and implementing agencies are in place
   - making available materials for implementing the MISP and ensuring their use

2. Prevent sexual violence and provide appropriate assistance to survivors by:
   - ensuring systems are in place to protect displaced populations, particularly women and girls, from sexual violence
   - ensuring medical services, including psychosocial support, are available for survivors of sexual violence

3. Reduce transmission of HIV by:
   - enforcing respect for universal precautions
   - guaranteeing the availability of free condoms
   - ensuring that blood for transfusion is safe

4. Prevent excess maternal and neonatal mortality and morbidity by:
   - providing clean delivery kits to all visibly pregnant women and birth attendants to promote clean home deliveries
   - providing midwife delivery kits (UNICEF or equivalent) to facilitate clean and safe deliveries at the health facility
   - initiating the establishment of a referral system to manage obstetric emergencies

5. Plan for the provision of comprehensive reproductive health services, integrated into primary health care (PHC), as the situation permits by:
   - collecting basic background information identifying sites for future delivery of comprehensive reproductive health services
   - assessing staff and identifying training protocols
   - identifying procurement channels and assessing monthly drug consumption

1. In mass natural disasters, an Ob/Gyn team is invaluable and serves as a beacon of hope to the disaster victims, even if its resources are scarce.
2. The mix of cases that the Ob/Gyn team will confront requires that they are specialists who are prepared to treat mostly complicated cases and be trained in dealing with emergencies in a suboptimal environment.
3. The delivery "suite" should be prepared for emergent cesarean sections, partly to avoid the need to transfer the woman in labor to an OR, which may or may not be immediately available.
4. Once the Ob/Gyn team has arrived at the disaster zone, the likelihood of readily obtaining additional equipment and medications is low. The team should therefore prepare a sufficient inventory of supplies in advance (Table 20.1).
5. An outreach Ob/Gyn team with a portable mobile ultrasound, including vaginal and abdominal probes, can detect problematic pregnancies and bring enormous psychological comfort to pregnant victims who are unable to reach the hospital.
6. Ob/Gyn teams working in postdisaster areas will confront a higher than usual number of preterm babies. Preparations for treating extreme prematurity should be made before the team arrives at the disaster zone.
7. Medical personnel may be overwhelmed in a mass natural disaster situation where intensive care resources are extremely limited. The medical staff may have no choice but to deal with ethical issues in determining how limited resources, such as NICU beds, will be distributed. Medical ethics discussion sessions are essential to prepare the relief teams for dealing with these and other ethical issues that will inevitably arise.
8. Ob/Gyn teams treating pregnant women under natural-disaster conditions should be especially sensitive to the catastrophic environment's impact on maternal mental health.
9. The most experienced professionals among the volunteers should be chosen, and predicted

scenarios and solutions should be analyzed before departure for optimal team preparation.

10. The team must be briefed by someone knowledgeable about local cultural sensitivities and taboos, and they must take great care not to inadvertently offend the female patient or her family.

References

1. Carballo M, Daita S, Hernandez M. Impact of the tsunami on healthcare systems. *Journal of the Royal Society of Medicine* 2005: **98**: 390–5.

2. Reproductive health care, in *Public health guide in emergencies*. Second edn. The Johns Hopkins and Red Cross Red Crescent; 2008: 136–197

3. Cooperative for Assistance and Relief Everywhere Inc. Moving from emergency response to comprehensive reproductive health programs: a modular training series. Washington, DC: CARE; 2002.

4. Bar-Dayan Y, Beard P, Mankuta D, Finestone A, Wolf Y, Gruzman C, et al. An earthquake disaster in Turkey: an overview of the experience of the Israeli Defense Forces field hospital in Adapazari. *Disasters* 2000: **24**: 262–70.

5. Nour NN. Maternal health considerations during disaster relief. *Expert Review of Obstetrics & Gynecology* 2011: **4**: 22–7.

6. Pinkert M, Dar S, Goldberg D, et al. Lessons learned from an obstetrics and gynecology field hospital response to natural disasters. *Obstetrics & Gynecology* 2013: **122**: 532–6.

7. Weissman A, Siegler E, Neiger R, Jakobi P, Zimmer EZ. The influence of increased seismic activity on pregnancy outcome. *European Journal of Obstetrics & Gynecology and Reproductive Biology* 1989: **31**: 233–6.

8. Sekizuka N, Sakai A, Aoyama K, Kohama T, Nakahama Y, Fujita S, et al. Association between the incidence of premature rupture of membranes in pregnant women and seismic intensity of the Noto Peninsula earthquake. *Environmental Health and Preventive Medicine* 2010: **15**: 292–8.

9. Tan CE, Li HJ, Zhang XG, Zhang H, Han PY, An Q, et al. The impact of the Wenchuan earthquake on birth outcomes. *PLOS One* 2009: **4**: e8200.

10. Hibino Y, Takaki J, Kambayashi Y, Hitomi Y, Sakai A, Sekizuka N, et al. Health impact of disaster-related stress on pregnant women living in the affected area of the Noto Peninsula earthquake in Japan. *Psychiatry and Clinical Neurosciences* 2009: **63**: 107–15.

11. Harville E, Xiong X, Buekens P. Disasters and perinatal health: a systematic review. *Obstetrical & Gynecological Survey* 2010: **65**: 713–28.

12. Chang HL, Chang TC, Lin TY, Kuo SS. Psychiatric morbidity and pregnancy outcome in a disaster area of Taiwan 921 earthquake. *Psychiatry and Clinical Neurosciences* 2002: **56**: 139–44.

13. Merin O, Ash N, Levy G, Schwaber MJ, Kreiss Y. The Israeli field hospital in Haiti – ethical dilemmas in early disaster response. *The New England Journal of Medicine* 2010: **362**: e38.

14. Ytzhak A, Sagi R, Bader T, Assa A, Farfel A, Merin O, et al. Pediatric ventilation in a disaster: clinical and ethical decision making. *Critical Care Medicine* 2012: **40**: 603–7.

15. Women's Commission for Refugee Women and Children (WCRWC). Field-friendly guide to integrate emergency obstetric care in humanitarian programs. New York: WCRWC; 2005: 84.

Chapter

21

Otolaryngology and Maxillofacial Surgery in a Field Hospital

Tal Marom, Haim Lavon, and Ariel Hirschhorn

Introduction

A field hospital is usually deployed to areas severely affected by natural disasters, in which local health-care systems would usually exhaust their resources, and would greatly benefit from any outside assistance. Maxillofacial and otolaryngology surgeons and head-and-neck (H&N) surgeons play a vital role in such field medical units due to their expertise in caring for acute trauma-care patients and treating emergent life-threatening conditions (i.e., airway injuries and H&N infections). In addition, field hospitals that arrive far beyond the "golden hour" of trauma are expected to treat daily routine H&N diseases that may exacerbate following the disaster, rather than focus only on trauma-related injuries.

Organization

Transport payload planning dictates which personnel and equipment will be eventually loaded onboard. Since space is limited, the exact surgical equipment and quantities will be determined by the hospital's general director, according to the expected burden of casualties and their nature[1]. Those unique logistic features are covered in other chapters. Consequently, the H&N surgeon should expect a suboptimal "surgical wish list" as the least important items, such as the otological microscope or endoscopic surgical set, are not likely to be available. The H&N surgeon should prioritize his or her designated surgical equipment in advance. Table 21.1 lists the recommended equipment for the H&N surgeon.

The main surgical focus and capabilities of the field hospital are procedures performed by general and orthopedic surgeons such as laparotomies and fracture fixations[2]. Therefore, the integration of other surgical disciplines is challenging in certain aspects. H&N surgeries are not routinely prioritized and assigned to specific time slots in the OR. Most of these surgeries can be regarded as nonurgent, semielective operations. In addition, these surgeries are time consuming, due to unique features of this body area, dealing with complex anatomy, aesthetic aspects, and the challenges of anesthesia.

Table 21.1 Recommended essential equipment for the H&N surgeon

Disposable materials

- sterile and nonsterile gloves
- drapes
- scrubs
- face masks
- scrub hats
- surgical gowns
- antiseptic solutions
- tongue depressors
- various materials for packing (including cotton wool and wicks)
- hemostatic agents and suturing
- swabs for cultures (if available)

Nondisposable tools

- headlamp
- portable otoscope
- forceps: Bayonet, Debakey, Brown–Adson, curved hemostatic mosquito forceps
- otologic instruments (ear speculum in different sizes, alligator forceps, microsuction tubes and adapter, hooks, curettes, cerumen irrigation tools, 512/1024 Hz tuning forks)
- nasal instruments (nasal speculum in different sizes, Baron or Ferguson–Frazier suction tubes, silver nitrate caustic pencils)
- laryngeal mirrors
- foreign-body loops
- abscess drainage kits
- percutaneous tracheostomy sets
- versatile fixation set
- globe protector
- Raney clips
- container for disposable medical sharps

Medications

- local anesthetic medications (including topical lidocaine spray)
- antibiotic agents in syrups, suspensions, and tablets: amoxicillin, amoxicillin–clavulanate, first- and second-generation cephalosporins, quinolones
- ear drops containing antibiotics, with or without steroids

Surgical personnel will be assigned to a general surgical department responsible for the surgical complex. Due to the limited number of surgical staff and the expected high volume of patients, H&N surgeons are expected to assist as scrubbed personnel in other surgeries while not operating. Hospitalized patients from all disciplines are admitted into mixed wards, which mandates meticulous follow-up by their surgeons.

If feasible, the location of the field hospital should be adjacent to a local hospital or clinic as it enables the use of local advanced resources if absent, or when the local resources are superior to the ones brought by the field hospital (e.g., a CT scanner for delineating maxillofacial or neck injuries, or an audiology clinic for assessment of hearing loss before treatment is planned).

Trauma

Facial injuries are incapacitating, and can cause major sequelae, including impaired perception, aesthetic disfigurement, and functional debilitation. Patients who require craniofacial surgery will usually need complex craniofacial reconstruction[3], which can pose a major challenge in a field hospital (Table 21.2).

In this setting, these operations are usually longer in their duration, compared to the regular hospital setting, due to several factors:

1. *Surgical staff*: the staff is usually composed of a leading H&N surgeon, surgical assistants, and an OR nurse; the latter two often not acquainted with such surgeries.
2. *OR setting*: the lack of specialized specific surgical instruments in the field hospital armamentarium may necessitate improvisation and adjustment of basic surgical instruments. When planned, and brought along, delicate surgical instruments such as suction tips, forceps, and sutures can be helpful in carrying out surgeries in the H&N region.
3. *Patient factors*: since every natural disaster is unique and they occur in different geographic locations, the surgeon should be acquainted with prevalent conditions in the disaster area; for example, submucosal fibrosis in Southeast Asia can adversely affect wound healing.

The mandible and the orbit are the most commonly involved in natural-disaster H&N trauma[4]. Hence, securing an airway tract and treating orbital injuries are the most important issues to be addressed, along with treatment and care of other facial skeleton fractures and soft-tissue injuries. The surgeon should opt for an immediate, definitive surgical correction of these fractures. Delayed reconstruction requires advanced equipment, augments the complexity of the operation, and usually will not be feasible in this type of setting.

The recommended treatment sequence must adhere to the advanced trauma life support (ATLS) protocol: gain control of the airway, gain control of any bleeding source, establish the state of consciousness, diagnose and treat any concomitant brain injuries, and carry out facial reconstruction.

Craniofacial reconstruction surgery requires establishing a wide surgical field, which enables exact visualization and exploration of fractures, precise fracture reduction, placement of internal rigid fixators, use of bone autografts, and treatment of soft-tissue injuries. Achieving the best aesthetic and functional results greatly depends on the use of internal rigid fixation materials and the use of bone autografts. However, the surgeon should balance aesthetic requirements against subjecting the patient to a double-site operation in such a suboptimal setting.

The surgical treatment must reconstruct the three-dimensional structure of the face – height or verticality, width and depth – restoring the aesthetic and functional pre-trauma status. This constitutes considerable challenges for the reconstructive surgeon in both planning treatment and surgical techniques. Usually panfacial fractures constitute a challenge for the reconstructive surgeon who not only should act as a surgeon but also as a leader of an interdisciplinary team composed of intensivists, neurosurgeons, ophthalmic surgeons, prosthetic dentists, and others. In the field-hospital setting, some of the abovementioned professionals will probably be absent, and the surgeon should conduct the surgery in a manner that will enable staged functional reconstruction later[5].

Table 21.2 Duration of facial surgeries in the Israel Defense Forces (IDF) field hospital, Nepal 2015 Gorkha earthquake

Diagnosis	Average duration of surgery
Compound zygomatic complex fracture	4 hours
Mandibular symphysis and angle fracture	5 hours
Nasoorbitalethmoid fracture, Le Fort type II fracture, maxillary midsplit	7 hours
Orbital rim fracture	1.5 hours

An important issue is the perioperative antibiotic coverage needed. In a regular hospital setting, H&N surgeries usually require coverage of Gram-positive cocci, such as *Staphylococci* and *Streptococci*. Yet, at a disaster scene, the pathogens may be different. For example, in an earthquake setting, the prevalent pathogens were reported to be Gram-negative *Enterobacteria*, originating from water and soil pollutions. Consulting with an infectious-disease specialist regarding the antibiotic coverage is recommended.

Pediatric patients will also present at the field hospital. The surgeon should always bear in mind the unique features of the pediatric population (e.g., greenstick fractures) and provide the best treatment (which can be nonsurgical), without compromising future growth and development of the facial skeleton. However, this more conservative treatment usually necessitates a prolonged follow-up period, which is not always feasible in these settings.

Delayed arrival of trauma patients to a properly equipped facility is characteristic of disaster scenarios. Unlike the usual medical route, where patients typically present minutes to hours after injury, in disaster situations, patients may arrive days afterwards; some partially treated and some not treated at all. Hence, the field hospital's H&N surgeon may encounter pathologies rarely seen in a regular hospital. Examples from the field hospital in Haiti included various foreign bodies, including concrete and wall-plaster remnants within deep lacerated wounds, soft-tissue necrosis, osteomyelitis in the H&N region in young and otherwise healthy patients, and even deep wounds with secondary healing processes, which concealed proper anatomical view during reconstruction.

Airway Management

H&N surgeries occasionally involve airway-management issues. The shortage in resources, such as OR time, intensive care unit (ICU) beds, and sometimes even a highly-trained anesthesiologist, dictates the careful planning of many of the operations, which need to be well synchronized with the corresponding surgical and anesthesiology departments.

In a mass-casualty disaster scenario, acute trauma-care patients presenting with major airway problems would either have their acute problem solved by the local medical personnel or die of their injury, if untreated. Hence, the H&N surgeon is expected to face three essential dilemmas concerning airway management: the "difficult airway anesthesia," delayed

postoperative extubation, and scheduling a planned, semielective tracheostomy for prolonged intraoral intubated ICU patients.

Maxillofacial surgeries, with an emphasis on trauma patients, often present with a "difficult airway anesthesia." While these injuries can be regarded as life-threatening situations, their management exploits important resources such as prolonged OR time and highly-trained anesthesiology personnel who may work elsewhere. To reduce the probability of unexpected events that may interrupt the hospital's coordinated team work, each H&N surgery should be considered a potentially "difficult airway anesthesia" surgery. This mandates the assignment of appropriate personnel, equipment, and time planning in the surgical log.

Similar dilemmas arise with the postsurgery extubation phase. Some of these surgeries eventually end up with the decision to extubate the patient later to keep a secure airway until the upper airway edema subsides or is ruled out. This requires the allocation of an ICU bed, a critical resource, for an OR-recovery alongside other critically injured and ill patients. This scenario is exacerbated when the ICU is at its full capacity. Greater awareness and anticipation of such planned or unplanned situations may increase patient safety and minimize the hospital's critical resource exploitation.

Planned tracheostomy is a procedure that aims to exchange ventilation from intraoral intubation to a tracheostomy cannula, which is a common procedure in prolonged ventilated ICU patients. In a field hospital, two major factors should be taken into consideration: (1) The site of operation. As in any regular hospital, transportation to the OR has been shown to increase morbidity, mortality, and ICU stay. In a field hospital, it also necessitates allocating critical OR time for a procedure that could be done elsewhere. For these reasons, proper equipment and ICU setup should be planned and brought along as part of the field hospital. (2) The patient's discharge poses an additional dilemma. In some natural-disaster scenarios, these patients would be discharged to a local hospital or a community-based medical system which is capable of supporting tracheostomy patients. In other situations, proper tracheostomy care is not guaranteed, thus the medical team should consider its decision accordingly, and even cancel the procedure.

H&N Infections

H&N infections require the establishment of airway patency, followed by the early and aggressive surgical drainage of all anatomical spaces affected by abscesses or collections. This sequence has dramatically decreased the mortality rate of H&N infections. Following a natural disaster, treatment of severe infections can be challenging due to the expected load on the local health system, which would normally shift to treating emergent conditions in the first few days following the disaster. This dictates a more aggressive management of H&N infections, due to the difficulty in routine patient evaluation, proper evaluation of host defenses, and the possible shortage of antibiotics.

Unusual severe and life-threatening infections might also be encountered. The H&N surgeon is expected to treat deep fascial space and deep neck infections, fascial hematomas, necrotizing fasciitis, and even osteomyelitis.

Routine, otherwise ordinary H&N infections may pose a dilemma; for example, children presenting with acute otitis media (AOM)[6]. According to the American Academy of Pediatrics guidelines on AOM diagnosis and treatment, antibiotic therapy should be prescribed in certain scenarios, most of them in severe cases, otherwise watchful waiting is recommended[7]. However, the follow-up option is not practical in a field hospital setting. For example, in the field hospital that operated in the Philippines, the chapter authors knew that the AOM burden is high in school-aged Filipino children, the pneumococcal conjugate vaccines were not in common use, and we were also unfamiliar with the incidence of bacterial antibiotic resistance. Consequently, we were more likely to be liberal in our management, and prescribed antibiotic therapy to most children with AOM.

Limitations

When no H&N surgeon is available, some H&N injuries can be treated by a general surgeon; for example, lacerations, control of bleeding, or reduction of nasal bone fractures. In more complex injuries involving the facial skeleton or the deep spaces of the neck, careful exploration can be done by a surgeon who is familiar with the complex neurovascular anatomy. Otherwise, stabilization of the patient and referral to a better equipped medical facility is warranted.

In the chapter authors' experience, we could not optimally handle combined H&N injuries that mandated a multidisciplinary team with surgical abilities beyond the ones available in a field hospital such as patients who needed complex facial reconstruction or free flaps. Also, patients presenting with advanced

H&N tumors to a field hospital should be referred to other facilities, unless a lifesaving (airway protection) or a palliative procedure (drainage of an abscess) can be performed in this setting. Other patients presenting to the field hospital who need elective procedures (e.g., cleft lip/palate, hearing loss) should also be referred elsewhere[8].

Aftermath

The array of physicians with various specialties constitutes the pillar of the advantage of the fully stocked field hospital with its ancillary services. In our experience, the large volume of patients, linguistic gaps, culture differences, complex logistics, and limited resources made the presence of the H&N surgeon extremely valuable. The synergic joint work was productive in terms of facilitating diagnoses, improving decision-making, carrying out surgical procedures, and augmenting the overall response of the field hospital to the disaster.

References

1. Peleg K, Kreiss Y, Ash N, Lipsky AM. Optimizing medical response to large-scale disasters: the ad hoc collaborative health care system. *Annals of Surgery* 2011: **253**(2): 421–3.

2. Kreiss Y, Merin O, Peleg K, et al. Early disaster response in Haiti: the Israeli field hospital experience. *Annals of Internal Medicine* 2010: **153**(1): 45–8.

3. Ray JM, Lindsay RW, Kumar AR. Treatment of earthquake-related craniofacial injuries aboard the USNS Comfort during Operation Unified Response. *Plastic and Reconstructive Surgery* 2010: **126**(6): 2102–8.

4. Tang YL, Zhu GQ, Zhou H, et al. Analysis of 46 maxillofacial fracture victims in the 2008 Wenchuan, China earthquake. *Oral Surgery, Oral Medicine, Oral Pathology, and Oral Radiology* 2009: **108**(5): 673–8.

5. Lin G, Lavon H, Gelfond R, Abargel A, Merin O. Hard times call for creative solutions: medical improvisations at the Israel Defense Forces Field Hospital in Haiti. *American Journal of Disaster Medicine* 2010: **5**(3): 188–92.

6. Marom T, Dagan D, Weiser G, et al. Pediatric otolaryngology in a field hospital in the Philippines. *International Journal of Pediatric Otorhinolaryngology* 2014: **78**(5): 807–11.

7. Lieberthal AS, Carroll AE, Chonmaitree T, et al. The diagnosis and management of acute otitis media. *Pediatrics* 2013 (3): e964–99.

8. Marom T, Segal D, Erlich T, Tsumi E, Merin O, Lin G. Ethical and clinical dilemmas in patients with head and neck tumors visiting a field hospital in the Philippines. *American Journal of Disaster Medicine* 2014: **9**(3): 211–19.

Chapter 22

Ophthalmology in a Field Hospital

Erez Tsumi

Introduction

There are many events that require a field hospital: some are natural disasters while some are human made. Although ocular injuries are not the most common injuries in these incidents, acute eye injuries during a disaster can result in considerable disability and often require the care of an ophthalmologic surgeon. In some areas in the world, especially in developing countries, blindness resulting from untreated eye injury can cause serious economic burden and even the loss of life. This is why the first objective in the management of eye injuries is to save sight and to prevent the progression of conditions that could produce further damage. Field hospitals are deployed most often in countries with low-level medical infrastructure.

This chapter covers the preparation for treating ocular injuries in the field hospital during disasters. The role and the importance of the ophthalmologist during disasters is to provide services for both victims and relief workers during the end of the emergency phase and ongoing rehabilitation. Specific ocular patterns of injury will be described according to the type of the disaster, its geographical area, and the time elapsed from the disaster.

The ophthalmology field is a high-technology area with the need for expensive equipment and therefore is not fully established in developing countries, causing a significant gap between the needs and the treatment capabilities. This gap intensifies during a disaster and dictates the ophthalmologist's work environment and functional capabilities in the field hospital, which are very different to those existing in a hospital in developed countries. For example, there is an absence of diagnostic tools for ocular injuries such as CT or MRI scanners, which are basic tools in modern ophthalmology, as well as more advanced diagnostic tools, such as the fluorescein angiography, optical coherence tomography, and so on.

While in other medical disciplines, basic equipment in the field hospital is sufficient, ocular trauma care relies largely on the OR. The ophthalmology instruments are very advanced and expensive, and include microscope, phaco and vitrectomy machines, and laser. The field hospital is not prepared in terms of equipment and staff, which often dictates "damage-control" treatment in penetrating ocular injuries. After the initial treatment, patients with severe injuries should be transferred to a regular medical center for definitive treatment. This difference between the ocular field and the other medical fields is even greater with the passage of the first wave of trauma victims and the arrival of the patients with chronic ocular problems. The field-hospital resources are limited in those cases, especially for elective eye surgery requiring advanced equipment. This sharp transition between the ophthalmologist's everyday work at his or her hospital and the work at the field hospital is dramatic and therefore requires, first and foremost, a change in mental attitude. This limited framework, beyond the need for a change in mindset, also raises significant ethical questions. However, even with these limitations, the goal of the field hospital remains the provision of optimal care possible under these circumstances.

Understanding the characteristics of ocular injuries during various types of disasters in different geographical areas is important to be able to prepare for them properly, both mentally and practically[1,2]. The type and the location of the disaster dictate the needs of the affected population and the medical mission preparation[3–5].

Epidemiology

The field hospital is usually ready for work a few days after a disaster. As time passes following the disaster, the nature of the referrals to the field hospital changes. Initially, most of the referrals are trauma or disaster related, but later in the deployment the ocular

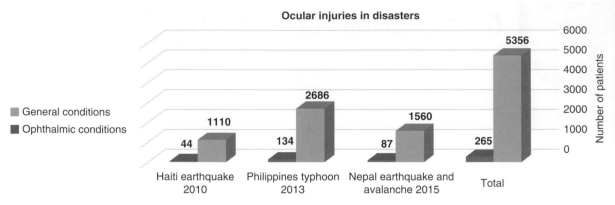

Figure 22.1 Ocular injuries in disasters

problems are chronic conditions such as cataract, pterygium, dry eye, and refractive errors.

The epidemiology of ocular injuries during mass-casualty events differs significantly in terms of extent, type, and severity of the injuries, and depends on the nature of the event and its location. There are differences between the injuries sustained during the various types of disasters, as well as those made by humans. It is vital to understand the characteristics of ocular injuries during various types of disasters in different geographic areas to be able to prepare for them properly[6,7]. The type and the location of the disaster dictate the needs of the affected population and the medical mission's preparation[8–10].

The eyes account for only 0.1% of the total body surface area, yet during an explosion as many as 10% of survivors may suffer eye trauma[11]. On September 11, 2001 – the attacks on the World Trade Center – the incidence rate for ocular injury was higher than any other type of injury, with a rate of 59.7 injuries per 100 worker-years[12]. During some types of disasters, ocular injuries may be among the most commonly encountered morbidities [6–10,13–15].

During three different disasters, the Israeli field hospitals saw a similar rate of ocular injuries: 3.96% at the Haiti earthquake, 4.98% at the Philippines typhoon, and 5.58% at the Nepal earthquake and avalanche (Figure 22.1)[16]. The ocular injuries during disasters can be divided into two main categories: disaster related and nondisaster related, since the ophthalmologist is replacing the basic infrastructures that have been destroyed as a result of the disaster.

The ocular injuries that are typical to disasters are foreign bodies, eyelid laceration, blunt trauma, and penetrating eye injuries[17–21]. The nature of the disaster and its location dictate the type of the acute ocular injuries treated in the field hospitals. There are more ocular foreign bodies and intraocular foreign bodies in urban areas compared to rural areas. Moreover, the kind of natural disaster affects the nature of the injuries: in earthquakes, face and eyelid laceration and ocular blunt trauma are usually the most common due to the collapse of buildings[22]. Typhoons, due to the strong winds, usually cause injuries characterized by ocular foreign bodies, penetrating eye injuries, and blunt trauma (Table 22.1)[23].

The geographical location of the disaster affects the type of chronic ocular problems the field hospital will deal with in the second phase of the nondisaster-related injuries. In the tropical maritime climate with high ultraviolet light exposure (the pterygium belt), cataract and pterygium are the most frequent presenting pathologies[24–26]. In underserved regions suffering from poverty and poor sanitary conditions, acute and chronic conjunctivitis are very common causes for patients to turn to the field hospitals[27].

Although one must suspect ocular injuries when a patient suffers from facial injuries, sometimes the presentation of these conditions can be more subtle, and it is often difficult to diagnose and appropriately triage these ocular conditions during the acute phase [28–30].

Preparing for Disasters

Proper preparation of the field hospital to treat ocular injuries requires meticulous planning. The field hospital's success depends on its ability to cope with the field demand. The lack of advanced eye surgical

Table 22.1 Chief disaster-related ocular injuries

Diagnosis	Haiti earthquake 2010	Philippines typhoon 2013	Nepal Earthquake and avalanche 2015
Face/scalp laceration	40%	0	4.8%
Eyelid/eyebrow laceration	13.3%	7.1%	0
Loose sutures/need for suture removal	13.3%	0	0
Orbital fractures	0	7.1%	9.5%
Exposure keratitis	0	14.3%	19%
Foreign body	3.3%	42.9%	28.6%
Subconjunctival hemorrhage	6.6%	7.1%	19%
Preterm retinopathy of prematurity	3.3%	0	0
Blunt trauma	20%	21.4%	19%
Penetrating ocular trauma	0	0	0

equipment imposes a very conservative management policy for ocular injuries and a damage-control approach. Moreover, field-hospital resources, which are restricted due to transport limitations, may cause a depletion of supplies. This makes prioritization and triage the cornerstones on which the field hospital is built. Precise and accurate preparation, and selecting the right medical personnel and equipment suitable to the exact disaster guarantee the mission's success.

Personnel

During disasters, the number and disciplines of the medical staff in the delegation are limited. However, the inclusion of an ophthalmologist is essential if significant ocular injuries are to be treated, as no other specialist is capable of treating these injuries. Ophthalmologists will be found in type 2-plus and type 3 emergency medical teams (EMTs). In lower-level facilities, ocular care will be provided by other physicians. During a disaster, the field hospital provides not only urgent care but also everyday medical care for the population. Considering the high prevalence of ocular injuries, the emergency response teams must include an ophthalmologist. Although the number of ophthalmologists needed will be determined according to the nature and the extent of the specific disaster, usually one ophthalmologist will meet the field hospital's needs. There is a need for an ophthalmologist who is a surgeon with a preference for an oculoplastic surgeon who can treat orbital and ocular trauma, and facial and eyelid laceration. Ideally, the ophthalmologist will have previous experience in treating ocular injuries in a field hospital during disasters. If possible, it is advisable to include an

ophthalmologist with no previous field hospital exposure to enlarge the pool of experienced personnel. There is also a need for close cooperation between the various medical disciplines such as an otolaryngologist for combined treatment of orbital fractures and a plastic surgeon when there is a need for wound coverage.

Paramedical personnel are very important and can assist in testing visual acuity, applying dressings, keeping the medical records, and serving as an interpreter if possible.

Other available personnel who should be taken into consideration if available are the local medical paramedical personnel, who can assist in providing medical help, and in mediating with the local population and the local authorities.

Equipment

A list of medical equipment for the ocular clinic must be created as part of the requirements of the field hospital. The list should include necessary basic equipment and options for additional equipment depending on the type of disaster. Because of weight restrictions and the amount of equipment required for the field hospital, the list of required equipment must be carefully planned and adapted to the type of disaster and the expected injuries. Furthermore, the ophthalmologist's assumption must be that there will be no extra equipment or reinforcements and therefore the use of the equipment should be planned with careful thought and restraint. The priority is equipment to treat urgent ocular injuries that are disaster related such as foreign bodies, eyelid lacerations, and penetrating injuries. The second priority is equipment for treatment of chronic and nondisaster-related conditions such as dry eye and eye infections. The amount of equipment brought will dictate the extent of help and care the ophthalmologist can provide during the disaster. One major limitation of the field hospital is the inability to perform complex eye surgery, in part because of the lack of equipment needed for those operations.

Recommended ophthalmologist equipment

- Examination room:
  1. Direct ophthalmoscope
  2. Indirect ophthalmoscope
  3. Diagnostic lenses: 78 D or 90 D lens for slit lamp, 20 D lens for indirect ophthalmoscope
  4. Slit lamp with Goldmann applanation tonometer (and spare light bulbs)
  5. Rechargeable, cordless slit-lamp microscope
  6. Snellen near and distance vision charts: full sized and pocket sized
  7. Tonometer: Tono-Pen tonometer and tip cover protection
  8. Fluorescein sodium ophthalmic strips: thin strips of fluorescein sodium 0.6 mg
  9. Eye plastic shields
  10. Contact lenses
  11. Eye pads
  12. Plastic/Transpore tape
- Operating theater:
  1. Ophthalmic loupes
  2. Speculum
  3. Lacrimal cannula
  4. Micro-needle holder
  5. Forceps
  6. Scissors: corneal scissors
  7. Punctum dilator
  8. Scalpel
  9. Needle: 25 g
  10. Sutures: coated VICRYL suture: 7–0, 6–0, 5–0. 10/0 nylon double armed
  11. Desmarres eyelid retractor
  12. Slit blades (keratome)
  13. Retrobulbar needle
  14. Surgical eye sponges
  15. 5 ml disposable syringes luer lock; 2 ml disposable syringes luer lock
  16. Eye drape

- Ocular medication:
  1. Acute treatment: disaster related
     a. Eye drops and ointments
        i. Antibiotics: eye drops gentamicin sulfate 0.3%, eye drops ofloxacin 0.3%, ophthalmic ointment chloramphenicol 5%
        ii. Steroids: eye drops dexamethasone sodium phosphate 0.1%, ophthalmic ointment polymyxin B sulfate 6000 U/ml
        iii. Mydriatics: eye drops tropicamide 0.5%
        iv. Cycloplegics: eye drops cyclopentolate HCl 1%, eye drops phenylephrine HCl 10%
        v. Antiglaucomatous: eye drops brimonidine tartrate 0.15%, eye drops pilocarpine HCl 2%, eye drops latanoprost 50 µg/ml, eye drops dorzolamide HCl 2%, eye drops timolol maleate 0.5%
        vi. Tear substitute: eye drops hydroxypropyl methylcellulose 0.3%
  2. Ophthalmic betadine 5%
  3. Anesthesia
     a. Localin eye drops (eye drops benoxinate HCl 0.4%)
     b. Lidocaine
     c. Marcaine
  4. Uramox: blister tablets acetazolamide 250 mg

- Chronic treatment: disaster nonrelated:
  1. Eye drops diclofenac sodium 0.1%
     a. Antiherpetic
     b. Acyclovir 3%
  2. Vernal conjunctivitis
     a. Topical antihistamines
     b. Cyclosporine A
  3. Chronic blepharitis treatment
     a. Blephamide
     b. Tea tree oil
     c. Oral tetracycline

Ophthalmology Layout in the Field Hospital

Ocular treatment will be given in three areas in the field hospital: triage, the ocular department, and the OR. The treatment of ocular injuries should start with ocular triage, prioritizing interventions that assure timely resolution of eye injuries. At this first stage, a plastic protective eye cover will be put on the injured eye to prevent more injury during the second survey. After the first assessment and stabilization of the patient's systemic physical condition, his or her ocular area will be examined. The ophthalmologic clinic will include an examination area and outpatient and waiting areas. The field hospital should be ready to assign hospitalization beds for ocular injuries according to the volume and the type of the disaster. Patients with injuries other than ocular ones will be admitted to a department according to their major injury. Preferably, the clinic location will be close to the medical fields related to ophthalmology such as ENT and plastic surgery. According to medical priority, ocular operations will be performed in the field hospital operating theater: there is no need for a designated OR. Regional anesthesia will be given by the ophthalmologist, while general anesthesia and appropriate monitoring will be available as part of the field-hospital services. Complicated surgeries, such as intraocular foreign bodies and penetrating injuries, can be operated on in collaboration with the local hospital and surgeons depending on their availability.

Although there is a need for an ocular clinic, the field hospital ophthalmologists and their examination equipment must be mobile so that they can provide consultations around the hospital.

The Role and Importance of the Ophthalmologist During Disasters

The main role of the ophthalmologist as part of a field hospital is to diagnose and treat ocular injuries during the disaster. However, he or she has many other different roles as part of the hospital staff and as the only ophthalmologist in the area. Moreover, the field hospital's ophthalmologist provides medical care for chronic ocular problems of the population whose medical infrastructure was damaged in the disaster.

Trauma Care

The primary, and perhaps the most important, role of the ophthalmologist in the field hospital is the identification and treatment of ocular trauma. Although eye injuries are not life threatening, they can cause major disabilities. In the first days after the disaster, most of the referrals to the field hospital will be trauma related. The ophthalmologist must be able to diagnose and treat

ocular emergencies such as ocular perforation and penetration, and ocular trauma including orbital fractures, eyelid lacerations, and foreign bodies. Furthermore, he or she will need to know who can perform reconstruction of the lacrimal drainage system, canthotomy, cantholysis, and orbital decompression.

Consultant

One part of the ophthalmologist's role in the field hospital is as a consultant to other disciplines: firstly in trauma and disaster-related injuries such as complicated facial trauma. In cases of head trauma, the ophthalmologist will perform a fundoscopic examination to rule out papilledema. There will be a close follow-up with the plastic surgery and ENT patients as needed. In chronic or nondisaster-related conditions, especially in emergency situations, examinations such as fundoscopic examinations are necessary to rule out meningitis, preeclampsia, and fat emboli. But examinations are also necessary in chronic conditions such as the diagnosis of diabetic and hypertensive retinopathy.

Community Physician

During disasters, local medical infrastructures, such as hospitals and ophthalmological outpatient clinics, can be severely damaged. With limited transportation capabilities, the local population cannot reach basic medical care. Therefore, as time passes, ocular problems will become chronic conditions (nondisaster related), such as cataract, pterygium, dry eye, and refractive errors. Treating these injuries can become, with time, the major role of the ophthalmologist and sometimes his or her most important work in the delegation. The field-hospital ophthalmologist will have to function as an ocular community physician while treating ocular trauma.

Surgeon

One of the roles of the ophthalmologist in the field hospital will be performing surgeries, such as ocular, eyelid, and orbital, on trauma patients. Due to the basic equipment and the lack of an ocular microscope, most of the surgeries will be damage control in nature. In complicated injuries such as perforations or intraocular foreign bodies, a first closing of the eye will be performed, and the patient will be transferred to a medical center with the ability to treat those injuries.

The ophthalmologist may often be part of a multidisciplinary team including a maxillofacial surgeon and a plastic surgeon treating complex injuries such as face and eye lacerations and orbital fractures.

As time passes from the disaster, and there are fewer trauma surgeries, more elective ocular procedures can be done such as correction of pterygium.

Ocular Referrals to the Field Hospital During a Disaster

After the first phase in which patients with injuries related to the disaster arrive at the field hospital, many patients with problems unrelated to the disaster are expected. The most influential factor on this type of chronic illness is the geographic area and the ocular illnesses that characterize it. Only a deep understanding of these variables will allow accurate preparation for the existing challenges in the field.

According to the Disaster Type

Conflict Zones

Ocular injuries during conflicts are highly dependent on the combat characteristics and the types of weapons used. While with the use of cold weapons, the eye injury rate is expected to be low, the use of modern weapons is characterized by a high rate of severe eye injuries. The changes in warfare during recent years involving the ever-expanding use of explosive weaponry have resulted in an increase in the risk of eye injuries on the battlefield. These injuries are usually accompanied by lacerations involving the eyelids and the lacrimal tract. The most common eye injuries in explosions are foreign bodies and penetrating ocular injuries, which are the most difficult to treat, especially since they often accompany other multisystemic injuries. Beyond the challenge of treatment, these injuries are characterized by multiple casualties and insufficient treatment capabilities.

Natural Disasters

The nature of the disaster is the most important factor that affects and dictates the type of acute ocular injuries treated in the field hospitals[3]. The type of disaster determines not only the types of injuries but also their scope. Referred injuries vary depending on the different types of disasters such as typhoon, earthquake, avalanche, and mass-casualty event due to an explosion. In the field hospital following the Haiti earthquake in 2010, face and eyelid lacerations (53.33%) and ocular blunt traumas (20%) were the most common injuries due to the collapse of buildings as result of the earthquake. The strong winds, with flying debris and collapse of houses, during typhoon Haiyan in the Philippines in 2013 caused injuries characterized by ocular foreign bodies (42.85%) and blunt trauma (21.42%). Following the earthquake and avalanche in 2015 in Nepal, the most common ocular traumas were blunt trauma (28.57%), as at Haiti, and foreign bodies (19.04%)[16]. Complex and multisystem injuries are to be expected during earthquakes.

Timeline Dependence

It is clear that the purpose of the ophthalmologist's mission is first and foremost to treat ocular injuries as a result of the disaster. In the first phase – within the first two weeks after the event – most patients will present with disaster-related injuries such as eyelid lacerations, ocular perforations, and orbital fractures. In the later phases, the predominating ocular problems presenting in the field hospital will be chronic conditions such as cataract, pterygium, dry eye, and even refractive errors. This shift can be very dramatic and, as time passes after the disaster, most, if not all, the referrals to the field hospital are chronic in nature. During three disasters – the Haiti earthquake in 2010, the Philippines typhoon in 2013, and the Nepal earthquake and avalanche in 2015 – of the patients treated in the deployed Israel Defense Forces (IDF) field hospitals, 75.47% required ocular medical care for chronic conditions[16]. This is consistent with the data from the mission vision van after the east Japan earthquake in 2011, where mostly preexisting ocular conditions, rather than trauma or disaster-related injuries, were treated[2]. Understanding the difference in the nature of ocular injuries – related and nonrelated to the disaster – according to the timeline is important for the success of the mission. It is therefore clear that the time when the field hospital starts to operate in the field has a great impact on the type of ocular injuries treated in it.

Geographical Factors

The location of a disaster affects the referrals to the field hospital. The same disaster can cause different damage depending on where it occurred. For example, the damage caused to a rural place will be different to that caused to an urban, heavily populated area. In densely populated areas, a greater morbidity and outbreak of contagious diseases is expected. The geographical location of the disaster has a great effect on the type of chronic ocular problems treated in the field hospital. For example, in the tropical maritime climate with high ultraviolet light exposure (pterygium belt), cataract and pterygium are the most common presentations. In places with poor sanitary conditions and poverty, chronic conjunctivitis is very commonly seen in the field hospitals.

Infrastructure-Related Factors

The medical infrastructure in the disaster area, including hospitals and available ORs, affects the referrals of ocular injuries to the field hospital. In addition, the extent of damage to transportation and communications in the disaster area plays a crucial role in the volume of injuries that must be addressed by the field hospital. The extent of the damage should be assessed, and collaboration with local health professionals should be established to enable continued care, especially for the patients with more complex ocular injuries.

Summary

During a disaster, the field hospital faces many difficulties. Not only does it function as a trauma center and treats the disaster-related injuries, it also needs to take the place of local medical infrastructures damaged in the disaster. The most important consideration when preparing for deployment to a disaster zone is the location and type of the disaster: as with other injuries, ocular injuries seen in the field hospital are affected by the geographic location of the disaster and the nature of the disaster: the ophthalmologist should be prepared accordingly.

The role of the ophthalmologist in the field hospital is important and irreplaceable. Eye injuries during disasters are very common and, although ocular injuries may not be as life threatening as other injuries, they can still cause the patient to suffer from permanent disability. The ophthalmologist's role during a disaster changes as time passes. In the first phase, his or her role will be mostly treating disaster-related injuries. In the later phases, this changes to treatment of chronic ocular problems of the local population.

As a doctor in the field hospital, the ophthalmologist has to deal with ethical dilemmas regarding the need to work with limited resources and make life-changing decisions in difficult circumstances.

References

1. Doi H, Kunikata H, Kato K, Nakazawa T. Ophthalmologic examinations in areas of Miyagi Prefecture affected by the great east Japan earthquake. *JAMA Ophthalmology* 2014: **132**(7): 874–6.

2. Yuki K, Nakazawa T, Kurosaka D, et al. Role of the vision van, a mobile ophthalmic outpatient clinic, in the great east Japan earthquake. *Clinical Ophthalmology* 2014: **8**: 691–6.

3. Birnbaum ML, Daily EK, O'Rourke AP. Research and evaluations of the health aspects of disasters, part V: epidemiological disaster research. *Prehospital and Disaster Medicine* 2015: **30**(6): 648–56.

4. Zhong S, Clark M, Hou XY, Zang YL, Fitzgerald G. Development of hospital disaster resilience: conceptual framework and potential measurement. *Emergency Medicine Journal* 2014: **31**(11): 930–8.

5. Born CT, Briggs SM, Ciraulo DL, et al. Disasters and mass casualties: I. General principles of response and management. *Journal of the American Academy of Orthopaedic Surgeons* 2007: **15**(7): 388–96.

6. Tokuda Y, Kikuchi M, Takahashi O, Stein GH. Prehospital management of sarin nerve gas terrorism in urban settings: 10 years of progress after the Tokyo subway sarin attack. *Resuscitation* 2006: **68**: 193–202.

7. Sobaci G, Akyn T, Mutlu FM, Karagul S, Bayraktar MZ. Terror-related open-globe injuries: a 10-year review. *American Journal of Ophthalmology* 2005: **139**: 937–9.

8. Odhiambo WA, Guthua SW, Macigo FG, et al. Maxillofacial injuries caused by terrorist bomb attack in Nairobi, Kenya. *International Journal of Oral and Maxillofacial Surgery* 2002: **31**: 374–7.

9. Negrel AD, Thylefors B. The global impact of eye injuries. *Ophthalmic Epidemiology* 1998: **5**: 143–69.

10. Mimran S, Rotem R. Ocular trauma under the shadow of terror. *Insight* 2005: **30**: 10–2.

11. Mines M, Thach A, Mallonee S, et al. Ocular injuries sustained by survivors of the Oklahoma City bombing. *Ophthalmology* 2000: **107**(5): 837–43.

12. Berrios-Torres SI, Greenko JA, Phillips M, Miller JR, Treadwell T, Ikeda RM. World Trade Center rescue worker injury and illness surveillance, New York, 2001. *American Journal of Preventive Medicine* 2003: **25**: 79–87.

13. Holmes S, Coombes A, Rice S, et al. The role of the maxillofacial surgeon in the initial 48 h following a terrorist attack. *British Journal of Oral and Maxillofacial Surgery* 2005: **43**: 375–82.

14. Centers for Disease Control and Prevention. Rapid assessment of injuries among survivors of the terrorist attack on the World Trade Center – New York City,

September 2001. *Morbidity and Mortality Weekly Report* 2002: **51**: 1–5.

15. Ari AB. Eye injuries on the battlefields of Iraq and Afghanistan: public health implications. *Optometry* 2006: **77**: 329–39.

16. Osaadon P, Tsumi E, Pokroy R, Sheleg T, Peleg K. Ocular morbidity in natural disasters: field hospital experience 2010–2015. *Eye* 2018: **32**(11): 1717–22.

17. Gossman MD, Roberts DM, Barr CC. Ophthalmic aspects of orbital injury. A comprehensive diagnostic and management approach. *Clinics in Plastic Surgery* 1992: **19**: 71–85.

18. Kuhn F, Halda T, Witherspoon CD, Morris R, Mester V. Intraocular foreign bodies: myths and truths. *European Journal of Ophthalmology* 1996: **6**: 464–71.

19. Manolidis S, Weeks BH, Kirby M, Scarlett M, Hollier L. Classification and surgical management of orbital fractures: experience with 111 orbital reconstructions. *Journal of Craniofacial Surgery* 2002: **13**: 726–37, discussion 738.

20. Roncevic R, Roncevic D. Extensive, traumatic fractures of the orbit in war and peace time. *Journal of Craniofacial Surgery* 1999: **10**: 284–300.

21. Cakanac CJ. Orbital fractures. *Optometry Clinics* 1993: **3**: 57–65.

22. Cai YS, Zhou GJ. Compressive eye injuries caused by earthquake. *Chinese Medical Journal* 1983: **96**(10): 731–6.

23. Lubeck D. Penetrating ocular injuries. *Emergency Medicine Clinics of North America* 1988: **6**(1): 127–46.

24. Detorakis ET, Spandidos DA. Pathogenetic mechanisms and treatment options for ophthalmic pterygium: Trends and perspectives (Review). *International Journal of Molecular Medicine* 2009: **23**: 439–47.

25. Coroneo MT. Pterygium as an early indicator of ultraviolet insolation: a hypothesis. *British Journal of Ophthalmology* 1993: **77**: 734–9.

26. McCarty CA1, Taylor HR. A review of the epidemiologic evidence linking ultraviolet radiation and cataracts. *Developments in Ophthalmology* 2002: **35**: 21–31.

27. Mariotti SP, Pascolini D, Rose-Nussbaumer J. Trachoma: global magnitude of a preventable cause of blindness. *British Journal of Ophthalmology* 2009: **93**(5): 563–8.

28. Steinsapir KD, Goldberg RA. Traumatic optic neuropathy. *Survey of Ophthalmology* 1994: **38**: 487–518.

29. Larian B, Wong B, Crumley RL, Moeinolmolki B, Muranaka E, Keates RH. Facial trauma and ocular/orbital injury. *Journal of Cranio-Maxillofacial Surgery* 1999: **5**: 15–24.

30. Jones WL. Traumatic injury to the lens. *Optometry Clinics* 1991: **1**: 125–42.

31. Merin O, Nachman A, Levy G, Schwaber MJ, Kreiss Y. The Israeli field hospital in Haiti – ethical dilemmas in early disaster response. *The New England Journal of Medicine* 2010: **362**: e38.

Chapter

23

Anesthesia and Pain Management in Field Hospitals

Ralf E Gebhard, Asima Iqbal, and Mohamed Koronfel

Introduction

Anesthesiologists play a pivotal role controlling airways, performing resuscitation and providing anesthesia and analgesia, not only in the ORs with relatively controlled settings but sometimes also extending to practicing in austere environments or field conditions where care has to be provided on site[1]. Anesthesia delivery in below-standard conditions with limited resources is indeed challenging[2]. Field hospitals are usually established when natural disasters (earthquakes, hurricanes, and floods, and so on) occur or in the battlefields during wars[3,4,5]. Such events result in mass casualties as well as hospital damage and local infrastructure insults, compromising electricity, transport, and supply chains.

In the aftermath of natural disasters, local hospitals may need to be evacuated into temporary field hospitals due to building collapse or imminent collapse. Later on, main field hospitals are established and they usually start running within days. Foreign medical providers historically volunteer for humanitarian missions to help local medical staff to establish and operate field hospitals, as in the major earthquakes that occurred in Armenia (1988), Japan (1995), Pakistan (2003), China (2008), and Haiti (2010).

The medical system of the USA military provides five levels of care, between which patients are transferred. Level I occurs at the battlefield aid station, focusing mainly on providing advanced trauma life support, stopping blood loss, and evacuating the wounded soldiers. Level II occurs in main field hospitals near the frontline, in which surgical interventions are conducted. Level III facilities are known as combat evacuation or support hospitals, where more surgical subspecialties are available. The level IV service is being served at facilities located in USA allied countries, in which evacuated soldiers are evaluated and treated. Lastly, level V are hospitals in the USA, where soldiers are transferred to be treated depending on their wounds, screened for post-traumatic stress disorder (PTSD), and treated for any chronic pain they might be experiencing.

Most disaster or combat casualties present with acute traumatic injuries, in the form of lacerations, bone fractures, gunshot wounds, and injury to brain, spinal cord, and other organs requiring urgent surgical intervention. The predominant injury pattern reported in the literature involves a high incidence of limb injuries. Consequently, operations for traumatic limb injuries and for penetrating trauma rank among the most common interventions in austere environments, while endoscopic and cardiac procedures are rare and infrequently performed.

The field environment is often associated with limited medical supplies, equipment, and space, as well as shortage of electricity, oxygen, and trained personnel. Therefore, a combination of problems, anticipation, proper planning, and coping with difficult situations is required for a successful anesthesia care model. The number of patients in need often overwhelms the capacity. Thus, the key role is selection and triage. The surgeon has to identify and prioritize eligible patients and choose the adequate procedure that results in the desired outcome without unnecessary draining of resources or personnel. The anesthesiologist must develop an anesthetic plan and choose a modality that allows for effective anesthesia and analgesia, while avoiding unnecessary risks to the patient. The goal is to attempt to provide the safest anesthetic possible for surgeries to be performed, despite the constraints and limitations of technical equipment and supplies.

Anesthesia Options and Considerations

Many advances have been made in anesthesia delivery at the time of wars and disasters, from using ether, chloroform, thiopental, and halothane, to the more modern drugs and agents being used nowadays.

Choosing the right anesthesia management type or modality is of paramount importance. Multiple anesthetic techniques have been successfully used in field hospitals, from monitored anesthesia care (MAC) to general anesthesia. Anesthetic management in this special population is not an easy task as most patients suffer from intravascular volume depletion secondary to bleeding and dehydration, electrolyte derangements, coagulopathies, and/or sepsis. Therefore, maintaining hemodynamic stability is imperative.

The various limitations in an austere environment always favor the utilization of compact, lighter weighted, reusable, and easily mobile items. Given the constricted availability and interruptions of supplies, the required anesthetic system should ideally be simple to operate, able to withstand extreme conditions, and rely minimally on electrical supplies and compressed gases.

General Anesthesia

General anesthesia is used in many cases and can be provided parenterally, via inhalation, or a balanced combination of both.

Inhalation Anesthesia

In general, mechanical ventilators have limited portability, and their use requires the availability of electricity, compressed gas, suction, and scavenging systems, which all add to the constraints of its utility in postdisaster scenarios. In response to these limitations, manual ventilation is frequently used, especially during the early phases of surgical interventions. Many devices have been developed along the continuous search for a durable, dependable, and portable system, which can minimize the logistical footprint. In military fields, the draw-over anesthesia system, Ohmeda Universal Portable Anesthesia Complete (UPAC), has been one of the most reliable devices for inhalation anesthetics since the 1970s[6]. The UPAC does not require power or gas flow for operation. It is designed to deliver volatile inhalation agents to spontaneously breathing patients using their inspiratory efforts to draw ambient air through the vaporizer, but it can be used with a portable ventilator, such as the lightweight, battery-powered Impact Uni-Vent 754 Eagle, and supplemental oxygen can be added if necessary. Despite being a dependable device, it is very difficult to find replacement parts as the UPAC is no longer being manufactured. Other examples of draw-over anesthetic vaporizers used in

austere conditions include the Oxford Miniature Vaporizer, the Diamedica Draw-over Vaporizer, and the vaporizer of the Universal Anesthesia Machine. Military forces are now increasingly using conventional compact anesthesia machines, such as Dräger Fabius Tiro M, Narkomed M, and others, which are more sophisticated, a lot heavier than draw-over devices, and require electrical power for operation. The need for oxygen supply adds to the logistical burden[7]. Compressed gas cylinders are heavy to be ported from one place to another, require refill or replacement, and carry some explosive hazards. Consequently, portable oxygen generators that can be used to fill oxygen cylinders and concentrators that can generate oxygen via room air concentration were developed. Many oxygen concentrators, such as Saros, Eclipse, and DeVilbiss, are able to provide uninterrupted supply of oxygen in harsh environments. However, with all the progress and advancements in anesthesia delivery over the years, inhalation anesthesia is still considered a challenge in an austere environment[8].

Total Intravenous Anesthesia

Total intravenous anesthesia (TIVA) is becoming a more desirable method for the induction and maintenance of general anesthesia in deployed settings[9]. It can be used to provide sedation, amnesia, analgesia, and akinesia without the use of volatile anesthetic gases. Its small logistical footprint and the lack of need for bulky anesthesia machines, sophisticated vaporizers, heavy equipment, or power supply make TIVA preferable over inhalation anesthesia on the battlefield, where space, electricity, and resupply are potential issues. The main limitation of TIVA is that its administration requires anesthesia providers who are familiar with TIVA. In addition, existence of an adequate intravenous access is mandatory.

TIVA provides more hemodynamic stability, does not trigger malignant hyperthermia, decreases the incidence of nausea and vomiting, and carries less waste-disposal burden compared to volatile gas anesthetics. Other advantages of the total intravenous technique include easy titration due to predictable pharmacokinetics and dynamics, and reduction of recovery time. Many induction agents, such as propofol and etomidate, can be bolused or continuously infused through pumps to maintain anesthesia. Benzodiazepines, narcotics, and muscle relaxants are often used as adjuncts in intravenous anesthesia. The ability to maintain patients on the same intravenous agents without interruption allows easier en route control during patient transport. A popular infusion recipe is the mix of propofol and ketamine. This admixture (ketofol) results in relevant reduction in postoperative nausea, vomiting, and pain compared to inhalation anesthesia. The high-quality emergence and decreased recovery are also among the most documented benefits of TIVA. All these previously stated desirable qualities lead to fewer postoperative interventions, reduced cost, and lowered workload on medical personnel, thus making TIVA a very reliable technique in an austere environment.

Ketamine

Ketamine is one of the most unique agents used in TIVA or MAC. It is a noncompetitive antagonist of the N-methyl-D-aspartate receptor, with rapid onset and short half-life that can provide analgesia, amnesia, and hypnosis while maintaining hemodynamics, airway reflexes, and spontaneous ventilation. The increase in heart rate and blood pressure caused by ketamine can be beneficial in hypotensive patients and can also be neuroprotective by improving cerebral perfusion. It helps in temperature conservation by causing peripheral vasoconstriction. In addition to potentiating the effects of opioids, ketamine can provide significant pain relief itself and therefore spares narcotic use and decreases the potential risk of opioid-induced hypotension and respiratory depression, which can be lethal in polytrauma patients. Its use can have some potential side effects, which providers need to be aware of, particularly with higher doses, such as the tendency for causing excessive salivation, and psychotomimetic effects like hallucinations and nightmares. Ketamine is traditionally believed to cause a possible increase in intracranial cerebrospinal fluid pressure and intraocular pressure. Therefore, despite conflicting evidence, ketamine should be used with extreme caution in patients with traumatic brain and eye injuries. Ketamine can be administered orally, intramuscularly, or intravenously, either as a sole agent or in combination with other medications, especially when ventilators are unavailable. It can also be used in supplementation of regional anesthesia in some cases. Ketamine MAC is well tolerated in general, with a low rate of complications or adverse events, making it a very useful drug in the field environment[10].

Regional Anesthesia

In an environment with limitations in equipment, oxygen, and electricity, regional anesthesia appears to be an optimal option for many surgical procedures as an anesthetic technique or for acute perioperative pain management[11]. It permits spontaneous ventilation without the need for airway instrumentation, maintains consciousness and reflexes, and does not require cumbersome machines. Regional anesthesia teams are easily mobile, allowing rapid and efficient field dispatch. The required equipment can be transported without limitation on planes and helicopters, and can be promptly assembled in a very reasonable timeframe.

Depending on the surgical site and the nature of the intervention, regional anesthesia can be performed via peripheral nerve or plexus blocks, field blocks, or neuraxial techniques to block pain pathways. It can be combined with general anesthesia or with multiple intravenous agents such as ketamine or midazolam for sedation. Anesthesia providers often utilize anatomical landmarks to perform a blockade, with or without the help of ultrasound or nerve stimulators. Nerve stimulators are of small size, battery operated, and consequently ideally suited for an environment that requires a high degree of mobility. Portable ultrasound machines allow for relatively objective target identification and visual needle guidance. Since ultrasound-guided nerve block techniques have been demonstrated to be associated with a lower risk for local anesthetic system toxicity[12], this methodology should be utilized whenever possible to avoid such a dangerous complication. Regional anesthesia usually provides highly efficient surgical anesthesia and perioperative pain control, as well as reduced postoperative complications. However, it is not appropriate for all surgical procedures and requires relatively experienced practitioners. In particular, neuraxial techniques, such as spinal or epidural anesthesia, can be somewhat troublesome in field hospitals. The resulting sympathectomy can lead to severe hypotension, which is worsened by the intravascular volume depletion that typically is highly prevalent in this specific patient population, requiring fluid resuscitation before and during placement. Furthermore, as a result of their trauma, patients frequently present with severe coagulopathies. The practitioner may not have the necessary laboratory resources available to determine coagulation parameters or may lack the blood products required to

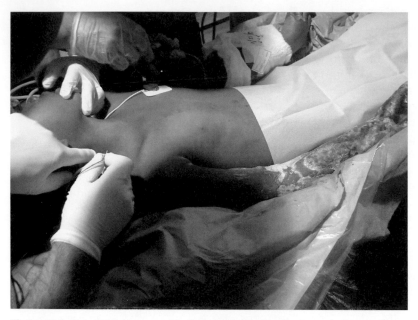

Figure 23.1 Wound debridement under interscalene block in the aftermath of the 2010 Haitian earthquake (A black and white version of this figure will appear in some formats. For the color version, please refer to the plate section.)

correct a coagulopathy. Since neuraxial techniques carry the risk for spinal or epidural hematoma, these techniques may not be safe to be performed if a patient's hemostasis is severely altered. Nevertheless, a peripheral nerve block (PNB) can be an excellent choice in austere environments. PNBs provide optimal operating conditions with stable patient hemodynamics and minimal side effects. Their effective neural blockade has a rapid onset and can be extended by using long-acting local anesthetics, which in turn can help decrease postoperative pain, reduce the need for frequent redosing of narcotics, and hence lower the burden on the medical personnel, as well as decreasing the incidence of opioid-associated complications such as nausea, vomiting, and respiratory depression. The use of ketamine MAC in combination with PNB is a great option in a field environment, especially for limb surgeries, as it can be fulfilled by using small, lightweight, portable equipment or carry-on kits, which are ready for rapid deployment. However, when utilizing PNBs as the anesthetic technique, the practitioner is well advised to select the technique with the most favorable safety profile. For instance, choosing an axillary block over a supraclavicular block when providing anesthesia for a hand or forearm procedure eliminates the risk of a pneumothorax. This may represent a significant and

potentially lifesaving advantage in an environment in which chest tubes and suction equipment may not be readily available. During the 2010 Haitian earthquake, many upper extremity surgeries were safely carried out under single-shot interscalene or axillary nerve blocks (Figure 23.1), while patients undergoing lower-extremity procedures typically received a combination of single-shot femoral and sciatic blocks[13].

Pain Management

In addition to the unfortunate traumatic injuries, acute and chronic pain are among the major consequences associated with surviving wars and natural catastrophes. Pain has been recognized as a pathophysiologic process that, if inadequately treated, can lead to many physical and psychological morbidities such as loss of function and depression. It has multiple components and many factors can contribute to it such as PTSD, which might complicate pain and make it persist and become chronic, even after treating the initiating trauma. Contributing factors for development of chronic pain also include older age, female gender, bigger injuries, and poor management of acute pain. More than 60% of survivors of the battlefield develop chronic pain affecting their quality of life[14]. Historically, opioids have been used in field hospitals as a tool for pain management as monotherapy for many decades, with morphine being the gold standard. Initially strictly administered via intramuscular injection, it became quickly apparent the intravenous route has multiple advantages such as faster onset and independency from absorption. The addition of patient-controlled analgesia allowed for decreased response time and reduced the workload and burden of health-care providers, allowing them to attend to other duties. Opioid monotherapy is highly efficient in controlling pain, but, especially in higher doses, opioids are associated with significant side effects such as respiratory depression, nausea and vomiting, and constipation. These side effects may require additional monitoring or medical intervention, which in a field environment may not always be readily available due to lack of either supplies or personnel. In addition, opioids carry the potential for tolerance, dependence, and abuse.

Due to the aforementioned reasons, a more modern and efficacious pain management approach, in which different treatment modalities – pharmacologic and nonpharmacologic – are included in a multimodal concept, may be advantageous in a field hospital. The overall goal of such an approach would be to deliver highly effective and predictable pain control while reducing any unwanted side effects to a minimum. Pain is transmitted and modulated via different pathways, humoral transmitters, and various receptors in the peripheral and central nervous system. Consequently, targeting pain at multiple stages of transmission, at different receptor sites, and via inhibiting pathways appears to be promising. This is being achieved by combining several different classes of analgesics with individual mechanisms of action such as opioids, nonsteroidal antiinflammatory drugs, Tylenol, ketamine, and, more recently, gabapentinoids. Targeting pain from multiple angles allows decreasing the dose of each individual agent to a level where serious side effects are relatively rare. In addition to optimizing medication therapy with oral and intravenous agents, local anesthetics can be added either for surgical site infiltration or in the form of regional anesthesia techniques whenever possible.

Regional anesthesia plays an important role in the improvement of perioperative pain management, providing excellent analgesia and resulting in an opioid-sparing effect. PNBs are frequently used not only to provide surgical anesthesia but also to extend the analgesic effects into the postoperative period.

However, even if long-acting local anesthetics are utilized for PNBs, the duration of analgesia is typically exhausted within 12–16 hours. To provide longer lasting pain control with these techniques, continuous PNBs (CPNBs) need to be applied via catheter placement. Infusion pumps can then be attached, allowing extension of the analgesic effects for several days.

In combat environments, CPNBs are being integrated as part of the standard of care of the wounded [15]. However, they are less frequently used during natural disasters. In such settings, infrastructure collapse and the consequent shortage of supply often preclude their implementation. Besides, the unusual surrounding conditions in field hospitals can increase the likelihood of site or even systemic infection associated with indwelling catheters. Other obstacles include the need for the availability of experienced providers for placement, equipment such as infusion pumps, and trained medical staff for follow-up management and troubleshooting.

Overall, multimodal pain management, including regional anesthesia, is becoming more standardized due to its positive favorable effect on long-term health, enhancing recovery, and reducing lifelong morbidities secondary to the inadequacies in traditional pain relief methods.

Summary

Field hospitals established during wars or after natural catastrophes are challenging environments for medical providers to practice in. Anesthesia delivery continues to evolve in a continued pursuit of an ideal anesthetic, which can be delivered safely and effectively. The limited resources and the harsh surrounding conditions impose a treatment strategy that can depend as little as possible on electricity, heavy supplies, equipment, and technology to meet most of the clinical needs and compensate for the effects of the austere environment. The choice of the anesthetic technique is also dictated by the availability of medical personnel and their expertise and training. Due to the limitations of the use of inhalational methods, TIVA appears to be one of the most reliable techniques for delivery of general anesthesia in field conditions. TIVA is a very promising alternative for the future of field anesthesia given its safety, simplicity, rapid set-up, and small logistical footprint. Therefore, more anesthesia providers need to be trained and educated to be familiar and comfortable with administration of

TIVA. Whenever regional anesthesia use is appropriate, it can be another excellent choice to provide better pain control and decrease postoperative complications in austere environments. There is no perfect analgesic, and hence a multimodal approach for pain management is imperative. Early pain treatment has been proven to decrease chronicity, improve functionality, and reduce the risk of subsequent development of psychological morbidities such as PTSD and depression[16].

References

1. Mellor AJ. Anaesthesia in austere environments. *Journal of the Royal Army Medical Corps* 2005: **151**: 272–6.

2. Dobson MB. *Anaesthesia at the district hospital.* Second edn. World Health Organization; 2006.

3. Grathwohl KW, Venticinque SG. Organizational characteristics of the austere intensive care unit: the evolution of military trauma and critical care medicine: applications for civilian medical care systems. *Critical Care Medicine* 2008: **36** (7 Suppl): S275–83.

4. Bartels SA, VanRooyen MJ. Medical complications associated with earthquakes. *The Lancet* 2012: **379**: 748–57.

5. Wilson J, Barras P. Advances in anesthesia delivery in the deployed setting. *US Army Medical Department Journal Archives* 2016: (**2–16**): 62–5.

6. Reynolds PC, Furukawa KT. Modern draw-over anesthetic vaporizers used to deliver anesthesia in austere and battlefield conditions. *Military Medicine* 2003: **168**: ii–iii.

7. Szpisjak DF, Lamb CL, Klions KD. Oxygen consumption with mechanical ventilation in a field anesthesia machine. *Anesthesia & Analgesia* 2005: **100**: 1713–17.

8. Jiang J, Xu H, Liu H, Yuan H, Wang C, Ye J. Anaesthetic management under field conditions after the 12 May 2008 earthquake in Wenchuan, China. *Injury* 2010: **41**(6): 1–3.

9. Barras P, McMaster J, Grathwohl K, Blackbourne L: Total intravenous anesthesia on the battlefield. *US Army Medical Department Journal Archives* 2009: 68–72.

10. Mulvey JM, Qadri AA, Maqsood MA. Earthquake injuries and the use of ketamine for surgical procedures: the Kashmir experience. *Anaesthesia & Intensive Care* 2006: **34**: 489–94.

11. Missair A, Pretto E, Visan A, et al. A matter of life or limb? A review of traumatic injury patterns and anesthesia techniques for disaster relief after major earthquakes. *Anesthesia & Analgesia* 2013: **117**(4): 934–41.

12. Barrington MJ, Kluger R. Ultrasound guidance reduces the risk of local anesthetic systemic toxicity following peripheral nerve block. *Regional Anesthesia & Pain Medicine* 2013: **38**: 289–99.

13. Jaffer AK, Campo RE, Gaski G, Reyes M, Gebhard R et al. An academic center's delivery of care after the Haitian earthquake. *Annals of Internal Medicine* 2010: **153**(4): 262–5.

14. Croll SM, Griffith SR. Acute and chronic pain on the battlefield: lessons learned from point of injury to the United States. *US Army Medical Department Journal Archives* 2016: (**2–16**): 102–5.

15. Baker BC, Buckenmaier C, Narine N, et al. Battlefield anesthesia: advances in patient care and pain management. *Anesthesiology Clinics* 2007: **25**: 131–45.

16. Buckenmaier C, III, Mahoney PF, Anton T, Kwon N, Polomano RC. Impact of an acute pain service on pain outcomes with combat-injured soldiers at Camp Bastion, Afghanistan. *Pain Medicine* 2012: **13**(7): 919–26.

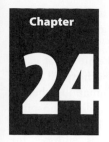

Chapter 24

Intensive Care Unit Buildup Within a Field Hospital Setting

Ami Mayo, Nisim Ifrach, Dekel Stavi, and Nimrod Adi

Introduction

A mobile hospital or field hospital, when activated in a disaster scenario, is generally guided by the principle of doing the greatest good for the greatest number[1]. This notion puts into question the allocation of a large amount of material and human resources to the treatment of a few critically injured patients.

Answering such a question must take into consideration the complexity of modern critical-care medicine. The development of the current concept of intensive care units (ICUs) has allowed the survival of patients with advanced illness and injury, although at a cost of substantial infrastructure. Since this discipline involves maximal lifesaving procedures and interventions, in the daily practice of the health system, it was usually not provided by most field hospitals deployed to disaster areas.

The capability to provide medical care to critically ill patients has evolved considerably since the 1970s. ICUs were developed where special expertise and equipment could be used to treat extremely complicated patients. Data suggesting that the presence of ICU staffing alone can affect a change in overall patient outcome (hospital mortality, length of stay) for the critically ill population, lends credence to the importance of adequate and aggressive ICU care, even in austere conditions[2]. As the field of critical care has developed, it has become clear not only that ICUs are effective tools for resuscitation and stabilization of the critically ill but also that the timing with which the treatment is initiated have lasting effects on the overall hospital course of the patient. A modern ICU represents a delicate assembly of skilled personnel and physical infrastructure. This infrastructure must include space to support patients and staff; temperature control; secure oxygen, electricity, water, and vacuum sources; medical supplies; pharmaceutical agents; and equipment. ICUs must also have ready access to surgical, radiographic, blood bank, and laboratory capabilities. Understanding the complex

infrastructure elements needed for the practice of critical-care medicine, and advanced monitoring and life-support technologies, enabled modern medicine to push forward ICU capabilities to austere situations. This can be a significant "pro" in the equation of "pros and cons" when considering the ICU integration in a deployed field hospital to a disaster area. Another aspect used in this equation of "pros and cons" is the modern approach to the concept of end-of-life decisions and limitation of care, practiced today more commonly in most modern critical care units in the Western world[3,4]. Combining these two aspects can offer a new notion to guide the ICU integration in a disaster event setting: *providing a limited number of predetermined critical care interventions to as many casualties as possible*, rather than maximal critical care to fewer patients.

Supportive elements for the decision whether to operate a critical care unit in a disaster scenario can be the nature of the disaster itself. Based on extent and severity of injuries, the literature classifies casualty level in disaster scenarios into two types: "mass-casualty event" versus "multiple-casualty event." These two types differ with respect to the balance between the scope and intensity of medical care required, and the numbers injured and their medical requirements[5]. In a "mass-casualty event," the medical system, which is supposed to provide medical services, is overwhelmed by the extent of the disaster and the number of casualties. In such a situation – for example, chemical-weapons attack or catastrophic nuclear event with mass radiation exposure – clear distinction is made between the walking wounded and casualties not able to move by themselves. Under such circumstances, medical resources should be directed to the walking wounded only, while other casualties receive minimal medical attention. Here, the strict guiding principle is to give the best possible treatment to the largest number of patients. Therefore, the individual patient requiring intensive care, including multisystem support, will not receive any treatment as this may divert treatment resources away from a wide group of more minor casualties having an acceptable outcome and a better prognosis. In this scenario, operation of an ICU should not be considered. In contrast, in a "multiple-casualty event," where the medical system is functional and its resources do meet the casualties' medical needs, high-quality medical care becomes possible and there should be aspiration to reaching the best available predefined standards of modern critical-care medicine. There is obviously a need for casualty triage and construction of an order of therapeutic priorities, but in this type of event, most casualties will receive medical attention, and establishment of an ICU within the framework of a deployed field hospital for such a scenario is completely indicated.

The medical response to recent disasters illustrates different ways in which critical care was provided during such events. A major earthquake struck western Turkey in August 1999, resulting in thousands of casualties and major damage to the region's medical infrastructure. The IDF deployed a field hospital to the city of Adapazarı, where 2627 people died and 5084 were wounded. This hospital included an ICU which was staffed with three physicians, three nurses, and five paramedics. Over the course of two weeks, this team managed a range of medical, trauma, and postsurgical patients[6]. To enhance their sustainability, they successfully integrated with the local medical system to augment their equipment and supplies.

In June 2001, Houston, Texas was struck by a tropical storm, causing major flooding. This resulted in compromise in emergency and critical care in the city. The US Air Force deployed a 25-bed portable field hospital, which, during an 11-day stay, successfully cared for 1036 patients, including 33 ICU patients[7]. This event validated the model of military response with a portable hospital/ICU for disasters within the USA.

In December 2003, an earthquake struck Bam, Iran, causing many thousands of casualties and disabling the city's medical system. An Iranian army-based team reported on their experience operating a portable field hospital with an ICU in the disaster area[8]. The authors faced a range of casualties from those suffering acute trauma to delayed complications (tissue infection, compartment syndrome, and rhabdomyolysis), as well as exacerbation of chronic illness. They emphasize the role of casualty

evacuation outside of the disaster area as a key for proper activation of a field hospital and especially the ICU.

In April 2015, a major earthquake hit Nepal, causing thousands of casualties. The field hospital of the IDF was deployed to the city of Kathmandu, where it was positioned beside the Nepalese military hospital, which was heavily damaged[9,10]. This deployment was unique since the field hospital was equipped for the first time with a full-scale critical-care unit. This added medical component allowed the teams to provide treatment to the most severe casualties, and allowed the surgical patients state-of-the-art post-operative care. After this deployment, numerous lessons regarding activation of a critical-care unit in such circumstances were learned. This chapter will review and summarize them.

Information Before Deployment

As discussed earlier, specific disaster event characteristics are to be assessed and analyzed to come up with a plan of action. Having this information prior to deployment of the critical-care unit can aid in defining three major elements, essential for the clinical activity of the unit: the nature of injuries and casualties to be anticipated, the scope and extent of treatment to be provided, and end-of-life decisions and limitations of treatment to be decided on. These three elements are, in turn, translated to the following variables:

- medical staff: training, seniority, and availability
- training and availability of nursing and other medical staff operating the unit
- extent of medical equipment available for operation within the framework of the unit

The "Donabedian model" for quality of care defines three domains: structure, process, and outcome[11]. In our case, structure of care specifies ICU infrastructure, equipment, and human resources. Process of care measures and monitors the process in which medical care is being delivered (daily rounds, bundles of care, and adherence to evidence-based guidelines). Outcome specifies the mortality and long-term morbidity of the patients being treated. In this chapter, we will focus on the structural component of the "Donabedian model." Our perception of ICU structure is based on a "module of four" ICU beds: this basic module can be extended as needed.

ICU Team

Building a field ICU team and delivering the appropriate level of care are challenged by two main issues. The first is the difficulty in practice arising from the lack of medical data available in a regular hospital ICU. The second is the fact that a field ICU team, based on the reserve forces (as in the IDF Medical Corps), is gathered from a few different-acting ICUs of regular hospitals. Bridging those two aspects is mandatory for a proper operation of a field ICU.

Medical Staff: Seniority, Diversity and Decision-Making in a Poor Evidence Environment

Patient medical data available in a critical-care unit operating in a field hospital are relatively limited. When compared to the continuous flow of information on patient history, lab results, or imaging studies results in a regular hospital setting, the field ICU is lacking a lot of data elements essential for numerous, daily, clinical decision-making processes. Under these circumstances, there is an inherent difficulty in undertaking therapeutic decisions. A team of senior physicians with a wealth of clinical experience and diverse expertise may compensate for the information deficit and enable modification of the well-established guidelines in such a way that assures best medical practice. A well-recognized notion in building an ICU team is that diversity in training of the medical staff is of great importance[12,13]. ICU capabilities of providing care to complex multiorgan-failure patients, the ability to support and stabilize life-threatening injuries, and deliver extracorporeal life support (ventilation or renal replacement therapy) are very well enhanced by recruiting critical-care specialists with different backgrounds. A variation of trained staff is likely to increase the efficiency of the ICU. Critical-care physicians with a specialty in anesthesia, pulmonology, surgery, and internal medicine can create a synergy within the ICU team. In addition, skills in performing abdominal and lung sonography and echocardiography, or in conducting regional nerve blocks, are of great importance. The basic "model of four" IDF field hospital's ICU in Kathmandu, Nepal, consisted of three ICU attendings (practicing in daily life as unit directors in three different facilities in Israel), one having a surgical background and two having anesthesiology backgrounds. This versatile team had the capability of making empirical decisions regarding delivery of maximal care, despite the scarcity of medical data. Therapeutic plans were continuously discussed, modified, and updated in accordance with the patient's changing clinical condition and flow of medical information. Clinical discussions must be conducted by professional medical staff, but other parties external to the unit, such as hospital directors or ethical authorities, can be involved regarding relevant issues as they arise. This empiric decision-making should drive the practice in which no admission request will be limited by clinical severity of the casualty presented. Only if the preadmission evaluation of the patient's severity, combined with the limitation of resources, leads to an estimate of nil survival chances, will patient admission be refused. During the deployment of the IDF field hospital in Kathmandu, only one incident of this type occurred. All the other patients were hospitalized "empirically." The scope of treatment administered was maximal without any technical limitations. "Treatment limitation" was put into effect only after comprehensive discussion: the staff's impression was that the patient would not survive. This occurred for one patient who presented with irreversible multiorgan failure.

Another aspect of the medical staff seniority is the presence of an attending physician 24 hours a day, 7 days a week, as all shifts are done by senior physicians (in contrast to regular critical-care practices, where shifts are done by residents). This allows safely shortening the time for medical procedures performed, like ventilation weaning or tracheostomy tube decannulation, since the ability to immediately and effectively address any procedural mishaps is present. In addition, it can offer the "pushing forward of medical conditions": rapid advancement of a patient's care plan, shortening of ICU stays, and faster discharge to the general wards, allowing for better utilization of the ICU beds. To be able to provide such high-level patient care for an uncertain amount of time, and preserve team capabilities in the long term, medical staff should start working in 12-hour shifts as soon as possible. Shifts should be started immediately with the initiation of field-hospital operation; usually within 12 hours of arrival on the scene.

Tasks that must be fulfilled by medical ICU physicians, apart from managing the most critical patients, also include consulting in the emergency room, the ORs, and the regular wards of the field hospital. The medical team must be versatile enough to support the pediatric ward in managing their most critical casualties. Other tasks to be covered by the team are the administrative aspects, military activities, and communication with the large framework of the field hospital. The core of three ICU attendings are essential for the basic "model-of-four" operability. In the chapter authors' experience, for every extension beyond four stations, another physician (not necessarily an ICU attending, but a general practitioner or a resident) should be added to the team.

Nursing Staff: Building-up, Routine Establishment, and Working Atmosphere

The wellbeing of the nursing-team is critical for the proper function of every ICU, especially in the extremes of operating in the framework of a field hospital[14,15]. The nursing team in the regular ICU is unified, well integrated, and highly skilled at working according to predefined protocols and routines. As with the physicians, the nursing team is based on reserve personnel who in everyday life work in various military and civilian facilities with different daily practices and routines. Unifying these in the short time available until the field ICU is fully operational is challenging. In the chapter authors' experience, protocol modifications were done rapidly, by the hour, and from shift-to-shift, until they were shaped into their final configuration. The team must be aware of patient safety issues during the first hour after unit activation. More medical and therapeutic mishaps can happen, and safety-related incidents may arise more frequently. Risk management should be a high concern, and preventive actions must be instituted until working routines and protocols are fully established.

The nursing team needed for the basic "model of four" comprises six nurses, all with a strong background of daily practice in taking care of critical patients. The nursing shifts should be eight hours – versus the 12-hour shifts for physicians – for better continuity of care. The nursing staff must be divided into three defined teams, with each team constituting a fixed organic unit. Only limited flexibility is allowed in terms of "switching" between teams. Each organic team is composed of two critical-care nurses and two additional nurse practitioners who can be replaced by paramedics if unavailable. The inclusion of nonregistered nurses, such as paramedics, mandates strict nursing and physician supervision. Their responsibilities and duties must be clearly defined, since in stressful moments – a frequent occurrence in the field ICU setting – they have to have

Table 24.1 Potential staff burnout factors

Knowledge and experience deficits
Lack of working procedures and inconsistency of protocols
Dangerous environment (e.g., aftershocks following an earthquake)
Challenging physical conditions
Physical fatigue
Uncertainty

full perception of what is strictly forbidden for them to do. Therefore, "two plus two" nursing personnel per shift are needed for activation of the "model-of-four" station's ICU.

There will always be an influx of volunteers with varying nursing experience offering assistance. These must be managed in an organized fashion and can only assist after strict evaluation of their credentials and capabilities. Tasks to be covered by the nursing team, aside from those in the critical-care unit, include supporting the emergency medicine department trauma bays, supporting the operating theaters with postoperative care in the recovery room, and the transportation of critical patients to and from the unit. This large workload places a huge burden of responsibility on the professional nursing team and can in turn lead to early burnout and fatigue. All factors potentially underlying staff burnout should be continuously searched for and, when identified, be resolved efficiently to avoid safety incidents and complications[14]. The main points to be anticipated are shown in Table 24.1.

Preventive measures should be planned, and action should be taken from day one of operation with frequent team meetings and multiple discussions:

- an opportunity to discuss subjects related to the establishment of medical procedures as rapidly as possible
- a forum for personal expression and venting
- daily multidisciplinary clinical discussions

As the team members may come from different backgrounds, the nursing staff daily schedule should be constructed from a synthesis of practice made by the various team members. A suggestion for an established daily schedule is as described in Table 24.2.

A method of coping with the expected physical and emotional load is to lead active team involvement in building an atmosphere of excellence, uniqueness, and precedent setting[14,15]. In the chapter authors' practice, this plan was extremely successful as the team was united within a short time, and a culture

Table 24.2 Nursing staff daily schedule: evolved by various team members

Suggested daily schedule for Field ICU operators in a disaster area	
Staff involved	**Activity description**
Nurse team	Morning nursing handover
Physician and nurse team	Comprehensive rounds: formulation of daily goals and therapeutic plan
Physician and nurse in charge	Individual confirmation of therapeutic plan for each patient
Physician and nurse in charge	Individual handover of medical instructions
Physician and nurse team	Evening rounds: confirmation of daily goals' achievement and therapeutic plan carried out
Nurse team	Nursing handover to the night shift

Table 24.3 EMT roles and areas of responsibility for medical equipment and devices

Potential responsibilities for EMTs serving in the field ICU
Communication with staff in the medical equipment storeroom
Management of equipment inventory in the ICU site
Identification of equipment deficits
Medical equipment technician assistance in daily equipment checkup
Critical care admitting bay preparation (preadmission and postdischarge)
Obtaining and documenting vital signs

of mutual dependence was developed. It allowed maximal professional achievement by our small nursing team.

Other Professional Staff Training: Need and Utilization

The paramedic: The paramedic profession is becoming more centralized in the military medical corps, with new positions and tasks being carried out by paramedics. Positioning paramedics in the ICU of the field hospital is questionable since paramedic skills are distinct from those of a registered nurse. When considering the wide knowledge and expertise required to become a critical-care nurse, paramedic skills may seem even less applicable. As discussed earlier, the "model of four" comprises two registered critical-care nurses aided by two nurse practitioners. Paramedics can be used as alternatives to nurse practitioners[16,17]. Authorizations and tasks must be strictly defined prior to deployment to avoid, or at least minimize, uncertainty and confusion. Every nursing team has to define a "nurse in charge" for each paramedic. These organic pairs are essential for facilitation of the paramedic's training on unfamiliar issues. A significant task more suitable for a paramedic is the transporting of patients into and out of the ICU. This will be further discussed later.

The emergency medical team (EMT): EMT skills are even more remote from critical care nursing than those of the paramedic. The EMT profession is not appropriate for a significant clinical role in a field critical-care unit. EMTs can assist with medical equipment and devices, as shown in Table 24.3. As with the paramedic, defining the role's requirements and areas of responsibilities is crucial for optimum utilization of the available personnel and avoiding patient risks.

The medical equipment technician (MET): For every operative ICU, METs are essential for daily practice. METs are particularly needed in the field ICU, where backup equipment may not exist and, in most cases, units are supposed to handle their own malfunctioning devices. Therefore, METs should be constantly available. Ideally, two MET personnel should be present to maintain equipment and address the unit's requirements.

The social worker: Social workers in the ICU are uniquely qualified to assess and address many of the complex psychosocial circumstances that arise in the intense settings of every critical-care unit. These skills are extremely important in a field ICU setting deployed to a disaster area, where cultural differences and language barriers are significant obstacles. Social workers can clarify potential misunderstandings, and improve communication between patients, their families, and medical team members. This can not only help improve the quality of life for very sick and dying patients in the ICU and their families but may also reduce the likelihood of decision-making conflicts arising. As well as supporting patients and their families, the social worker must monitor the working atmosphere and stress among the ICU team [18]. Although the personnel restraints of a field hospital will not enable having a social worker dedicated to the ICU, these issues should be addressed within the psychosocial service of the hospital.

Building a field hospital ICU is challenging. To maintain it is even more demanding. The leadership team must ensure periodic training sessions and social meetings for team consolidation are undertaken, as well as practice of procedures.

Unit Location, Space Planning, and General Resources

Modern medicine critical-care units are regarded as the "beating heart" of their facility. This obviously originates from the various services provided by the ICU team. This concept should be reflected in field hospital planning. The field ICU should be geographically centralized within the hospital, with proximity to the different units it is supposed to serve. The operating theater, recovery room, the emergency department, resuscitation bays, and the admitting wards should encircle the ICU, with predefined and clearly marked routes of transporting patients into and out of the unit (Figure 24.1).

The working space allocated for the field ICU operation (generally a tent) has to be divided into admitting stations and the administration working area such as medical equipment storage and medications shelves with cooling storage. A registration desk and a place for the "point-of-care" laboratory must be taken into consideration as well. The ICU space must be flexible, adjustable for patient volume and capacity, according to the extent of the disaster. As mentioned earlier, the "model of four" can be used as a basic building block, multiplying it if needed. Doubling or tripling it, if needed, is feasible after appropriate preplanning of staff and equipment.

Environmental temperature control can be a significant challenge in the setting of a field ICU. Alteration of the inherent body-temperature control mechanism described among critically ill patients means those patients are markedly influenced by the ambient temperature[19]. In previous experience, patients suffered significant fluctuation in body temperature during their stay in the ICU tent. Hyperthermia was recorded during the day, changing to hypothermia during the night. Treating patients with uncontrolled body temperature is a great challenge in ICU common practice, and can be even more challenging in field conditions. The "lethal triad of trauma" – a combination of hypothermia, acidosis, and coagulation – is a well-known and devastating condition, which needs to be prevented, and treated

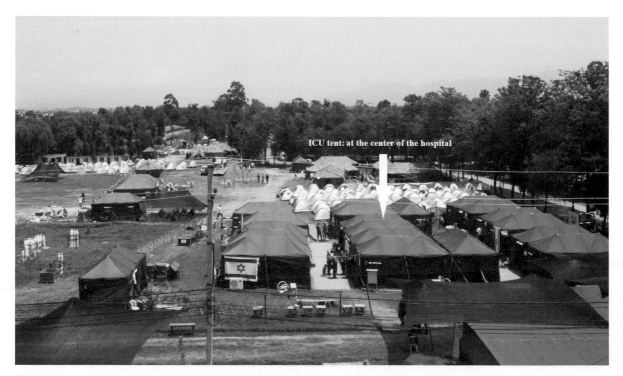

Figure 24.1 The ICU tent positioned in the center of the field hospital, in proximity to the different units it serves (A black and white version of this figure will appear in some formats. For the color version, please refer to the plate section.)

urgently when diagnosed[20,21]. Avoid hypothermia by minimizing patient undressing, and body exposure to ambient temperature should be kept to a minimum. Patients should be covered as soon as possible.

Heating can be provided either by passive or active measures. Passive heating can be achieved using blankets, while active heating can be achieved by applying warm air and/or infusion of warmed IV fluids to normal body temperatures.

Hyperthermia can develop before patient evacuation to the ICU after long exposure to the daily climate. It can also be caused during an ICU stay due to weather conditions combined with altered body temperature regulation, as discussed above. Since hyperthermia may cause significant damage to the already critically ill or wounded patient, active cooling measures should be taken to keep body temperature normalized. Cooling can be achieved by environmental control (air conditioners), and by direct patient-cooling measures. These can either be noninvasive, such as ice packs applied to the axilla or groins or water-cooled blankets, or invasive measures such as providing cold fluid infusions or applying cold water to the nasogastric tube. Neutralizing the ambient temperature effect by constantly activating an air conditioning system can keep a stable environment inside the field ICU tent. It is a highly significant measure of preventing the morbidity and mortality related to the body temperature altered regulation. An air conditioning system is required for every admitting bed in the field ICU tent.

Imaging modalities: Imaging studies are one of the most used tools during ICU practice. When planning for the field setting, sonography and planar X-ray modalities are easily applicable. Point-of-care ultrasound has been established as an ideal imaging modality when used by trained physicians in the ICU setting[22,23]. It can rapidly and accurately diagnose life-threatening conditions including hemoperitoneum, pericardial effusion, cardiac tamponade, pneumothorax, and abdominal aortic aneurysm. In addition, ultrasound machines are commonly used during procedures like IV-line insertion, drainage of fluid collections, and other therapeutic measures such as regional blocks. Sonography has become the imaging modality of choice in the critically ill patient due to its portability, ease of use, speed, and provision of dynamic real-time information, avoiding patient exposure to ionizing radiation. These attributes make ultrasound imaging an attractive tool for decision-making in the field ICU setting.

The simple planar X-ray remains a staple of medical diagnostic imaging. While more advanced imaging modalities such as CT and MRI, so commonly used in a regular ICU setting, can offer the clinician enhanced diagnostic insights, these 3D imaging methods come at the expense of increased size and weight, preparation, acquisition time, and complexity. Until proper portability is achieved, these exclude them from the field hospital and ICU settings. Planar X-ray imaging is still the workhorse of medical imaging, offering the most rapid and simplest diagnostic modality for a wide range of medical conditions. It is often the first-line imaging technique in many emergency situations. Today, new classes of portable X-ray sources are available, having reduced and much more focused radiation exposure. It makes planar X-ray imaging more easily accessible to the point of care, even for the field ICU, where protecting patients and staff from radiation is complicated. Its use can improve outcomes and reduce mortality, as described for portable ultrasound.

Laboratory: The ICU requires immediate and extensive laboratory services. Providing the team with an ability to conduct "point-of-care" examinations is a standard operating practice almost universally in all civilian hospital ICUs. It should be available in the field ICU as well. Capabilities required are blood gas analysis, blood count, and electrolyte levels. The addition of coagulation profiling and metabolic profiling may also be considered.

General documentation and patient medical records: There are a variety of computerized documentation systems that serve ICUs around the world, but one that is stable and easy to use, which can endure the field ICU environment, is lacking. A disaster event is characterized by disorder. One of the major challenges facing a medical facility deployed for such an event is preventing the extension of the surrounding chaos into the functional hospital units. Documentation and writing orders using plain-paper patient charts is possible, but as with previous experience, it is a source for medical mistakes and misunderstandings among the ICU teams. A computerized ICU medical information system, with the ability to gather information quickly and accurately, helps to ensure the adequacy of care[24]. In addition, an electronic medical record system contributes to an effective patient discharge by produ-cing a clear and easily readable medical summary. This is crucial for maintaining the continuity of care in all medical settings and especially in the setting of an ICU operated within a field hospital. The IDF Medical Corps field hospital has implemented a specially tailored IT solution[25]. The solution includes a hospital administration system and a complete electronic medical record for all wards. As of writing, a tailored ICU application is under development and is to be deployed. Nevertheless, since electronic medical-record systems have a risk of failure, plain-paper records must be ready as a fallback solution.

Station Buildup, Medical Devices, and Equipment

Planning a field ICU station uses similar principles as for a regular ICU. Building the station will need max-imal functionality for admitting the most severely injured casualty.

The austere environment in which the critical-care medicine is being practiced presents obstacles like limited space, which drives modifications from a regular ICU planning (Figure 24.2). Following are main points to be considered:

Patient beds and mattresses: Stretchers commonly used in the field-hospital setting are not satisfactory

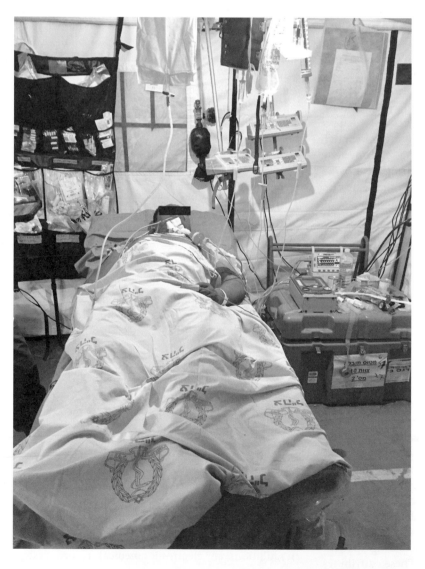

Figure 24.2 A critically injured casualty in the ICU station; equipment is smaller for efficiency and space saving (A black and white version of this figure will appear in some formats. For the color version, please refer to the plate section.)

and even present patient risk when used in the field ICU. They do not allow patient position changes and are associated with increased risk of the patient falling out. Stretchers are also suboptimal because they do not allow patient to be placed in a sitting position, which is essential for the critically ill patient's recovery and weaning from mechanical ventilation. Patient beds selected during field ICU buildup should allow for these issues: allow for patient rotation and position change to avoid pressure ulcers, have side rails to prevent the patient from falling out, but be lightweight and transportable. The ability to provide a sitting position is a great advantage. Pressure ulcers are a danger for all critically ill patients, and are accelerated in the case of the field ICU. Being equipped with proper beds and mattresses is a significant measure in preventing this morbidity.

Oxygen supply: Traditionally, the oxygen source of the field hospital is based on cylinders. These have some limitations, such as heavy weight and being difficult to transport. Refills are repeatedly and frequently needed, and in unstable disaster conditions, oxygen cylinders can pose a real danger. Another aspect of the complexity of oxygen supply to the field ICU is that the total oxygen amount required for the unknown time period of unit deployment may be difficult to calculate and preplan. Solutions can be to rely on oxygen supply streaming from local resources within or outside the disaster zone, dependent on availability. However, one must be prepared for incompatibility of tubing, connectors, and adaptors, between one's home standards and the local ones. For this reason, it is highly recommended to become familiarized with the local oxygen system prior to deployment. Refilling one's own cylinders may cause the same difficulty since local compressors, if functional, can be incompatible with the oxygen connectors. Another solution for these oxygen-supply limitations can be to switch to oxygen concentrator machines. The US Army has demonstrated that low-pressure, portable oxygen concentrators can deliver high FiO_2 during mechanical ventilation in austere locations, and oxygen concentrators could be sufficient to support forward-area mechanically ventilated patients and surgical procedures, and positively impact logistics[26]. Modern concentrators can provide oxygen up to a flow rate of 10 L/min. In previous reports, even the most complicated patients (e.g., acute respiratory distress syndrome [ARDS], lung contusion), did not demonstrate oxygen dependency on a flow rate higher than this value [27]. In light of the adopted concept of "permissive hypoxia" and targeted oxygen saturation of 88–92%, patients may even be supported by minimal FIO_2 of 21%; that is, room air. Switching usage of oxygen cylinders to oxygen concentrators offers an elegant solution for the complex field ICU oxygen supply burden. One must ascertain that the ventilators in use in the ICU are capable of working with low pressure oxygen supply and/or room air only.

Mechanical ventilators: Mechanical ventilation is needed in the field ICU, both for respiratory support in the critically ill and for wounded patients suffering respiratory failure. The postoperative patient group, in need of mechanical ventilation during the recovery phase, should be less challenging. Respiratory pathologies can range from ARDS, lung contusion, and flail chest, requiring extreme ventilation parameters, to patients suffering pneumonia after inhalation injury or aspiration. Patients in need of respiratory support can present late in their disease course; for example, after extrication from prolonged entrapment under ruins following an earthquake. Thus, ventilators with sufficient versatility to overcome high resistance and low compliance should be selected. Basic ventilators aimed at short ventilation and simple support, found in most field hospitals, may be incompatible with the field ICU needs. Small, compact, but still robust ventilation devices available today (Hamilton T1, CareFusion ReVel, and others) are the ones with which to equip a modern field ICU. Having these kinds of ventilators will ensure the ability to provide the best ventilatory support to the most severely injured patients, and avoid ventilator-associated lung injury and the morbidity associated with it. Obviously, all ICU teams should undergo thorough training sessions on operation of the different devices, and be fully acquainted with them.

Monitoring devices: Monitoring devices should be equipped with all the transducers that are also used in a regular ICU. These include noninvasive blood pressure, oxygen saturation, heart rate, respiratory rate, EKG, end tidal carbon dioxide level, invasive blood pressure monitoring, and body temperature. Continuous temperature recording using an esophageal, rectal, or a urinary probe is of high importance for early recognition and real-time response to environmental body temperature dependency, as described earlier. More advanced monitored parameters like cardiac output, stroke volume variation, electroencephalogram, and others are nice to have but not mandatory. Compact, battery-operated monitors are a great advantage due to transportability issues.

Syringe pumps, volumetric pumps, and enteral feeding: To provide adequate treatment in a basic field ICU, operating 4 stations, 12 syringe pumps (3 per station), should be provided. In addition, to ensure precise administration of fluids and medications, at least 8 volumetric pumps (2 per station) are mandatory. Volumetric enteral feeding pumps should be available for every station as patients will need to get early enteral feeding according to nutritional guidelines in intensive care.

Negative pressure suction devices: Negative-pressure suction devices are extensively used in daily practice throughout the field hospital ICU. They are useful in clearing respiratory system secretion, preferentially done using closed systems for better protection of the patient, the caregiver, and the adjacent environment. Continuous negative pressure is applied for other therapeutic purposes, such as chest cavity drainage and VAC dressings. For the purpose of respiratory suctioning, a "foot pump" can be used, but for continuous negative pressure, a specific electricity-operated vacuum pump device is required.

Electricity infrastructure: After counting the diverse devices needed for each station, the "model-of-four" field ICU mandates six to eight electric sockets to be installed. Assigning an electrical technician to the team during the buildup period is important. This technician will establish the complex electrical network needed for a proper operation of the field ICU, and should connect it to the local electricity system, should this be an option. Automatic backup generators are mandatory for the field ICU, so that in the event of an electricity failure, ventilators and other life-support machines will continue to be operative.

Medications and disposable equipment: Space constraints in the field ICU limit the possibility for proper well-organized equipment storage and pharmacy rooms, which are considered essential in regular ICUs. Additionally, the option to build a per-station personal disposable equipment storage, such as a cart or even a shelf, is not feasible. These limitations can be a significant risk for cross-infections in the unit since it creates a common reservoir for infection to spread from patient to patient due to staff members sharing the common equipment shelves. A possible solution

for this is the use of a textile packaging modality – the "unique disposable equipment packaging" – developed by the IDF Medical Corps. This device, which can be hung on the tent wall adjacent to patient's bed, stores all necessary disposable equipment in a slim, space-saving method. The same packaging solution was developed for medications and fluids. The importance of using a per-station "unique disposable equipment packaging" concept should be stressed to the staff during training and drills. Prepacked, specific procedure kits, such as percutaneous tracheotomy, CVC insertion, and others, widely adopted in today's practice of critical care, are highly recommended for use in austere field ICU settings. Using those can ensure a safer and more sterile performance of all procedures.

Only immediate and minimal equipment should be kept in the station itself. The field hospital equipment storeroom must be the source for all medical supplies, while supply routes can be managed by the auxiliary personnel of the ICU (medics and EMTs). Deficiencies in ICU equipment may sometimes be complemented with equipment found in the local medical system or adjacent EMTs. This solution is risky and can be unsatisfactory as the items of equipment may not fulfill modern standards and/or can have expired date when sent to a low-income country. The same is true for medications, where there can be uncertainty over whether drugs available at a local pharmacy have been kept under the appropriate conditions, and they may be expired as well.

Application of these guidelines when planning the field ICU will ensure a properly functioning station, with the ability to admit casualties from all possible scenarios. Ready-to-admit stations, as in a regular ICU, will lead to achieving the goal of providing the best possible care, even in these austere circumstances.

Unique Aspects of Operating a Field ICU

Communication With Local Facilities and Teams

Understanding the full extent of the disastrous event is mandatory for the decision process regarding the establishment of a critical-care unit within the deployed field hospital. An important element of this evaluation is the degree in which the local medical system is overwhelmed. Preliminary data will be available prior to deployment, but detailed information will be available only on arrival at the scene. Locating local medical system leaders and understanding their capabilities can have a significant impact on the field hospital performance as a whole and especially on the ICU operability. Essential information regarding missing medical components or other known gaps of the field ICU equipment or capabilities should be identified and efforts to bridge these using local system resources should be attempted.

Once contact is established with local ICU professionals, a collaboration may be established between the EMT and a local medical facility, as was done during the IDF deployment in Nepal in 2015. In such a case, a triage round is required to evaluate the number of casualties requiring ICU intervention.

Main Local Medical Resources to be Sourced

Even the most advanced field hospital with the most well-equipped ICU will lack advanced imaging modalities and therapeutic capabilities. A lack of these may create significant gaps and become a major obstacle when taking care of injured casualties. Such gaps can be a lack of CT or MRI scanners, essential for diagnoses and clinical decision-making. If one can locate these devices in a local facility and operate them, using local medical personnel or one's delegation personnel, this would greatly improve the diagnostic capabilities in the field hospital and in the ICU. In the chapter authors' experience, during the IDF Medical Corps field hospital deployment to Kathmandu, Nepal, locating an operable CT machine in the local military hospital had a significant impact on the critical care provided, as well as on patients' morbidity and mortality.

An active blood bank can impact clinical outcome. Blood products available in the setting of a field ICU are scarce. In addition to a "Walking blood bank", which is usually found in an EMT, locating even remnants of the local blood bank and pushing it to full operability, gaining the ability to transfuse patients with units of blood, can be a huge step toward better patient care.

A further gap when deploying a field ICU is the limited ability to provide renal replacement therapy. A type 3 EMT may have the capability to provide peritoneal dialysis, but only to a limited degree. The scope of other solutions is limited. The local medical system dialysis services, if present, should be made

operational and available to patients in the field ICU. Closing this therapeutic gap was of high importance during the deployment to Nepal. As expected, in the setting of a major earthquake, numerous casualties suffering from severe crush injuries were treated, some of them presenting with rhabdomyolysis. The ability to locate hemodialysis services in the damaged local hospital and get them to an operable condition had a remarkable impact on those patients' outcome.

Patient Transport Outside the ICU

A plan for locating and utilizing local medical system resources mandates preparing for complex transport of unstable patients outside the unit. Moving away from the relatively safe environment of the field ICU to a medical facility that may be partially damaged exposes these unstable patients to risk. Within a regular, stationary ICU, this risk is weighed each time an ICU patient is transported for a diagnostic or therapeutic procedure within the hospital. Disaster-area transport adds a significant degree of difficulty to those risks, even considering the transport distance to the functional local facility. The potential complications of transport are well known. These include accidentally dislodging life-sustaining devices, diverting attention from vitals to attend to the transport, suspending access to treatment capabilities, and the risk of a mishap directly related to the transport[28]. Guidelines for the transport of critical-care patients should be well defined in the field ICU, and every patient move should be carefully considered and be in the patient's best interest. A pretransport plan, which meets the patient's ongoing and anticipated needs, must be completed[29]. The plan execution must be carried out by a well-trained, well-equipped team, composed of a physician trained in a critical care-related specialty, a critical-care nurse, and a paramedic. In the chapter authors' practice, due to shortage of critical-care physicians, available anesthesiologists offered to carry out those transport missions.

Infection Control

An easily overlooked issue of practicing critical care in a field hospital setting is infection control. The challenge of maintaining infection control in a field ICU; that is, control of environmental contamination from the exterior, as well as the risk of cross infection between patients, is huge. The admitting conditions,

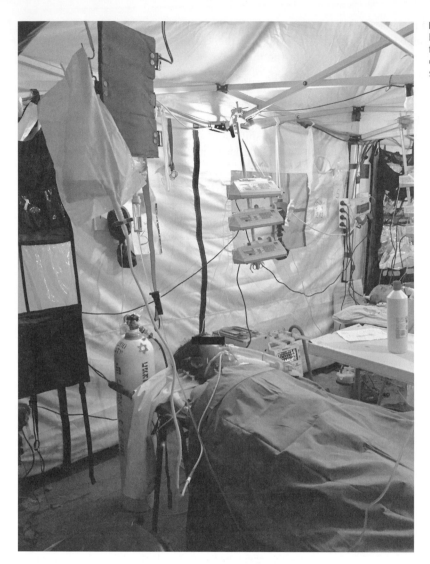

Figure 24.3 Proximity between patient beds (A black and white version of this figure will appear in some formats. For the color version, please refer to the plate section.)

with proximity between patient beds (Figure 24.3), and infection control supplies limitation, mandate extreme awareness of this highly significant issue.

As part of infection control and antimicrobial stewardship activities, analyzing the microbial flora and its unique susceptibility profile in the region deployed to is of major importance. Having this information prior to deployment can be used for the preplanning of the antimicrobial arsenal you will equip your ICU with. Due to the high impact of infections on the outcome of critical care patients, these principles should be adhered to, especially in countries where antimicrobial stewardship programs are not widely practiced, and the population may be highly colonized with multiple drug resistant (MDR) bacteria. During the IDF deployment following the Nepal earthquake, the incidence of MDR superbug isolation from blood and sputum cultures was extremely high. Preparedness led the team to be equipped with suitable broad-spectrum antibiotics, significantly affecting critically injured patients' morbidity and mortality.

Ethical Issues

An ethical committee should be an integral part of a field hospital, serving the ICU within it. Difficult ethical issues will occur in the triage period, both during ICU admission and in decision-making during the ICU stay. In the case of deployment to a foreign country, a suitable local representative, familiar with local culture habits and perception of disease conditions, should be included. As practiced in every regular ICU, in the case of a patient succumbing to extreme illness, a staff discussion with the ethics committee should lead to end-of-life decision, and treatment limitation with palliative measures only should be provided. The local ethical representative is crucial for communicating this decision to the patient's family members[30,31].

Summary

Providing critical care in the setting of a field hospital is possible in a type 3 EMT. Awareness and a proper anticipation of the complex medical, social, ethical, and technical issues, as described earlier, enable the delivery of the best medical care possible in a disaster scenario. For certain disasters, the response timing is critical to ensure optimal casualty outcome. Preparedness is key. Equipping and training critical-care personnel to be rapidly deployed within the field hospital framework can make a great change in the ability to deliver appropriate care to the most seriously injured or sick patients. One must keep in mind that, in general, enhancing capabilities, capacity, or sustainability increases complexity and decreases agility and portability. Considering the design characteristics of an ideal stationary ICU, deploying an ICU in a field hospital will require making significant adaptations and some compromises. From a critical-care perspective, the team must be prepared not only to address trauma or the direct effects of a disaster but also to treat preexisting disease and decompensation of patients with comorbid conditions.

References

1. Richman A, Shapira SC, Sharan Y. Medical response to terror threat. IOS Press; 2010. Published in cooperation with NATO Science for Peace and Security.

2. Grathwohl KW, Venticinque SG. Organizational characteristics of the austere intensive care unit: the evolution of military trauma and critical care medicine; applications for civilian medical care systems. *Critical Care Medicine* 2008: **36**(7 Suppl): S275–83.

3. Graw JA, Spies CD, Kork F, et al. End-of-life decisions in intensive care medicine – shared decision-making and intensive care unit length of stay. *World Journal of Surgery* 2015: **39**(3): 644–51.

4. Morgan CK, Varas GM, Pedroza C, et al. Defining the practice of "no escalation of care" in the ICU. *Critical Care Medicine* 2014: **42**(2): 357–61.

5. Smith SP, Cosgrove JF, Driscoll PJ, et al. A practical approach to events medicine provision. *Emergency Medicine Journal* 2017: **34**(8): 538–42.

6. Bar-Dayan Y, Beard P, Mankuta D, et al. An earthquake disaster in Turkey: an overview of the experience of the Israeli Defence Forces field hospital in Adapazarı. *Disasters* 2000: **24**(3): 262–70.

7. D'Amore AR, Hardin CK. Air Force expeditionary medical support unit at the Houston floods: use of a military model in civilian disaster response. *Military Medicine* 2005: **170**(2): 103–8.

8. Abolghasemi H, Poorheidari G, Mehrabi A, et al. Iranian military forces in the Bam earthquake. *Military Medicine* 2005: **170**(10): 859–61.

9. Bar-On E, Blumberg N, Joshi A, et al. Orthopedic activity in field hospitals following earthquakes in Nepal and Haiti: variability in injuries encountered and collaboration with local available resources drive optimal response. *World Journal of Surgery* 2016: **40**(9): 2117–22.

10. Glick Y, Baruch EN, Tsur AM, et al. Extending a helping hand: a comparison of Israel Defense Forces Medical Corps humanitarian aid field hospitals. *The Israel Medical Association Journal* 2016: **18**(10): 581–5.

11. Donabedian A. The evaluation of medical care programs. *The Bulletin of the New York Academy of Medicine* 1968: **44**(2): 117–24.

12. Scales DC, Rubenfeld GD. The organization of critical care: an evidence-based approach to improving quality. New York: Humana Press; Springer science + Business media; 2014.

13. Yoo EJ, Edwards JD, Dean ML, et al. Multidisciplinary critical care and intensivist staffing: results of a statewide survey and association with mortality. *Journal of Intensive Care Medicine* 2016: **31**(5): 325–32.

14. Benner P, Hooper-Kyriakidis P, Stannard D. *Clinical wisdom and interventions in acute and critical care.* New York. Springer Publishing Company; 2011.

15. Tawfik DS, Phibbs CS, Sexton JB, et al. Factors associated with provider burnout in the NICU. *Pediatrics* 2017: **139**(5).

16. Gershengorn HB, Xu Y, Chan CW, et al. The impact of adding a physician assistant to a critical care outreach team. *PLOS One* 2016: **11**(12): e0167959.

17. Costa DK, Wallace DJ, Barnato AE, et al. Nurse practitioner/physician assistant staffing and critical care mortality. *Chest* 2014: **146**(6): 1566–73.

18. Høye S, Severinsson E. Multicultural family members' experiences with nurses and the intensive care context: a hermeneutic study. *Intensive and Critical Care Nursing* 2010: **26**(1): 24–32.

19. Shigeki K, Satoshi Y, Tomoyuki E, et al. Body temperature abnormalities in non-neurological critically ill patients: a review of the literature. *Journal of Intensive Care Medicine* 2014: **2**(1): 14. Published online.

20. Peres BD, Lopes FF, Vincent JL, et al. Body temperature alterations in the critically ill. *Intensive Care Medicine* 2004: **30**(5): 811–6.

21. Tsuei BJ, Kearney PA. Hypothermia in the trauma patient. *Injury* 2004: **35**(1): 7–15.

22. Cardenas-Garcia J, Mayo PH. Bedside ultrasonography for the intensivist. *Critical Care Clinics* 2015: **31**(1): 43–66.

23. Lichtenstein D, van-Hooland S, Elbers P, et al. Ten good reasons to practice ultrasound in critical care. *Anaesthesiology Intensive Therapy* 2014: **46**(5): 323–35.

24. Prgomet M, Li L, Niazkhani Z, Westbrook JI, et al. Impact of commercial computerized provider order entry (CPOE) and clinical decision support systems (CDSSs) on medication errors, length of stay, and mortality in intensive care units: a systematic review and meta-analysis. *Journal of the American Medical Informatics Association* 2017: **24**(2): 413–22.

25. Levy G, Blumberg N, Kreiss Y, et al. Application of information technology within a field hospital deployment following the January 2010 Haiti earthquake disaster. *Journal of the American Medical Informatics Association* 2010: **17**(6): 626–30.

26. Rybak M, Huffman LC, Danielson PD, et al. Ultraportable oxygen concentrator use in US Army special operations forward area surgery: a proof of

concept in multiple environments. *Military Medicine* 2017: **182**(1): e1649–52.

27. Chiumello D, Brioni M. Severe hypoxemia: which strategy to choose. *Critical Care* 2016: **20**(1): 132.

28. Grathwohl KW, Venticinque SG. Organizational characteristics of the austere intensive care unit: the evolution of military trauma and critical care medicine; applications for civilian medical care systems. *Critical Care Medicine* 2008: **36**(7 Suppl): S275–83.

29. Rice DH, Kotti G, Beninati W. Clinical review: critical care transport and austere critical care. *Critical Care* 2008: **12**(2): 207.

30. Pankaj B, Sanjiv N, Bishnu P, et al. High prevalence of multidrug resistance in bacterial uropathogens from Kathmandu, Nepal. *BMC Research Notes* 2012: **5**: 38.

31. Narayan P, Pooja M, Hridaya P, et al. High rates of multidrug resistance among uropathogenic *Escherichia coli* in children and analyses of ESBL producers from Nepal. *Antimicrobial Resistance & Infection Control* 2017: **6**: 9.

32. Narayan P., Subhash P, Shyam K, et al. High burden of antimicrobial resistance among gram negative bacteria causing healthcare associated infections in a critical care unit of Nepal. *Antimicrobial Resistance & Infection Control* 2017: **6**: 67.

33. Meyer-Zehnder B, Albisser-Schleger H, Tanner S, et al. How to introduce medical ethics at the bedside – factors influencing the implementation of an ethical decision-making model. *BMC Medical Ethics* 2017: **18**(1): 16.

34. Merin O, Ash N, Kreiss Y, et al. The Israeli field hospital in Haiti – ethical dilemmas in early disaster response. *The New England Journal of Medicine* 2010: **362**(11): e38.

Chapter

25

Infectious Diseases and Public Health in a Field Hospital

Paul Reed and Boris Lushniak

Introduction

Field hospitals can play a key role in the clinical treatment and public-health management of infectious diseases during various emergency situations. An infectious disease outbreak itself may in fact represent the reason for the establishment of a field hospital and the facility's primary mission may be directly related to that specific infectious disease; that is, an infectious disease disaster. Such was the case for many field hospitals established as Ebola treatment units (ETUs) in the 2014–2015 public health emergency of international concern associated with the epidemic of Ebola virus disease (EVD) in Western Africa[1–5]. This same scenario can effectively occur with other contagious pathogens, which lead to epidemics or pandemics that overwhelm established health-care systems in various parts of the world (e.g., a regional epidemic of cholera or pandemic influenza). This scenario is not likely to be unique to sub-Saharan Africa or even isolated to solely lower resourced countries. The same considerations for setting up field hospitals in the context of an overwhelming contagious disease outbreak may become necessary in the developed world, as well.

More commonly in other disaster scenarios, a field hospital is established for reasons unrelated to infectious disease, primarily. These include emergency situations caused by war and conflict, natural disaster, famine, population movements, and resettlement: all of which may, and often do, manifest outbreaks of infectious diseases as secondary concerns.

Infectious Diseases in Emergencies

Within the emergency phase of crises, and not uncommonly in periods of recovery from disaster, morbidity and mortality rates can surge because of infectious diseases, with over half of the mortality in refugee situations, for example, caused by measles, diarrheal diseases, acute respiratory infections, and malaria[6]. Refugee populations are at higher risk for outbreaks of many diseases including measles, cholera, shigellosis, meningitis, and typhus[6].

The conditions following acute and chronic disasters often include displaced populations, compromised water supplies and sanitation, nutritional vulnerability, and limited access to health-care services including diminished access to immunizations [7]. Disasters routinely influence the personal hygiene practices of a population and can result, secondarily, in wounds and injuries that become infected (via tetanus, *Staphylococci*, *Streptococci*, waterborne organisms such as *Aeromonas, Vibrio* and *Pseudomonas* species)[8]. Diseases often occur at a higher rate in the wake of disasters due to these other environmental conditions, such as infections resulting from contaminated food and water, including cholera, diarrheal diseases, hepatitis A, hepatitis B, parasitic diseases such as amebiasis, cryptosporidiosis, and giardiasis, rotavirus, shigellosis, and typhoid fever[8]. Animal bites (leading to secondary infections, including rabies) as well as vector-borne diseases could be of concern, including West Nile virus, encephalitis, dengue, Zika, and malaria[8]. Diseases associated with crowding such as measles, meningitis, and acute respiratory infections can also be major issues of concern in the field-hospital setting [7]. Exposure to dead bodies in the midst of disaster is usually not a source of outbreaks of disease, although exposure to blood-borne and other bodily fluid-related pathogens for those handling corpses is a potential concern and precautions need to be taken[7]. This was a significant element needing to be addressed by field hospitals throughout the Ebola crisis in West Africa. Generally, infection control practices can be a challenge in any field-hospital environment, with a broad range of issues needing to be addressed to include those associated with field-hospital design, the placement of patients, food and water supplies, waste disposal, toileting, and vector and pest control[9,10].

Planning

There are numerous considerations that need to be entertained in planning for the deployment of a field hospital under any circumstances during crises or following disaster. There is no such thing as the routine deployment of a field hospital, but in planning for operations under conditions associated with a high threat of a contagious pathogen there are even more extraordinary considerations that must be addressed. Site selection and the characteristics of the facility to be employed, as well as expertise and training of personnel are several issues that are normally looked at when mobilizing a field hospital to provide surge capacity in crises. These issues are of no less concern in an epidemic scenario and may, in fact, require added scrutiny. Additionally, issues related to medical intelligence (e.g., epidemiology of disease, bioterrorism threats), information sharing, and risk communications all may be heightened concerns to build into the planning for circumstances related to an epidemic outbreak, which may not be part of more typical planning cycles in preparation for mobilizing a field hospital[11].

Site selection for the deployment of a field hospital for any purpose and under any conditions demands attention to many details. Vehicle and pedestrian access, proximity to the population served, and vulnerability to flooding are examples of the many generic concerns that must be addressed in planning. When considering the location for a field hospital in the midst of or at risk for an infectious outbreak, added attention should be paid to the choice of geographic location that ensures security of the site, more controlled access, vector control, and which mitigates the environmental spread of contagion. Particularly, site selection should focus on effective and manageable clean water and sanitation, as well as possibly prevailing wind patterns, which may influence the spread of disease. If quarantine measures are in practice for the field hospital, the added burden of security may become paramount in deciding where to locate a facility.

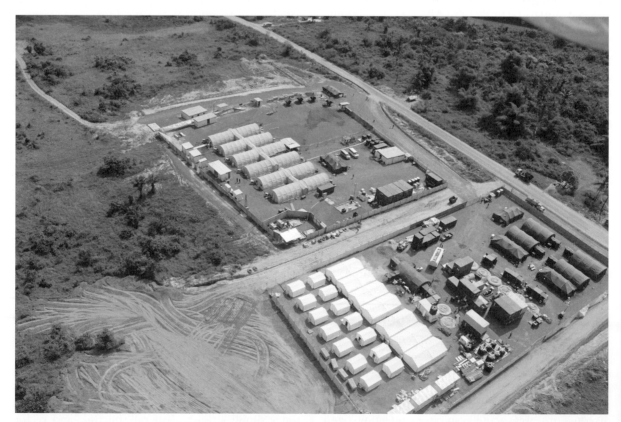

Figure 25.1 Aerial view of the US public-health service Monrovia Medical Unit, 2015 (A black and white version of this figure will appear in some formats. For the color version, please refer to the plate section.)

The physical structure, organic supplies, and mobility of a field hospital are all characteristics that must be considered when planning for a facility's deployment for surge bed capacity during a contagious outbreak. Not all types of deployable field hospital platforms are amenable to be configured for adequate infection control, both in terms of physical barriers and standard operating procedures (SOPs). Thoughtful and deliberate consideration of how a particular field hospital platform can accommodate such measures must be conducted and ideally exercised in contingency planning scenarios; if at all possible, well in advance of an actual event. One important physical attribute that should be addressed is whether the layout can be adapted to ensure patient isolation, for instance. SOPs for infection control that many clinical providers are familiar with in routine practice within fixed hospital or clinic facilities may not be readily translated to the field-hospital setting. In part, this may be due to the physical layout of the field hospital or it may relate to the inherent supplies of the field hospital under normal, noncontagious threat conditions. Most notably, more aggressive standards for personal protection may be required in the field-hospital setting under a contagious epidemic threat than are usually accounted for in supplying a field hospital under other disaster conditions. Additionally, certain higher levels of care including field surgery or intensive care unit (ICU) level cardiovascular and respiratory support may be deemed very high risk or yield very low reduction in patient mortality in the context of certain contagious pathogens and associated morbidities; and, therefore, the field hospital supplies routinely stocked to support these clinical activities may be deemed unnecessary as clinical care is focused on more basic supportive care. Such was the case in the setting of ETUs in 2014–2015 in West Africa[12].

The profile of the personnel employed to staff a field hospital requires equal scrutiny to that of the platform. It is not uncommon for field hospitals deployed to disaster situations to be more heavily weighted in terms of clinical personnel and materiel toward acute, emergent, and surgical care. Primary-care medicine is often adjunctive to the focus of care that is directed toward emergent lifesaving efforts. While that balance of clinical skills may be appropriate in disaster scenarios of a certain type (e.g., immediately post-earthquake), in the setting of a clinical and public-health concern mainly for infectious disease, clinical staffing of the field hospital ought to reflect predominantly primary care skills. Depending on the scale of the epidemic crisis and the availability of resources to address the clinical needs, the extent of medical and surgical care rendered may be limited to attempts to help the greatest numbers of patients to survive[13]. Selection of staffing for the field hospital should therefore appropriately balance clinical skill sets with the parameters for the delivery of care that have been defined. Generally, for a larger scale infectious outbreak, clinical care (and therefore the profile of the field hospital staffing) would be directed toward basic supportive care, ensuring adequate hemodynamic and respiratory support commensurate with bed capacity, patient volume, and available resources. Resource constraints and infection control measures may dictate limited, if any, ventilator support or renal replacement therapy, as cases in point. Nevertheless, expertise of clinical providers from certain specialty fields, such as infectious disease, intensive care, pediatrics, and obstetrics, may be value-added if the parameters for delivering care afforded more aggressive management strategies and/or the patient population served was expected to weigh toward children and pregnant women.

Additional focus on staffing of the field hospital in circumstances of an infectious-disease threat needs to be directed toward ensuring skills sets in infection control, preventive medicine, epidemiology, and environmental engineering. In addition, given the importance of early diagnosis of infection for certain pathogens in helping to determine isolation procedures and clinical management strategies for patients, more unique laboratory skills and resources may be required than is typical of most field-hospital deployments. Laboratorians skilled and resourced to diagnose pathogens and their differential counterparts can contribute greatly to all other aspects of patient regulation in the field-hospital setting under contagious threat. It may be necessary to ensure a significant proportion of staffing overall is exclusively focused on infection control, decontamination, safety, and preventive-medicine strategies for the field hospital; benefitting patients and providers equally. Epidemiologists and other public-health specialists may be valuable for the mission of the field hospital under such conditions to provide effective case definitions, tracking, and support contact tracing to relevant public-health agencies. In providing clinical care to Ebola patients in West Africa, extraordinary attention was paid to nonclinical staffing, as much as to those providing beside care directly to patients (Table 25.1).

Consistent with the staffing of a field hospital under any conditions, appropriate training of personnel is

Table 25.1 ETU staffing model

10 physicians/midlevel providers

20 nurses

4 pharmacists

1–2 lab technicians

10–15 safety officers (preventive medicine, environmental health, engineers)

5 behavioral health providers

10 administrators, logisticians, planners

imperative for them to adequately function in the more austere conditions. Generically, there are many aspects of clinical care in the field-hospital setting that demand nuanced training in contrast to how professionals might otherwise be trained to deliver care in their normal work environments. Such nuanced training may become all the more important in the situation of a deployed field hospital responsive to a crisis with an epidemic contagious threat. Inherent in the planning for such field-hospital conditions is the need for appropriately focused training toward the biological threat, in terms of its epidemiology, its clinical presentation, and relevant clinical management protocols, and perhaps most importantly, its attendant risk of transmission and the management strategies for infection control within the field hospital. The psychological stress of working in an environment where there is a real risk of personnel acquiring disease must be addressed overtly when preparing staff for such a scenario. The requirement for such specific training was made clear in the Ebola outbreak of 2014–2015. It was readily apparent that very few responders were adequately prepared to safely and effectively deliver clinical care in tertiary care centers in developed countries, much less in the conditions in West Africa within field hospitals. An enormous effort was made to rapidly develop and deliver appropriate training in clinical care and infection prevention and control to ensure responders were available to function in field settings and to do so with as little risk as possible[14–16].

The nature and extent of clinical care delivered in a field-hospital setting varies tremendously with the scope and scale of the crisis or disaster confronted. As has been discussed, the inherent capabilities and capacities of a field hospital platform and its personnel are factors that define the limits of care that need be applied. However, in the context of a contagious pathogen impacting a community, and particularly impacting that community in a manner that exceeds the resources available to normally respond to clinical and public-health demands, the parameters for the delivery of clinical care may be greatly influenced by balancing the risk of transmission of disease with the impact of clinical interventions on morbidity and mortality. An infectious agent that is causing disease in a larger and larger number of patients, and one that has a high attack rate (degree of transmission from one person to another) with a mechanism of spread difficult to control, potentially places significant limitations on the manner in which care can be safely rendered in the field-hospital setting. The extreme example of a highly infectious, highly virulent, airborne-spread virus would put an enormous burden on a field hospital in terms of standards of infection control and the required material and personnel skills to safely care for patients. Even in the less severe example of a contagion that is spread via contact with bodily fluids, the burden on resources in a field-hospital setting can be extraordinary. No matter how grave the infectious risk is, planning for the delivery of care in the field hospital must take into consideration the appropriate level of personal protection and environmental controls. It is not clear from recent global experience or existing planning considerations that an adequate availability of resources exists to support a large-scale field hospital response for surge bed capacity in a global pandemic scenario[17].

The adequacy and timeliness of information in periods of crisis is critical to effective disaster medical assistance. The epidemiology of various types of disasters in different populations in different environments can and has been modeled[18]. For more static events leading to disaster, such as a bombing or earthquake, predictive modeling has demonstrated to have some benefit[19]. How predictive those models are to accurately plan for requirements for field hospitals in all scenarios is debatable, however. As was realized in the evolving Ebola epidemic in West Africa, predictions for the spread of epidemic disease and therefore assessments of the commensurate burden on clinical bed capacity are potentially more problematic. The accurate planning for and deployment of field hospitals to a particularly dynamic situation such as an evolving epidemic crisis is therefore dependent on real-time data and analytics. Medical and epidemiologic information should be sought early in planning for field hospital operations to best align the physical requirements of a facility as well as the requirements for personnel and training against the mission. A field hospital's success will depend significantly on planning that addresses accurate information regarding the infectious agent, specifically its clinical and epidemiologic profile.

Equal to the need for accurate data up front in the planning for field-hospital operations in the face of a contagious outbreak is the need to plan for data collection within the facility. Beyond the value in improved clinical care for patients, accurate and complete data collection in the field-hospital setting can provide important health data to the larger public-health response during a crisis. Clinical and demographic data obtained from patients in the field hospital can be applied discretely and aggregated to help inform the broader public-health picture of an epidemic crisis and direct public-health interventions to control for the further spread of disease. In planning for a field-hospital engagement under such circumstances it behooves medical planners to develop systems of data collection which can easily be shared with public-health authorities. As well, such an approach of information sharing needs to be built into planning for training purposes for field hospital staff.

A final planning consideration for field hospitals in the context of an infectious outbreak is in appropriately managing information sharing with the public. Given the prominent role that strategic and risk communications play in public-health crises, information sharing regarding the spread of disease ought to be appropriately vetted and controlled. An accurate representation of the epidemiology and clinical aspects of the disease, which is evidenced-based, is necessary to minimize public distrust and uncertainty in such crises. Field-hospital planners must account for how information relating to their operations and their patients is integrated into the larger public-health-risk communications strategy.

Preparation

Rarely, if ever, in emergent disaster response situations will the planning cycle for the deployment of a field hospital to a particular scenario be fully realized before establishment of the facility is necessary. The issues on the ground more often define the timeliness of executing the mission of a field hospital than does the completeness of planning activities. Given this limitation, contingency plans need to be entertained well in advance of crises where field hospitals may be

employed to help manage unique contagious threats. Failing such comprehensive advanced planning for varying field-hospital configurations and operating procedures, quick and deliberate preparation for operations must often be conducted in real time while finalizing elements of the planning for a given situation. In practice, this demands flexibility and innovative skills to further planning considerations along while actually laying out the physical platform of the field hospital and rehearsing SOPs, focused on the known clinical and infection control issues at hand.

In the context of infectious disease risks, including to the patient population served and the personnel rendering care in the field hospital, appropriate preparation of the facility and practiced operational procedures are imperative. The effectiveness of clinical-care practices to treat patients and preventive medicine strategies to mitigate the spread of contagious disease within the facility is directly correlated with the design of the field hospital and the procedures employed by staff[20]. While appropriate immunization status should be demanded of all field-hospital personnel under any conditions as a best preventive medicine practice, situations where there is risk of a contagious pathogen present additional impetus for targeted vaccination. When feasible, relative to the specific infectious threat, directed vaccination of staff should be sought. In the case of emerging biological threats, where fully validated vaccines may not be available, but a vaccine may exist that is under study, a unique sociopolitical and clinical/scientific set of considerations needs to be weighed to entertain the protection of those personnel, many of whom are volunteers.

The design of the field hospital, relative to infectious risks and clinical requirements for managing patients, will vary considerably with the nature of the pathogen, or pathogens, that are prevalent. Low-risk versus high-risk contact isolation necessitate different considerations for patient triage, segregation, and movement through the facility, as well as movement of staff. These considerations could directly impact the layout of the field hospital in profound ways. The selection of the type of platform to be used for the field hospital should be considered early on in planning given the limitations of certain facilities to adequately accommodate these requirements. The design of ETUs in West Africa in 2014–2015 is a demonstrative example of the importance of layout and patient and staff movement. In this example of extreme contact isolation, design was influenced in every conceivable way to minimize droplet spread of disease – unidirectional flow of patients and staff through the facility, segregation of suspect versus confirmed patients, placement of decontamination stations, distancing of beds, and complete separation of high-risk and low-risk zones are but a few examples of measures taken.

While there are subtleties that need to be addressed with many different types of contagious pathogens, one major discriminator in the design of a field hospital during a contagious threat is whether there is risk of airborne spread. Very few platforms exist for field-hospital deployment that can accommodate the limitations of a facility attempting to control for the airborne spread of a highly infectious contagion, particularly under exaggerated conditions with large numbers of patients necessitating significant bed capacity. There remain little data on the adequacy of physical or procedural barriers to minimizing airborne pathogen spread in the field hospital setting[21].

Beyond the choice of platform and the configuration of a facility to accommodate the physical barriers needed to manage infectious disease risk, the preparation of SOPs to control for disease spread while maximizing patient care demands equal or greater attention. Like advanced planning for the physical design of a field hospital under various contingency scenarios with infectious disease risk, advanced development of SOPs should be sought. SOPs for fixed medical treatment facilities under nonemergent or disaster conditions can be modified for the field hospital setting. Early planning that accounts for the potential limitations of a field hospital in more austere circumstances can help minimize the real-time preparations required once a field hospital is deployed. Nevertheless, any preplanned SOPs must be exercised in the setting of the deployed field hospital prior to receipt of a first patient, whenever possible. There will always be unforeseen limitations to the application of SOPs within a field hospital that are situation-dependent and that require modification of the SOPs to ensure good clinical care and safe infection control measures.

Just-in-time training of personnel will always be required in considering infectious disease risk in a field hospital setting. It is unlikely that any or all personnel deployed to support a field hospital will have the complete knowledge, skills, and abilities to address a given communicable disease scenario, including awareness of the type of platform being employed for the field hospital, the logistical limitations for the field hospital, the specific steps of the SOPs being applied, the characteristics of the pathogen(s) that are prevalent, the pathophysiology and epidemiology of the disease being addressed, or the cultural variations that are relevant to the population being served. All these issues need to be raised in the consciousness of personnel staffing a field hospital under such a contagious disease threat. This demands that a great deal of attention is paid, at the time of preparation of a facility, to innovative means of training and education. Much of the just-in-time training will need to be developed in a notional sense. However, whenever possible, additional real-world experience for personnel should be sought before executing the mission of the field hospital. This can be conducted with aligned partners in the crisis, if there are other actors conducting similar operations ahead of the mission at hand.

Medical record keeping, by whatever means, is always a necessity and often a challenge in the field hospital setting. However, in the context of a communicable disease outbreak, either as the primary or secondary issue in a crisis situation, accurate health records can also be vital to the larger public-health concerns. Patients with infectious disease who are clinically cared for in a field hospital represent part of the broader picture of the health-related event. Information that addresses how a patient acquired the disease, their clinical status, and response to therapy could inform public-health measures for contact tracing, control of further spread of disease, and future clinical management strategies for the care of other patients. Therefore, establishing an effective and efficient system of record keeping, and one that can be accessed by the public-health community, for the field hospital in the scenario of a contagious disease outbreak becomes essential.

Operations

Application of standard clinical and infection control procedures in the field-hospital setting impacted by a large-scale infectious disease outbreak necessitates constant review and frequent adjustment. Following a routine of planning (plan), carrying out (do), analyzing the effectiveness of (check), and refining (act) (PDCA) procedures will help ensure the best clinical outcomes for patients while optimizing infection control and mitigating risk to patients and personnel, alike. As thorough as a series of rehearsals prior to the initiation of clinical operations may be, applying procedures with real patients while a field hospital is under stress, especially in the face of large numbers of patients in a short period of time, will often elucidate inefficiencies or issues of safety that need to be addressed. Therefore, a routine application of the PDCA model will help manage those efficiencies with little disruption to clinical operations.

A key to efficient patient management in the field-hospital setting of a contagious outbreak is optimized patient regulation, from referral into the facility to discharge or transfer from the field hospital. Above and beyond the normal concerns of patient movement in crisis scenarios (i.e., bed capacity, mass triage, discharge rates, logistical limitations regarding patient transport, and others), the added considerations relating to an infectious disease outbreak can be quite complicated and constraining. Isolation of patients by means of physical barriers and standard practices to minimize spread of disease will impact the pace with which patients are able to be triaged into a facility and accommodated with appropriate clinical bed space, and the timeliness with which they may be discharged. Aspects of decontamination of transport vehicles, beds, and reusable supplies, for example, will all potentially influence a field hospital's bed capacity and throughput of patients, over time. Of unique concern with patients recovering from contagious disease is their management at the point when they are clinically stable for discharge but remain a communicable risk to the community. These considerations could significantly impact the movement of patients and field-hospital bed capacity. Depending on the nature of the infectious pathogen and public-health measures in the community, field hospitals in a crisis situation may be burdened with demands for ongoing isolation of persons as part of the overall management of the spread of disease.

A contagious pathogen evident in patients being rendered care in the field-hospital setting represents a source of nosocomial infection for other patients who may otherwise be receiving care for an unrelated illness or injury. Depending on the virulence and attack rate of the pathogen, this may pose an extraordinary risk to noninfected patients and staff. Therefore, once recognized (if not the prevalent concern itself), an infected patient should be managed carefully to ensure minimal risk of spread of disease. Once such a contagious threat is established in a field hospital, particularly with increasing

numbers of patients being infected, clinical operations should be modified to ultimately prevent spread of disease. Such preventive infection control measures may obviate the ability to deliver any other medical or surgical care in the facility, beyond that directed at patients infected. In the extreme example of such epidemic disease during the Ebola crisis, field hospitals (ETUs) exclusively cared for patients with Ebola, taking great care to establish differential diagnoses and rule out patients without Ebola, to minimize their risk of exposure.

Commensurate with evolving epidemic disease in the field hospital setting, as in any medical treatment facility, is the inherent risk for the development of antibiotic resistance. Depending on the nature of the infectious agent, the attendant appropriate or inappropriate use of antibiotics, and the duration of the epidemic, there may be significant risk for such resistance to develop. Accurate diagnosis of those patients presenting with an aligned case definition should be sought, whenever possible. If laboratory resources for accurate diagnosis are not available, an accurate case definition to drive clinical decision-making toward judicious use of antibiotics ought to be applied.

Public-health practices and environmental management strategies employed routinely in hospital settings are no less important in the field-hospital setting for the control of spread of disease than are individual patient care protocols. Such practices should be closely tied to clinical protocols as seamless SOPs for the mitigation of environmental spread of disease. While not specifically clinically care driven, procedures for waste management, the provision of clean water including for effective sanitation practices, handling of food and potable water, cleaning of bodily fluids, and handling of human remains all demand attention. Procedures should be integrated between clinical and nonclinical staff functioning in patient care areas, such that bedside care and environmental hygiene practices appear one and the same. Relative to a specific infectious agent's behavior in the environment, particular attention may be necessary to manage effluent from patient-care areas or ventilation procedures for air entry and exit. Such environmental considerations likely will overlap with patient care procedures and both should be adapted accordingly.

Public Health and Prevention

Depending on their specific missions, jurisdictions, and capabilities, field hospitals can play an important role in public health and the prevention of spread of disease beyond the facility itself. The mission of field hospitals to provide direct clinical care can be expanded to help stabilize epidemics, as required, to ensure that basic living conditions are available to communities, including the provision of adequate food, clean water, sanitation, and shelter. These basic human services may be just as critical, or even more so, than direct medical care for the broader public health interests. The public-health activities of a field hospital can also include community-based prevention and health-promotion activities, nutritional support, and disease surveillance and control.

In the emergency phase of any complex crisis, the top-ten public health priorities that can be undertaken by a field hospital include the following: (1) an initial assessment of the population and its health and human services needs with an emphasis on rapid assessment for immediate action, (2) measles immunization and distribution of vitamin A to at-risk populations, (3) assessment of and assistance with water and sanitation, including solid waste and contaminated medical-waste control, disposal of the dead, personal hygiene, and vector control, (4) food and nutrition, including supplementary and therapeutic feeding programs, (5) shelter and site planning or integration for displaced populations, (6) the provision of direct clinical care, with an emphasis on respiratory infections, malaria, and diarrheal diseases, where indicated, (7) control of communicable diseases (CDs) and epidemics through patient isolation, contact tracing, and potentially quarantine of exposed persons, (8) public-health surveillance to measure the health status of the population and to detect new epidemic diseases as soon as they appear, (9) human resources and training, realizing that the skill sets needed may include varied expertise in public health, epidemiology, water and sanitation, nutrition, administration, and logistics, and (10) coordination among operational partners[22].

Prevention of epidemic disease is critical and a field hospital should be involved in prevention activities before an infectious disease becomes a larger communicable threat to the community. Once outbreaks occur, public-health interventions tied to field hospital operations become even more important. The objectives during an outbreak include minimizing the number of cases through preventive measures and reducing the morbidity and mortality among cases through early detection and treatment[23].

Early involvement of local, regional, and national health authorities, if available, as well as international partners in relevant crises, is a key component of effective field-hospital public-health assistance. Accurate clinical diagnosis and laboratory confirmation, if feasible, targeted treatment of cases meeting a case definition, identification of a specific pathogen and the sources of infection, as well as the application of appropriate preventive measures are all critical elements in field hospital operations in an infectious disease outbreak. Measures to control outbreaks vary and are directly related to the pathogen in question and the environment of the affected population, but they should focus on reducing contact with the sources of infection, protecting vulnerable groups, and ultimately interrupting transmission. Epidemiologic and pathophysiologic factors to consider include the occurrence of the disease process, its reservoir, mode of transmission, incubation period, duration of communicability, susceptibility and resistance, and specific methods of control[23]. Based on these factors, methods of control can include blocking transmission through measures such as hygiene and handwashing, proper disposal of contaminated materials, prevention of food and water contamination, control of patients, contacts, and the immediate environment (isolation, quarantine, immunization, disinfection), and specific epidemic and international measures[23]. Many of these measures can and should be taken in the field-hospital setting.

Public education and crisis emergency risk communication are vital tools in the midst of public-health emergencies[24]. Public education must take into account the concerns of the community and consist of culturally appropriate messaging, community engagement, and social mobilization[25,26]. Infection prevention and control mandates an engagement with the community and its leaders using multimethod communications to create an environment of trust[27]. Effective risk communication includes the following six principles: (1) be first – if the information is yours to provide, do so as soon as possible, (2) be right – communicate what you know when you know it, what you do not know, and if you will know more later, (3) be credible – tell the truth, rumors are more damaging than hard truths, (4) express empathy, (5) promote action – give people things to do which can calm anxiety, (6) show respect [28]. As direct agents for clinical-care delivery and public-health monitoring and intervention during crisis, field-hospital administrators should be well

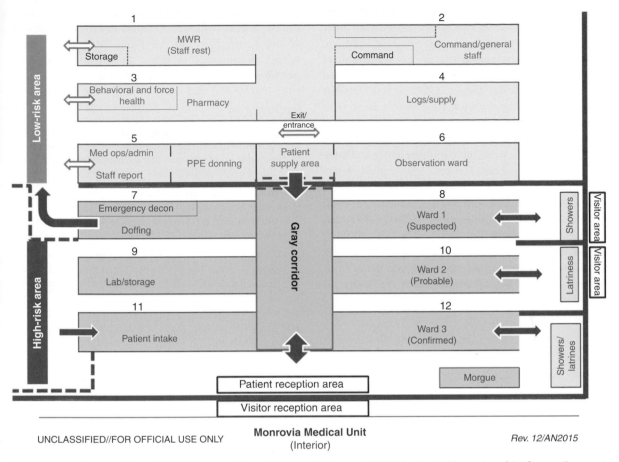

Figure 25.2 Schematic of US public-health service Monrovia Medical Unit Layout, 2015 (A black and white version of this figure will appear in some formats. For the color version, please refer to the plate section.)

prepared to address risk communications as part of the larger public-health campaign strategy.

Decommissioning and Redeployment

Decommissioning of any field hospital mandates an emphasis on disinfection and sterilization of medical and surgical material, if possible, or proper disposal of all material and equipment that may be contaminated.

Redeployment and reintegration of staff are critical steps to consider in the planning for and administration of personnel. Proper medical clearance of staff prior to redeployment ensures that potentially ill staff are not traveling back from a mission. Just as crucial is the establishment of a system of appropriate medical monitoring once redeployment has taken place to ensure that all signs and symptoms of potential disease are investigated. Decisions regarding the quarantine of exposed individuals need to be made wisely. Redeployment

needs to consider not just the physical health of the staff but also their mental health and social wellbeing. Redeployment also opens up issues surrounding social interactions with family, friends, workplace colleagues, and others. The transparent sharing of factual, scientifically based information regarding the mission of field-hospital staff and the disease in question can provide a clearer path to alleviate the concerns of others.

Patient and Staff Movement

In the context of the depicted ETU, redesigned from a deployable field hospital doctrinally intended for combat medical/surgical purposes, careful consideration was made for patient and staff movement through the facility to minimize the risk for spread of the contagious pathogen. Standard procedures for patient intake, isolation relative to their known infected status (suspect, probable, or confirmed), and limitation of movement during hospitalization optimized infection control. Laboratory confirmed Ebola patients are kept segregated from other suspected but yet unconfirmed patients by this design. Additionally, procedures to maximize unidirectional movement of staff from suspect through to confirmed patient areas, with modified decontamination stations (boot, handwashing stations) in between areas were employed. Segregated areas for patients' latrine and shower use, as well as visitation with families (across a defined barrier), were built into the design to keep confirmed Ebola patients isolated. A unique characteristic of this particular facility was the intersecting "gray" zone. Due to structural limitations of the platform used, this main corridor was a necessary obstacle with which to contend. Procedures for hand and boot washing, in and out of the "gray corridor," were intended to mitigate cross-contamination when staff were traversing from confirmed patient areas to other areas of the facility.

Summary

Field hospitals can play a key role in the clinical treatment and public-health management of infectious diseases during emergency situations, in the setting both of disasters primarily of an epidemic nature and of outbreaks that result secondarily in the midst of other crises. Planning and preparation are key components to successful operation in these settings and present unique issues compared to more routine field-hospital scenarios absent a contagious threat. Special consideration needs to be given to site selection, the physical structure of a facility, infection prevention and control measures, personal protection, selection and training of staff, data collection and sharing, and clinical SOPs. The mission of field hospitals can be expanded beyond clinical care to help stabilize epidemics through ensuring basic living conditions are available, including the provision of adequate food, clean water, sanitation, and shelter. The public-health-focused activities of a field hospital should include community-based prevention and health-promotion activities, risk communication, and disease surveillance and control; all of which may provide invaluable contributions to broader public health response efforts during crisis.

Disclaimer

The content of this publication is the sole responsibility of the authors and does not necessarily reflect the views, assertions, opinions or policies of the Uniformed Services University of the Health Sciences, the University of Maryland, the US Public Health Service, the Department of Defense (DoD), nor the departments of the Army, Navy, or Air Force. Mention of trade names, commercial products, or organizations does not imply endorsement by the USA government.

References

1. Lamb LE, Cox AT, Fletcher T, McCourt AL. Formulating and improving care while mitigating risk in a military Ebola virus disease treatment unit. *Journal of the Royal Army Medical Corps* 2016: 2–6.

2. Mosquera A, Braun M, Hulett M, Ryszka L. US Public health service response to the 2014–2015 Ebola epidemic in West Africa: a nursing perspective. *Public Health Nursing* 2015: **32**(5): 550–4.

3. Vetter P, Dayer J-A, Schibler M, Allegranzi B, Brown D, Calmy A, et al. The 2014–2015 Ebola outbreak in West Africa: hands on. *Antimicrobial Resistance & Infection Control*. 2016: **5**(1).

4. Wilson D. Inside an Ebola treatment unit: a nurse's report. *American Journal of Nursing* 2015: **115**(12): 28–38.

5. Lushniak BD. The hope multipliers: the US public health service in Monrovia. *Public Health Reports* 2015: **130**(6): 562–5.

6. Toole MJ, Waldman RJ. Prevention of excess mortality in refugee and displaced populations in developing countries. *JAMA* 1990: **263**(24): 3296–302.

7. Watson JT, Gayer M, Connolly MA. Epidemics after natural disasters. *Emerging Infectious Diseases* 2007: **13**(1): 1–510.

8. Ligon BL. Infectious diseases that pose specific challenges after natural disasters: a review. *Seminars in Pediatric Infectious Diseases* 2006: **17**(1): 36–45.

9. Sullivan SM, McDonald KW. Post-Hurricane Katrina infection control challenges and the public health role at a mobile field hospital. *American Journal of Infection Control* 2006: **34**(5): E11–12.

10. Lichtenberger P, Miskin IN, Dickinson G, Schwaber MJ, Ankol OE, Zervos M, et al. Infection control in field hospitals after a natural disaster: lessons learned after the 2010 earthquake in Haiti. *Infection Control & Hospital Epidemiology* 2010: **31**(9): 951–7.

11. Murray CK, Yun HC, Markelz AE, Okulicz JF, Vento TJ, Burgess TH, et al. Operation united assistance: infectious disease threats to deployed military personnel. *Military Medicine* 2015: **180**(6): 626–51.

12. Lamontagne F, et al. Evidence-based guidelines for supportive care of patients with Ebola virus disease. *The Lancet* 2017: **391**(10121): 700–8.

13. Torabi-Parizi P, Davey RT, Jr., Suffredini AF, Chertow DS. Ethical and practical considerations in providing critical care to patients with Ebola virus disease. *Chest* 2015: **147**(6): 1460–610.

14. Hageman JC, Hazim C, Wilson K, Malpiedi P, Gupta N, Bennett S, et al. Infection prevention and control for Ebola in health care settings – West Africa and United States. *MMWR Supplements* 2016: **65**(3): 50–6.

15. A review of the role of training in WHO Ebola emergency response/Examen du role des formations dispensees dans le cadre de la reponse de l'OMS a la crise Ebola. *Weekly Epidemiological Record* 2016: **91**(181).

16. The National Ebola Training and Education Center (2017). Website. https://netec.org/

17. Dasaklis TK, Rachaniotis N. Epidemics control and logistics operations: a review. *International Journal of Production Economics* 2012: **139**: 393–410.

18. Guha-Sapir FV. Earthquakes, an epidemiologic perspective on patterns and trends, in Spence R, So E, Scawthorn C (eds.) *Human casualties in earthquakes.* New York: Springer; 2011: 13–24.

19. Bar-On E, Peleg K, Kreiss Y. Coping with the challenges of early disaster response: 24 years of field hospital experience after earthquakes. *Disaster Medicine and Public Health Preparedness* 2013: 7: 491–8.

20. Forrester JD, Hunter JC, Pillai SK, Arwady MA, Ayscue P, Matanock A, et al. Cluster of Ebola cases among Liberian and US health care workers in an Ebola treatment unit and adjacent hospital – Liberia, 2014. *MMWR Morbidity and Mortality Weekly Report* 2014: **63**(41): 925–9.

21. Li Y, Leung GM, Tang JW, et al. Role of ventilation in airborne transmission of infectious agents in the built environment – a multidisciplinary systematic review. *Indoor Air* 2007: **17**: 2–18.

22. *Refugee health – an approach to emergency situations* (Médecins Sans Frontières). Hanquet G (ed.) London and Basingstoke: Macmillan Education Ltd; 1997.

23. Heymann DL. American Public Health Association. *Control of communicable diseases manual.* Twentieth edn. (ed.) 2014.

24. Spengler JR, Ervin ED, Towner JS, Rollin PE, Nichol ST. Perspectives on West Africa Ebola virus disease outbreak, 2013–2016. *Emerging Infectious Diseases* 2016: **22**(6) 956–63.

25. Laverack G, Manoncourt E. Key experiences of community engagement and social mobilization in the Ebola response. *Global health promotion* 2016: **23**(1): 79–82.

26. Abramowitz SA, McLean KE, McKune SL, Bardosh KL, Fallah M, Monger J, et al. Community-centered responses to Ebola in urban Liberia: the view from below. *PLOS Neglected Tropical Diseases* 2015: **9**(4).

27. Marais F, Minkler M, Gibson N, Mwau B, Mehtar S, Ogunsola F, et al. A community-engaged infection prevention and control approach to Ebola. *Health Promotion International* 2016: **31**(2): 440–9.

28. Centers for Disease Control and Prevention (2016). Crisis & Emergency Risk Communication (CERC). Online article. www.emergency.cdc.gov/cerc

Primary and Ambulatory Care in a Field Hospital in Disaster Areas

Ilan Green and Shlomo Vinker

Introduction

Events like high-magnitude earthquakes or floods may cause humanitarian disasters especially in remote, poor, and underserved areas. In these areas, the pre-disaster health-care human resources and facilities are scarce. The constructions of public and private buildings as well as infrastructure are underdeveloped or poor and unable to give immediate as well as long-term services.

The ambulatory and primary-care units on scene may act as small outreach units that start their action as soon as international first-aid services are available. They may act for long periods with rotating volunteers and local health-care staff. Another mode of operation is as part of a larger body such as a field hospital. The deployment as well as the end of action on scene will depend in these scenarios on the aims and mission of the field hospital while the primary-care and ambulatory unit will act as an annex to the field hospital, receiving missions and responsibilities as a directive from the field hospital manager.

We aim to describe the primary care and ambulatory unit (PCAU) of such a field hospital in a disaster area.

Epidemiology

In a natural disaster there may be thousands of people who will die and many more will be injured, left homeless, and otherwise adversely affected by the loss of infrastructure. People displaced by structural damage to their homes or those afraid to return to their homes for fear of damage tend to go and live in tent camps, which spring up spontaneously or are organized by local authorities or international non-governmental organizations (NGOs). Displaced people, especially those without adequate shelter and without access to sanitation and other services, are at particular risk for immediate as well as long-term health problems.

In the hours and days immediately following a high-magnitude earthquake, it has been well demonstrated that injuries such as acute orthopedic injuries, head injuries, and crush injuries with subsequent rhabdomyolysis contribute to significant mortality. Illnesses resulting from poor shelter and lack of access to fuel, clean water, and sanitation will appear later.

Fernald and colleagues had been deployed with their MASH unit in response to the 2005 earthquake in Pakistan[1]. More than 20 000 patients received care during a four-month period. An initially high surgical workload decreased in about two weeks while the volume of primary-care patients increased, eventually accounting for 90% of the total patient visits. They estimated that 15% were < 5 years of age and about 50% of patients were < 18 years of age. A similar trend had been documented by one of the authors (Shlomo Vinker) in 2010 at Port-au-Prince, Haiti[2]. Figure 26.1 describes the relative workload in the ambulatory unit during the deployment of the Israeli field hospital in Port-au-Prince, Haiti.

Broach and colleagues collected data regarding the epidemiology in the tent camps of Port-au-Prince, Haiti on days 15–18 after the earthquake in 2010[3]. They note a preponderance of pediatric illness, with 53% of cases being patients younger than 20 years old and 25% younger than 5 years old. The most common complaints noted by category were respiratory (24.6%), gastrointestinal (16.9%), and genitourinary (10.9%). They also observed a high incidence of malnutrition among pediatric patients, noting that only a small number of cases of traumatic injuries were identified (less than 5%).

Operating Ambulatory Service in the Field Hospital or as an Outreach Mobile Unit

Service can be delivered as a department in the field hospital or by outreach to tent camps. It must be

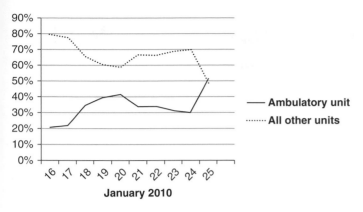

Figure 26.1 Visits to the Israeli field hospital in Port-au-Prince, Haiti – the relative workload in the ambulatory unit according to the date since deployment

coordinated with the local health-care authorities and/or other international bodies active in the arena.

The clinic should contain a triage area, an area for patient consultations, and a pharmacy area with medications to distribute.

Usually the PCAU should work in one shift in daylight and there is no need for night or afterhours shifts. The PCAU should work seven days a week. The workload is markedly decreased in local major holidays[1], and shifts and staff scheduling should take this into account.

Triage

Triage can be active – being performed by providers in the refugee camps – or passive, at the entrance to the field hospital. Triage medical officers may include family physicians or qualified nurses. Local translators should accompany all staff members, but are especially critical in the triage group.

The criteria for triage include factors such as age, nature of illness, and clinical appearance. The principle is to select those people who could most benefit from care while minimizing triage examinations.

Consultations and Treatment

After the triage, each patient should carry a medical record with his or her name, age, and chief complaint. The patient is then moved to wait in another area, separated from the triage area, where a provider will make a brief clinical note on each patient, including the symptoms, diagnosis, and treatment. In the pharmacy, medications will be provided free of charge.

The number of patients seen every day, the duration of time for which medications will be supplied,

and scheduling of follow-up visits all depend on the capacity of the PCAU in terms of staff, medications, and dressings supply.

It is recommended to give tetanus toxoid to each injured patient no matter what his or her vaccination status is.

An average consultation unit, which includes a family physician, a qualified nurse, and a translator, can treat 30–50 patients in a working day.

What Skills and Equipment Are Required by Physicians?

During routine operation, family physicians encounter complex medical, psychological, and social problems daily. These problems are intensified during disasters. As disaster responders, they face the unknown. The physician can be in an isolated, unfamiliar area with limited resources and patients with complex medical problems: acute, traumatic, and chronic illnesses.

Even in the most catastrophic event, the need for primary-care physicians in conjunction with trauma specialists is high since the local medical system is overwhelmed, especially in low-income countries[4]. The contribution of a family physician is crucial.

Health-care workers need some skills to cope with the consequences of devastating natural disasters and to provide successful intervention. Firstly, a health-care worker should prepare him- or herself to work long hours, usually in twelve-hour shifts. Teamwork ability is extremely important. And the physician should be ready to be exposed to suffering and agony. The level of suffering can be overwhelming.

The chapter authors' experience indicates that, during the first week, trauma injuries are predominant. Up to 80% of the patients have trauma injuries[2]. Primary-care physicians should therefore be skilled in emergency medicine and should be trained in basic and advanced trauma life support, especially first evaluation of severe traumatic injuries and treatment of minor trauma (closed fractures, wounds, and so on) [5,6]. Severe trauma will be treated by surgeons, orthopedic surgeons, and emergency-medicine specialists, but the triage and primary evaluation is often performed by the family physicians in the team.

Health-care teams should be prepared to treat infectious diseases[3], especially routine infections such as upper respiratory tract infections, gastrointestinal infections, and genitourinary tract infections. They should be familiar with the prevalence of different pathogens and their antibiotic resistance. It is very important to know what the endemic common medical problems are, and to learn about them before reaching the arena. For example, tropical diseases such as typhoid fever or malaria can be extremely rare in the daily clinic in high-income countries, but can be very common in the disaster area and physicians should be familiar with the signs, symptoms, and management of such diseases. It is recommended to consult an infectious diseases specialist about common infections in the disaster area. Another way to learn about the local infectious diseases is by using the Centers for Disease Control and Prevention (CDC) website: www.cdc.gov

One of the most crucial obstacles in treatment is communication with the local population. In the IDF field-hospital mission in Nepal after the earthquake in 2015, local medical students offered translation services. Translation services were also used in the field hospital of the refugee camp in Kosovo in 1999[7]. Every physician was accompanied by a medical student who helped to understand the medical problem and local cultural beliefs, and to explain the medical recommendations to the patients. The translation by medical staff facilitated the treatment and the stream of patients in the ambulatory clinic. Translation can be done by local medical staff like students or nurses, as well as local English teachers or other teachers or students.

The medical staff should be familiar with the local health care as well as public and religious facilities and with local approved medications. For example, in low-income countries, beta blockers are sometimes the first-choice treatment for hypertension because of their low cost. In such a scenario, prescribing an angiotensin converting enzyme (ACE) inhibitor would be worthless, since the patient cannot afford to buy the medication.

Recommendation for hemodialysis for chronic renal failure patient will be useless if the nearest dialysis unit is hundreds of kilometers away. Even simple recommendations such as drinking warm liquids or storing antibiotic syrups in a cold place can be unachievable to a patient who is discharged to a tent in a refugee camp.

There is a high risk of psychological problems such as acute stress disorder, depression, and anxiety after a disaster. The family physician should be familiar with assessment tools and brief interventions for mental problems to identify and treat patients at risk for mental problems[8].

Equipment

An ambulatory clinic needs all the equipment to diagnose and treat acute and chronic primary care problems. It includes ECG, otoscopes, stethoscopes, glucometer, intravenous infusions, liquids, suturing kits, birth delivery kits, sterilization and disinfection materials, and also commonly used medications for adult and pediatric population (analgesics, antibiotics, ointments, and so on) to provide the necessary medications for several days. As most deployments will be in underserved regions with a high incidence of poverty and malnutrition, there is a need for nutritional support such as multivitamins and infant milk substitutes. We must remember that the utilization of milk substitutes depends heavily on local beliefs and traditions.

Approach to Acute Illness Management

The lack of regular medical services causes increased demand for ambulatory medical services as a replacement for local primary-care clinics. There is a demand to treat routine acute medical problems as well as medical problems resulting from the disaster.

The emerging acute medical problems vary depending on the time elapsed from the disaster. The primary physicians in the field hospital are required to respond quickly to the changing caseload. Primary care medical problems can be divided into three main phases:

In the hours and days immediately following a high-magnitude earthquake, the role of the primary physician in the initial period following the disaster is to participate in the effort led by the orthopedic and surgical teams by treating minor trauma (wounds, fractures, etc.) and by preparing the patients for surgery after initial evaluation including X-rays, laboratory tests, and hemodynamic stabilization. The primary physician should be able to recognize and treat acute complications such as rhabdomyolysis and threatening acute renal failure.

The second type of problems are related to postoperative management such as wound treatment, pain evaluation and management, postoperative infection management, and prevention of pulmonary emboli after immobilization or orthopedic operation by prescribing venous thromboembolism prophylaxis[2,9].

The third type of acute problems are medical problems emerging because of poor sanitation, inadequate shelter, crowding, lack of access to fuel, lack of clean water, and emotional stress after the disaster, etc. These problems include infectious diseases, fatigue, dehydration, cardiovascular diseases (myocardial infarct, cerebrovascular accident), and psychiatric reactions. Previous studies have shown that the size and organization of the tent camp are crucial for the state of health. The less organized the camps, the greater the need for health services[1].

Khosaka and his colleagues who participated in the medical effort after the earthquake in Japan in 2011 found that those who came to the clinic with new complaints had mostly respiratory complaints, gastrointestinal symptoms, pain-related issues, and insomnia[4].

Malnutrition and anemia are other common problems in poverty-stricken areas where these disasters often occur. Chronic poor health due to protein and micronutrient deficiency before the disaster aggravates the health problems[10,11]. The nutritional status should be taken into consideration when planning the medications required for a field hospital.

Many patients may experience acute stress disorder for the month following the trauma. It is indicated that 3–58% of those exposed to trauma will develop PTSD. Grief over losses, uncertainty about family members' fates, frustration and stressors because of damaged houses, and the feeling of being a refugee predispose the victims to future development of PTSD [8]. The primary-care physicians should be proactive and assess the patients for mental-health problems using a short tool (for example, the case-finding and health-assessment tool).

Approach to Chronic Illness Management

As time passes, more efforts are directed at ambulatory primary care rather than emergency medicine. Fernald and colleagues[1] noted that, within the primary-care patients, there is evidence that patients with chronic medical problems are affected disproportionally to others after natural disasters.

The reasons for this include the following:

1. In rural deprived areas, even these predisaster health services are not accessible to all. After the disaster, local medical services function at an even lower level and the available health-care resources are redirected to emergency services[10].

2. Many victims cannot return to their homes since they are severely damaged or due to their fear of being in buildings following their earthquake experiences. A lot of them stay in temporary tent camps exposed to weather instability and without alleviating basic needs such as fresh water, hygiene facilities, and so on. Without their chronic medications (which were left at home), the chronic illnesses deteriorate. Inadequate food supply can also influence chronic disease states such as diabetes by worsening glycemic control[12,13].

3. Stress after a disaster can release stress hormones such as cortisol and adrenaline that worsen metabolic control, raise blood pressure, and expose the patients to risk for cardiovascular diseases.

4. Persons with chronic diseases are usually older and frailer. There is evidence that natural disasters affect chronic medical problems. Disruption of medical treatment for chronic conditions causes increase of 32% of adverse effects of medical outcomes[10].

A study in Japan, after the Hanshin-Awaji earthquake in 1995, showed an increase in the incidence of myocardial infarction and cardiac mortality in the four weeks after the disaster[14].

Earthquakes can adversely affect renal failure[15] and cause asthma exacerbations[16]. Of the patients with asthma, 11% had an exacerbation during the first month after the earthquake in Japan in 2000. Another study demonstrated an increase in the number of patients with newly diagnosed diabetes following the earthquake in Los Angeles[7].

All the abovementioned emphasize the importance of making chronic disease management part of the medical aid provided in the disaster area.

It is important that, during initial assessment of the patient, the chronic needs are targeted as well by active case finding.

We recommend that communication with local primary-care personnel be established as early as possible. This will facilitate the familiarization of the team with local guidelines and capabilities (medications, imaging, laboratory tests, costs and coverage, ministry of health guidelines, etc.).

The medications prescribed should be based on the available drugs in the local market and with the standard medical treatment present in the local health-care system in order that the patient will be able to continue the treatment thereafter. Diet recommendations should be based on local nutrition supply. A summary of the medical recommendations should be given to the patient for further treatment by his or her local physician. It is crucially important to work collaboratively with local health services and to give treatment and recommendations according to applicable local guidelines.

The aim should be to supply chronic medications for at least one month or even more, until the local health-care services can return to function. That fact influences the planning of the medications supply that is brought by the field hospital or the aid agency.

The field hospital preparations should address treatment of chronic medical conditions such as diabetes, hypertension, asthma, cardiovascular disease, and so on, and should take into account that primary care is one of the major needs in a disaster area, even in the initial period.

The collaboration with local medical teams can be an opportunity to teach and train the local health-care workers to identify risk factors, and to prevent and treat chronic medical conditions. It can also be an opportunity to learn from local teams about the local approach to treat local common diseases or tropical diseases.

Summary

- Acute injuries contribute to significant morbidity in the immediate time following high magnitude earthquake. Illnesses resulting from poor shelter and lack of access to electricity, clean water, and sanitation will appear later.
- The most common physical complaints are respiratory, gastrointestinal, genitourinary, and malnutrition. Acute stress disorder is also common.
- Ambulatory services can be delivered as a department within the field hospital or by

outreach. The triage is a crucial part of the clinic and the medical team should identify patients who could most benefit. Other parts of the ambulatory service should contain a consultation area, treatment area, pharmacy, and laboratory.

- In the initial period, the primary physicians will participate in the triage of trauma patients, treating minor trauma and preparing patients for surgery. Therefore, they should be skilled in emergency medicine, advanced trauma life support, and minor trauma.
- Later on, the primary physician may lead the postoperative management and their last efforts will be treatment of acute problems emerging due to poor sanitation and crowding and also management of chronic medical problems. For this purpose, they should be familiar with common infections in the disaster area and antibiotic resistance.
- Communication with local health-care services as well as public and religious facilities is mandatory.

References

1. Fernald JP, Clawson EA. The mobile army surgical hospital humanitarian assistance mission in Pakistan: the primary care experience. *Military Medicine* 2007: **172**(5): 471–7.

2. Ofer B, Hadar M, Miskin IN, Oded B, Shlomo V. Primary care in a disaster scenario: the experience of the family physicians in the IDF field hospital mission to Haiti. *Journal of Israeli Military Medicine* 2010: 7(2): 73–5.

3. Broach JP, McNamara M, Harrison K. Ambulatory care by disaster responders in the tent camps of Port-au-Prince, Haiti, January 2010. *Disaster Medicine and Public Health Preparedness* 2010: **4**(2): 116–21.

4. Kohsaka S, Endo Y, Ueda I, Namiki J, Fukuda K. Necessity for primary care immediately after the March 11 tsunami and earthquake in Japan. *JAMA Internal Medicine* 2012: **172**(3): 290–1.

5. Ushizawa H, Foxwell AR, Bice S, Matsui T, et al. Needs for disaster medicine: lessons from the field of the Great East Japan Earthquake. *Western Pacific Surveillamce and Response Journal* 2013: **4**(1): 51–5.

6. Fuday H, Trevino A. Primary health center disaster preparedness after the earthquake in Pandang Pariaman, West Sumatra, Indonesia. *BMC Research Notes* 2011: **4**(81).

7. Amital H, Alkan ML, Adler J, Kriess I, Levi Y. Israeli Defense Forces Medical Corps humanitarian mission

for Kosovo's refugees. *Prehospital and Disaster Medicine* 2003: **18**(4): 301–5.

8. Sullivan S, Wong S. An enhanced primary health care role following psychological trauma: the Christchurch earthquakes. *Journal of Primary Health Care* 2011: **3**(3): 248–51.

9. Crocker JT, Huang GC. Reflections on Haiti: the role of hospitalists in disaster response. *Journal of Hospital Medicine* 2011: **6**(2): 105–7.

10. Chan EY, Kim JJ. Characteristics and health outcomes of internally displaced populations in unofficial rural self-settled camps after the 2005 Kashmir, Pakistan earthquake. *European Journal of Emergency Medicine* 2010: **17**(3): 136–41.

11. Amundson D, Dadekian G, Etienne M, et al. Practicing internal medicine onboard the USNS COMFORT in the aftermath of the Haitian earthquake. *Annals of Internal Medicine* 2010: **152** (11): 733–7.

12. Sengül A, Ozer E, Salman S, et al. Lessons learnt from influences of the Marmara earthquake on glycemic control and quality of life in people with type 1 diabetes. *Endocrine Journal* 2004: **51**(4): 407–14.

13. Inui A, Kitaoka H, Majima M, Takamiya S, et al. Effect of the Kobe earthquake on stress and glycemic control in patients with diabetes mellitus. *JAMA Internal Medicine* 1998: **158**(3): 274–8.

14. Kario K, Ohashi T. Increased coronary heart disease mortality after the Hanshin-Awaji earthquake among the older community on Awaji Island. *Journal of the American Geriatrics Society* 1997: **45**(5): 610–3.

15. Erek E, Sever MS, Serdengeçti K, et al. Turkish Study Group of Disaster. An overview of morbidity and mortality in patients with acute renal failure due to crush syndrome: the Marmara earthquake experience. *Nephrology Dialysis Transplantation* 2002: **17**(1): 33–40.

16. Tomita K, Hasegawa Y, Watanabe M, et al. Seibu earthquake and exacerbation of asthma in adults. *The Journal of Medical Investigation* 2005: **52**(1–2): 80–4.

17. Kaufman FR, Devgan S. An increase in new onset IDDM admissions following the Los Angeles earthquake. *Diabetes Care* 1995: **18**(3): 422.

Chapter 27

Mental Health in a Field Hospital

Eyal Fruchter and Karen Ginat

Introduction

Any disaster – natural or human made – carries an urgent medical need. Most of the declared needs in the immediate aftermath of a mass trauma are physical, with surgical and orthopedic interventions in the immediate phase and medical problems with endemic epidemiological aspects in the next phase. Historically, the medical focus in disaster preparedness has been on injury, infection, and exposure related illness, but clinicians have been interested in postdisaster mental-health interventions since the 1940s[1].

Unlike physical injuries, adverse mental-health outcomes of disasters may not be apparent during the initial phases following the event, and therefore are often overlooked, but these mental outcomes due to exposure to a disaster are common. One-third or more of individuals severely exposed may develop posttraumatic stress disorder (PTSD) or other mental disorders – new or exacerbated. A systematic approach to the delivery of timely and appropriate disaster mental-health services may facilitate their integration into the emergency medical response[1,2] and improve their overall outcome. Among the mental disturbances, other than PTSD, the individuals might suffer from disorders such as adjustment disorder, major depression, and psychotic breakdown, as well as behavioral manifestations such as substance abuse, violence, helplessness, and suicidality.

The general society breakdown, personal and material losses, and physiological hardship (whether due to physical injury or to lack of food or shelter) make all the traumatic experiences severe and the chance of an unharmed long-term remission less probable.

Despite its severity, most victims of mass trauma tend to ignore the mental problem at first and most manifestations are those of the physical problems. As an example, during the post-tsunami medical care in Indonesia, evaluated at the Red Cross Hospital at Banda Aceh[2], the complaints were of the following:

(1) urological (19%), (2) digestive (16%), (3) respiratory (12%), and (4) musculoskeletal (12%). Although < 2% of patients were diagnosed with a mental-health problem, 24% had at least four or more of the seven depression/PTSD symptoms addressed in the study[3].

The responders – professional and nonprofessional, working in humanitarian delegations and field hospitals – are also a community at risk for mental disorders. PTSD and depression were the most studied diagnoses with prevalence of PTSD ranging from 0% to 34% and depression from 21% to 53%[4]. The variations in the morbidity rate are due to under reporting as well as the way the responders were screened for the mission[5], escorted during the work, and looked after when it was over[6]. In a large review paper, most samples of rescue and recovery workers showed remarkable resilience. Within adult samples, more severe exposure, female gender, middle age, ethnic minority status, secondary stressors, prior psychiatric problems, and weak or deteriorating psychosocial resources most consistently increased the likelihood of adverse outcomes[7]. Psychiatric outcomes are not the only mental ramification of trauma. Symptoms and unpleasant emotions not qualifying as a psychiatric disorder are referred to as psychological distress. Distress, at some level, is nearly universal after disasters and is far more prevalent than psychiatric disorders. The distinction between these two entities is critical for effective disaster response because different interventions are needed for them[8].

When trying to understand the specific needs from the MHPs in the field hospital, one must understand that, unlike any other crew member, the team must provide assistance to the victims of the disaster-acute phase and long term – in the emergency room as well as in the liaisons work in the departments – but not less important to the team, in the preparedness, actual work, and after the return to safety, in the psychiatric and psychological aspects[7–9].

The integration of psychosocial care into emergency and medical disaster response must occur prior to the disaster itself, and will depend on effective collaboration between medical and mental-health-care providers[8,10].

In this chapter, we will try to conduct an overview of the mental factors crucial for the hospital members, the MHPs needed for the team and hospital work, other missions that should be proposed by those professionals in a humanitarian mission to the area's population, and the basic screening and treating tools that should be implemented by them.

Field Hospital Team Care

The team must have as much knowledge as possible in regard to the nature of the disaster, the country's state after the disaster, the mission ahead, its probable length, specific cultural aspects, and specific epidemiological data. The preparedness is different when arriving at safe grounds of a clean area, with no epidemiological threat, like an organized country after a single terrorist attack, and when arriving in a country like Haiti immediately after an earthquake.

At the basis of all procedures taken are the international and national conventions and laws. This implies that the medical assistance is adjunct to the local capabilities and requirements. The treatment should be accessible to all. Treatment should be customized to the traumatic arena while standing on the highest clinical standards of care possible given the limitations[11]. The psychological intervention schemes of treatment are multivariable. The first consideration is the exact nature of the disaster as opposed to the local remaining infrastructure and treating capabilities. The flow of decision is dictated by moral obligation. The psychosocial intervention schemes are multivariable, depending mainly on the exact nature of the disaster and the local remaining infrastructure and treatment capabilities. The decisions will be dictated by moral obligation. They will be discussed according to the different phases of the deployment: pre-deployment, during, and post-deployment.

Prior to the Mission

From the chapter authors' experience, the three major reasons that people join an altruistic mission are as follows:

1. Leadership: Leadership in stressful situations should be as structured, concise, and trustworthy as possible. People need to feel that the commander is capable and reliable.
2. Camaraderie: The connection between people helps in building up courage. Team members are also willing to make sacrifices to help people they feel connected to. The strength of a group has been spoken of in literature, but its importance cannot be underestimated in a traumatic situation.
3. Meaning: The belief that there is something that is more important than themselves at this point of time. This can stem from ethics, religion, spirituality, beliefs, protecting of loved ones, and so on.

Therefore, the initial period while preparing for a mission should be dedicated to strengthening these three principles, and not "just" medical preparedness and equipment readiness.

The team members should meet before departure and engage in different, relevant missions such as preparing the gear for the mission and getting immunizations together. This enables the members to get to know each other on peaceful grounds and start feeling closer to each other before they feel tired and stressed. A team should be built with everyone knowing his or her specific role in the mission, and understanding that everybody has to take part in various combined missions such as erecting the hospital facility. Prior to leaving the country of origin, team members in the mission should be provided with information about the country they are going to and its condition after the trauma, and have people from past missions explaining what to expect. The main tool for this is psychoeducation and team building. This builds resiliency and puts the team at a better starting point for the mission. It is crucial to identify those not participating or those who tend to "cope by themselves." It is common for the commanding officers of the mission not to take an active part in the team buildup since they have a lot to do at the organization stage. It is important the MHP makes sure the commanders use this time for team building as well. The MHP's main focus at this point should be getting to know as many members of the team as possible. This includes members from all sectors: medical, paramedical, and logistic support personnel. They must attend as many team talks as possible as side participants, allowing the leadership team to lead the discussion, while taking part themselves. During these talks the MHP must ensure the participants understand that the MHP's main role in the mission is to help them.

The ideal professional team should include a psychiatrist equipped with medicine and either a social worker or a psychologist. Both should be familiar with different methods for the treatment of acute stress disorder, as well as having the ability for group sessions and leading a debriefing group.

The drugs recommended for a mission like this should include benzodiazepine (BZ), sleeping pills, and major tranquilizing drugs such as olanzapine (tablets and injections). The role of BZ should be minimal as it is known to help in the acute phases, but enhances the incidence of PTSD later on. Selective serotonin reuptake inhibitor medications do not help in early phases; thus, their role is minimal. The specific amounts of medications should be decided prior to the mission according to the nature and location of the disaster and the anticipated length of stay.

The Early Phases of the Mission

This is a crucial phase for the success of the mission, as well as the psychological outcomes of the whole delegation. This can be divided into two major fields of action: (1) a country with poor infrastructure in a large disaster, with a mission adjacent to the disaster, for example Haiti, and (2) a country with a well-established infrastructure in a large disaster, with a mission adjacent to the disaster, for example Japan.

A Country with Poor Infrastructure

In general, rehabilitation after a traumatic event can take years. The outcome heavily depends on the general rehabilitation of the infrastructure at a local area. The aim in long-term rehabilitation is to build a narrative of "survivors" as opposed to "victims." The empowerment of this shift in state of mind gives mastery and strength. What happened may be painful, but my choice is what I do with that pain and how it can help strengthen resilience, if implemented correctly. It is important to remember that, like any physical injury, the mind strives to repair itself. The MHP's goal is to enable the psychological environment needed to empower the natural course of recovery. A mission in a country with poor infrastructure demands intensive work with the mission team and, if possible, with the local population to build their coping skills.

The MHP's role with the emergency teams: The emergency teams do not tend to suffer from acute stress disorder nor any clinical sequelae. The teams are usually well prepared for the mission and have the necessary knowledge to fulfill their role.

Problems may arise in the early phase of the event in the following situations:

- Physical needs are not met. It is important to work with the commander to make sure shifts allow for sufficient food, sleep, and safety. When the body is weak, people are more susceptible to primary, instinctual, and emotional types of thinking patterns, focusing on the primal brain. The attempt to avoid PTSD or other traumatic psychological sequelae is the enactment of the prefrontal cortex and executive functioning. It is hard to think "logically" when one is hungry. The physical needs of the team – food, toilet, and a place to sleep – are all crucial to their ability to continue functioning. These missions are a "marathon" of physical hardships, and every member must find a way to balance his or her needs and resources.

- There is a big gap between the expected situation and that found on arrival. This can range from transportation problems to an overwhelming number of casualties with inadequate means to treat them. In this case, frustration and a feeling of helplessness can be detrimental to mental health. Frustration can also arise from other situations such as arriving to a "not-needed" scenario due to a paucity of casualties or an overabundance of local and foreign medical teams. It is important to abide by protocols and routine as much as possible. MHPs should encourage staff to share their difficulties with friends. Help the commander to phrase clear, precise, transparent, and hopeful messages to the staff.

- Previous training does not fit the specific needs required in the situation. Help integrate staff members into other useful situations in accordance with their capabilities. Help to cognitively build a narrative of their tremendous contribution to the new situation, helping them to understand the cohesiveness of the team and that success is measured by the overall assistance. Stress that there are no "small" jobs and that everyone is needed exactly where they are for the mission to succeed.

- The situation "hits home." Trained as the medical team is, different chords become very personal at times. To function in a disaster arena, a healthy amount of detachment is needed. MHPs need to empathize; not sympathize. When "the wall" is broken for any reason (shock, similarity to loved ones, previous experience, and so on) it will "hit home" for the team member. Lead and pace the team member gently back to the professional discussion. This should be done gradually and thoughtfully, restoring the confidence, mastery, and professionalism to the team member.

- Previous psychiatric problems are augmented or exacerbated by the physical or mental ordeal of the mission. In these situations, treat psychiatric problems as a psychiatrist would, taking into consideration: What do you have? How will it affect the team member? Side effects? The primary diagnosis and its implications on functioning? Always take into consideration lack of sleep as a major cause. If the psychiatric problem grows, consider evacuation home.
- Physical problems causing psychiatric disorders. A psychiatrist in an emergency medical team (EMT) must always be mindful of the medical aspects in diagnosis and treatment. The overlap between hypoxia and acute stress reaction can be settled by a pulse oximeter.

The MHP's role with the general population: The primary duty of an EMT is to understand the needs of the population and decide how the EMT can provide the best assistance to appropriately meet these needs.

Intervention in the population should involve working with local teachers, first responders, critical workers, and so on. This can have a secondary effect when these people work with wider circles of people in the population and alleviate suffering in a widespread manner. One must be familiar with the different stages societies may go through after a huge traumatic event.

Literature suggests that people and communities struck by disaster will generally go through four phases of response[11]:

1. Heroic phase: This first phase may begin prior to the event and last up to a week afterwards. People struggle to prevent loss of lives and they try to minimize property damage.
2. Honeymoon phase: The second phase may last from two weeks to two months. Massive relief efforts lift the spirits of survivors and hopes of a quick recovery run high, but optimism is often short lived.
3. Disillusionment phase: The disillusionment phase may last from several months to a year or more. Sometimes called the "second disaster," the realities of bureaucratic paperwork and recovery delays set in, outside help leaves, and the local population realize they have a lot to do themselves.
4. Reconstruction phase: The final phase may take several years as normal functioning is gradually reestablished.

There may be a place for the MHP in taking care of psychiatric and psychological reactions. Among the victims, one might find exacerbation of mental-health disorders, new and old, such as psychotic attacks, dissociation, affective disorders, anxiety disorders, and even withdrawal from different addictions.

A Country with a Well-Established Infrastructure

For a mission to a large disaster in a country with a well-established infrastructure, it is likely that the first phase again may be the most dangerous time for the team, since this is the phase where the team are needed the most. The first few days are the main buildup of the facility, which is typically extremely difficult – physically and mentally – yet one can run on adrenaline for the first 48 hours of the mission. In the previous section we identified this hardship to running a marathon. Here, it is a relatively short run, yet the expectations of the surrounding population and their municipal leadership put a high burden on the team to provide a high-level service as early as possible. On the mental-health side, it is crucial to ensure that everybody gets at least some rest, food, and most importantly, a connection with their families. Phone or an internet connection enable most team members to share the experience and relieve part of the burden. The main psychological tool at this point is joining and avoiding exhaustion. This is important for all the team and particularly so for the commanders of the mission. It is generally not spoken of, or even thought of, yet a tired commander may give a bad example and may show bad decision-making. The MHP should work alongside others, participating as part of the team, yet on the lookout for detached people, people who are argumentative, and those who seem more tired than the others.

During the Mission

When the facility is built and working, team members face hardship from three different areas: (1) working long hours in challenging surroundings, (2) witnessing traumatic sights and having to make difficult moral decisions, and (3) being far away from home and normality.

All three are true for hospital personnel as well as supporting or rescue teams, usually more so in underserved countries. Since the work in the field hospital is a long-distance struggle, one should make sure personnel get some rest, a place and time during the day for refueling their resources, and a place to share their thoughts about the traumas they have seen and the moral questions encountered.

The best tool to use in these three areas is to have a rigid daily routine or timetable. It should start in the morning with a structured meeting, where information is updated and operational plans are made for the day. The day should end at a reasonable time (based on demands and staffing). At the end of each day, all the teams should have a debriefing talk to share and learn from each other, and to discuss plans for improvements for the next day.

The hospital should have a "relaxation zone", where team members can have a snack, a hot or cold drink, and have a chat with colleagues. The hospital should also have an ethical board to make sure difficult decisions are been taken together and not by a single person. This would enable team members to share the burden (see Chapter 32).

If the mission is a long one, it should include a "day-off" plan, in which members of each team get time off to recharge and take some time to mellow down. This can include a short tour in the area of operation so that team members get an idea of life in the country outside the field hospital.

Although the above are not part of the MHP's role, he or she is the one who should be working with commanders to make sure they happen. If these strategies are not put in place, it may accelerate burn-out and cause later postmission PTSD.

The MHP should also be a part of the ethical committee, take part in as many debriefing sessions as possible, and know where it's most important for him or her to participate. For example, he or she should be informed if a delivery of a baby failed and join the labor team for the talk that day. It is crucial that the MHP should "live the hospital" all the time.

As a professional in his or her field, the MHP should also consult in the psychiatric field for patients, taking part in difficult talks, such as with parents after losing their child, when necessary. They should also spend time in the relaxation zone to observe and listen to anyone who needs a friendly talk.

In some delegations, even in the later phase of the mission, the MHP could help to conduct group sessions and debriefing sessions with local groups such as teachers and other professionals in the community. It is important to take this opportunity to work with the trauma victims, yet also teach them how to conduct group work so they can do it later for others. This is best done through the local leaders in the educational boards or the local social work teams.

Before Coming Back Home

Again, this is often a period filled with energy; thus, is easier in the mental aspects. Sometimes ethical questions arise about the team's contribution in the face of a major trauma. The prospect of leaving a society in need and patients who need ongoing care may raise some other ethical issues. These should be discussed in the morning talks and at the team debriefings. The commander should consider a hospital talk to close open issues and to share information with everybody so rumors are minimal. The MHP should help team leaders to close the mission in a positive and optimistic manner, building a positive narrative for each team member. This is the narrative they go home with, so difficult situations should not be ignored; rather reframed in a more positive and "mindful" manner.

Arrival Home and Closure Points

Before departure, the MHP should remind team members that he or she is there for them if needed. The MHP should remind the team that sometimes it is hard to readjust and that traumatic memories sometimes return. If anybody has acute stress reaction, acute stress disorder, or any other mental-health issue, the MHP should make sure they have a meeting about two weeks after returning. For others, make sure they talk and do not avoid it, they get some rest, even though the usual work may have piled up, and most importantly, know how to get in touch with the MHP if needed in cases of lack of sleep, flashbacks, emotional flooding, or other aspects of trauma.

It is crucial to debrief the commanders as they tend to believe they are more resilient or need less taking care of, which is not necessarily true.

Returning from a Mission

The process of returning to home base and returning to "normal" is very important professionally and in terms of mental health. The switch from the high adrenaline felt in a mission to the mundane, routine work necessitates proactive building of a return process. This can include military ceremonies, operational investigations, and cognitive processing. It should be dealt with as a mission within itself.

The unique characteristics of each mission should be considered separately. The differential impact of the team characteristics, their job specifications, and feelings of pride and adequacy (as opposed to insufficiency) need to be addressed.

As a rule, cognitive processing should be done by the commander with the guidance of an MHP. The processing should be organized as a mission taking place a few days after return to home. The mission's organizer should not include the mental-health officers who joined the mission. Now is the time to care for the caregivers.

The talks should be in organic groups of approximately 10 to 15 people. People should be with the organic group of the mission. The talk is led by the commander with a mental-health officer present. In this way, the mental-health officer can also identify those in need of further mental assistance.

Each participant can only speak for him or herself and is limited to a certain amount of time to enable everyone to participate. Judgmentalism is prohibited. The participants are encouraged to help their comrades with positive reframing of the issues they brought up in the group.

The talk is divided into three different stages:

1. Opening: The opening should be about 5 to 10 minutes long. It consists of defining the purpose and rules of the talk. If this is not the first team talk that a specific organic team has gone through, then a quick reminder of the rules is usually enough.

2. The mission: This section of the team talk is divided into three separate rounds of participation from all members of the group:

    a. Fact phase: The purpose is to build a clear, realistic, and integrative picture of the overall situation in chronological order. Each participant describes factually, using the description of all five of the senses, what he or she experienced.

    b. Thought phase: In this phase, each participant describes what he or she thought throughout different situations in the mission. It is important to remain in the domain of "thoughts" and not "feelings" or "emotions," which encourage blood flow to the lower brain areas.

    c. Reaction phase: Each participant describes his or her new reaction to the integrative picture drawn by the group and commander.

3. Recruitment of strengths and summaries: At this point, each participant should leave with pride and a feeling of relevance to the mission. The last question that each of the participants answers in turn relates to personal meaning of the mission and the cohesive and protective factor of the group. For example: What are the important things you did for the team and for the mission? If a participant finds difficulty in answering, help him or her out. Positive reinforcement of purpose and being an integral part of a team is imperative. The commander should summarize the talk with the building of expectancies for the future.

Conclusions

The MHP in a humanitarian mission has multiple hats to wear: he or she is the therapist for the team, has to work with the hospital patients, and has to keep an open eye for missions with the local population outside the hospital missions. He or she should be active in the daily routine of the hospital, keep in touch with all the team members, make sure they know about both the positive and negative events occurring in the hospital, as well as the ethical issues arising. They should keep an eye on the commanders and listen to undercurrents within the team.

Mental-Health Team Members

The mental health team consists of two or more MHPs; one of whom is a senior psychiatrist and is the team commander. The MHPs should be experienced in dealing with disorders related to stress on an everyday basis, including pharmacotherapy and psychosocial treatments. It is important for the mental-health team to meet at least once a day at prescheduled, consistent times. The advantages are threefold:

1. Co-counseling: very often the challenges are surprising and sharing information, analyzing multi-professionally, and basically just thinking together creates a more open mind for opportunities and unique thinking of how to help in the unique situation.

2. Support: mental-health officers are human and as such are susceptible to feeling the strain too. Sharing with coworkers helps to share the burden and gives reassurance.

3. Modeling: "talk the talk and walk the walk". The chapter authors advise sharing as a coping mechanism and consultations are not just

professional. The mental health team should set an example regarding sharing their own problems, maintaining a routine and talking rests.

The mental-health team's abilities and tasks include the following:

- Giving psychological first aid, and referring to local high-level or chronic care for further treatment: the mental-health team approaches and treats patients who suffer from stress and disaster-related mental problems or other issues. The team tasks are to triage, deliver first aid, and to refer to mental-health centers. The field hospital cannot hospitalize patients who present only with mental-health problems. Connection with local mental-health services must take place as early as possible.

- Liaison psychiatry: the mental-health team gives psychiatric (e.g., delirium) and psychosocial consultations (e.g., interventions for patients and their families) to all hospital departments. Some of the patients in post-disaster situations are complex and need both physical and mental treatment. Since a disaster area affects mostly civilian populations, special consideration should be given to children and mentally ill patients.

- Prevention of stress reactions among hospital personnel and other members of the task force: mental preparation (primary prevention) and psychological first aid after personnel exposure to the disaster (secondary prevention). The humanitarian task force is at risk of developing stress and trauma-related problems. Mental preparation should begin before the task force arrives at the disaster scene as part of a preventive-medicine approach. Mental preparation should be the task of high-ranking officers with the support and consultation of the mental-health team. On ground, care should be given to the staff's well-being. The mental-health team should supervise these needs and advise the commanders. Briefings and debriefings should be held by the chain of command in all hospital departments. Time should be allocated for social, educational, and leisure activities. Once the mission is over, the mental-health team should take part in debriefings and pay special attention to any members of staff showing distress and trauma symptoms.

- Training and consulting local welfare and educational teams: training the local teams is more

effective than replacing them. The mental-health team should train and consult local welfare and educational teams (e.g., how to get back to school and routine).

- The field-hospital psychiatrist is a member of the ethics committee and takes part in headquarters decision-making.

References

1. Yum K, Lurie N, Hyde PS. Moving mental health into the disaster preparedness spotlight. *The New England Journal of Medicine* 2010: 1194–5.

2. Satcher D, Friel S, Bell R. Natural and manmade disasters and mental health. *JAMA* 2007: **298**(21): 2540–2.

3. Redwood-Campbell LJ, Riddez L. Health problems encountered in the International Committee of the Red Cross Hospital in Banda Aceh, Indonesia. *Prehospital and Disaster Medicine* 2006: **21**(1): s1–7.

4. Garbern SC, Ebbeling LG, Bartels SA. A systematic review of health outcomes among disaster and humanitarian responders. *Prehospital and Disaster Medicine* 2016: **31**(6): 635–42.

5. Nilsson J, Johansson E, et al. Disaster nursing: self-reported competence of nursing students and registered nurses, with focus on their readiness to manage violence, serious events and disasters. *Nurse Education in Practice* 2016: **17**: 102–8.

6. Pfefferbaum B, Flynn BW, et al. The integration of mental and behavioral health into disaster preparedness, response, and recovery. *Disaster Medicine and Public Health Preparedness* 2012: **6**(1): 60–6.

7. Noris FH, Friedman, et al. 60 000 disaster victims speak: part I. An empirical review of the empirical literature, 1981–2001. *Psychiatry* 2002: **65**(3): 207–39.

8. Nucifora FC Jr, Hall RC, Everly GS Jr. Reexamining the role of the traumatic stressor and the trajectory of posttraumatic distress in the wake of disaster. *Disaster Medicine and Public Health Preparedness* 2011: 5(Suppl 2): S172–5.

9. Norwood AE, Ursano RJ, Fullerton CS. Disaster psychiatry: principles and practice. *Psychiatric Quarterly* 2000: **71**(3): 207–26.

10. Ruzek JI, Young BH, et al. Integration of disaster mental health services with emergency medicine. *Prehospital and Disaster Medicine* 2004: **19**(1): 46–53.

11. Weaver JD. Disaster mental health: detailed information – assisting in the aftermath of disasters and other life crises. Operational Logistical Support. UN op log 060915.

Nursing in a Field Hospital
Planning, Organization, and Operations

Bronte Martin and Rebecca Weir

Introduction

Strong nursing leadership is pivotal in ensuring the effective and efficient running of a deployed field hospital with limited resources in an austere and environmentally challenging setting. In the context of overwhelming demand, limited resources, and a low-tech environment, there is a requirement for a flexible, adaptable, multiskilled nursing workforce to adequately meet the needs of the population at risk.

Delivery of care in an austere disaster environment creates many unique nursing challenges: operating in a resource-limited multidisciplinary team, identifying relevant scopes of practice, specialized skill sets and currency requirements, competency and skill mix considerations, human resource management, and patient flow.

In the ever-increasing age of technology in health care, a return to the foundation principles of nursing care and application of "clinical medicine" in the absence of many modern diagnostic tools is fast becoming the primary domain of the widely acknowledged aging generation of nurses. The absence of high-tech modern diagnostic tools in the disaster setting necessitates a return and emphasis on the basic clinical skills as foundation principles of nursing care.

Planning

Service Delivery/Roles

Ensuring safe and optimal quality standards of care to an affected population mandates broad and diverse areas for responsibility encompassing far beyond direct clinical care only; concurrently meeting unique, rapidly changing demands associated with delivering and maintaining an acute-care field hospital. Such responsibilities often require dual, complementary clinical and operational approaches to leadership, necessitating the designated nursing team leader to be highly flexible and adaptive in their leadership and

nursing practice when translated into in an austere, complex disaster environment.

A dual medical/nursing clinical operational co-leadership model jointly enables the holistic, interdisciplinary provision of leadership, management, and oversight of delivery of clinical field services:

- ensuring the highest standard of clinical care is delivered by the field facility
- ensuring compliance with global minimum technical standards related to patient and clinical care service delivery
- ensuring occupational work health and safety requirements are met in clinical areas
- coordination, rostering, and allocation of individual clinical staff duties
- identification of clinical infrastructure support requirements (water, power, lighting, environmental control) and communication to logistics
- monitoring and identifying patients presenting with specific, specialist care needs: infectious, obstetric, palliative, and so on
- identifying potential indicators of infectious disease outbreaks and communicating to taskforce leader
- oversight of team morale and welfare

Clinical team leaders (CTLs) require the expert knowledge, skills, and understanding of their respective professions to efficiently provide both clinical oversight and governance of the field facility, while also providing high-level support to the taskforce leader. A CTL should only engage in direct patient care where clinical load exceeds capacity and with the knowledge and agreement of the taskforce leader.

Role of the Nursing Team Leader

As is common practice in many modern health-care systems throughout the world, the nursing team leader in an austere field hospital environment is primarily responsible for the ongoing *operational management* of

Table 28.1 Overview of key clinical nursing lead roles and responsibilities by phase of deployment

Predeparture			
Ensure they have a thorough situational awareness of the deployment mission and destination environment	Support the taskforce leader in delivering mission briefings, and deliver a specific briefing on expected clinical case load and clinical service requirements	Familiarize themselves with the skillsets and competencies of all clinical staff	Create a roster to match anticipated clinical service requirements
On mission			
Support the team leader in delivering morning briefings with a focus on the clinical order of business for the day	Roster staff into clinical roles, including night shift and emergency on call if applicable	Ensure adherence to organizational clinical protocols	Act as a resource for treating clinicians as workload and operational requirements dictate
Actively monitor team welfare and report to the team leader regarding any specific points of concern	Oversee medical record keeping and data collection in conjunction with the nominated data collection officer	Convene the ad hoc "ethics committee" to assist with difficult ethical decisions surrounding individual patients	
Postmission			
Support the team leader in preparation and collation of postdeployment report	Participate in senior organization postdeployment debriefings	Act as a resource and support for returned team members where relevant	Monitor team welfare and report to the team leader regarding any specific points of concern

the clinical facility; working in tandem and close partnership with the medical team leader ensuring the delivery of optimal care. In contrast, however, the nursing team leader's role in the field hospital environment differs significantly and is extremely challenging and demanding; encompassing many diverse responsibilities including management, coordination, liaison, clinical, operational, and administrative tasks daily, which would not ordinarily be encountered by a sole practitioner during their standard nursing practice when not deployed into an austere field hospital environment (Table 28.1 and Figure 28.1). Each of these broad areas of responsibility requires the nursing team leader to be highly flexible and adaptive in their leadership and nursing practice and they are explored in further detail below.

Management Role

- rostering 24-hour clinical services: inpatient, outpatient, and emergency on-call services
- daily allocation of staff roles and rotations
- maintenance of skill mix across all clinical areas: primary health care, maternal/child health, triage, emergency clinic, resuscitation area, operating theater, medical/surgical, and pediatric wards

- ensuring staff occupational work health and safety in all clinical areas
- identifying and responding to critical incidents
- monitoring team morale and individual well-being; clinical facility rounds (minimum four times per day recommended)

Coordination Role

- clinical flow and referrals of patients between outpatient and inpatient areas
- inpatient bed management and allocation
- identifying and facilitating patient transfers: aeromedical and ground
- facilitation of discharge planning
- embedded external clinical staff, such as host ministry of health (MoH) staff and other emergency medical team (EMT) specialist cell teams (where applicable)

Liaison Role

- taskforce mission leader, EMT team leader, and clinical (medical) co-lead
- MoH

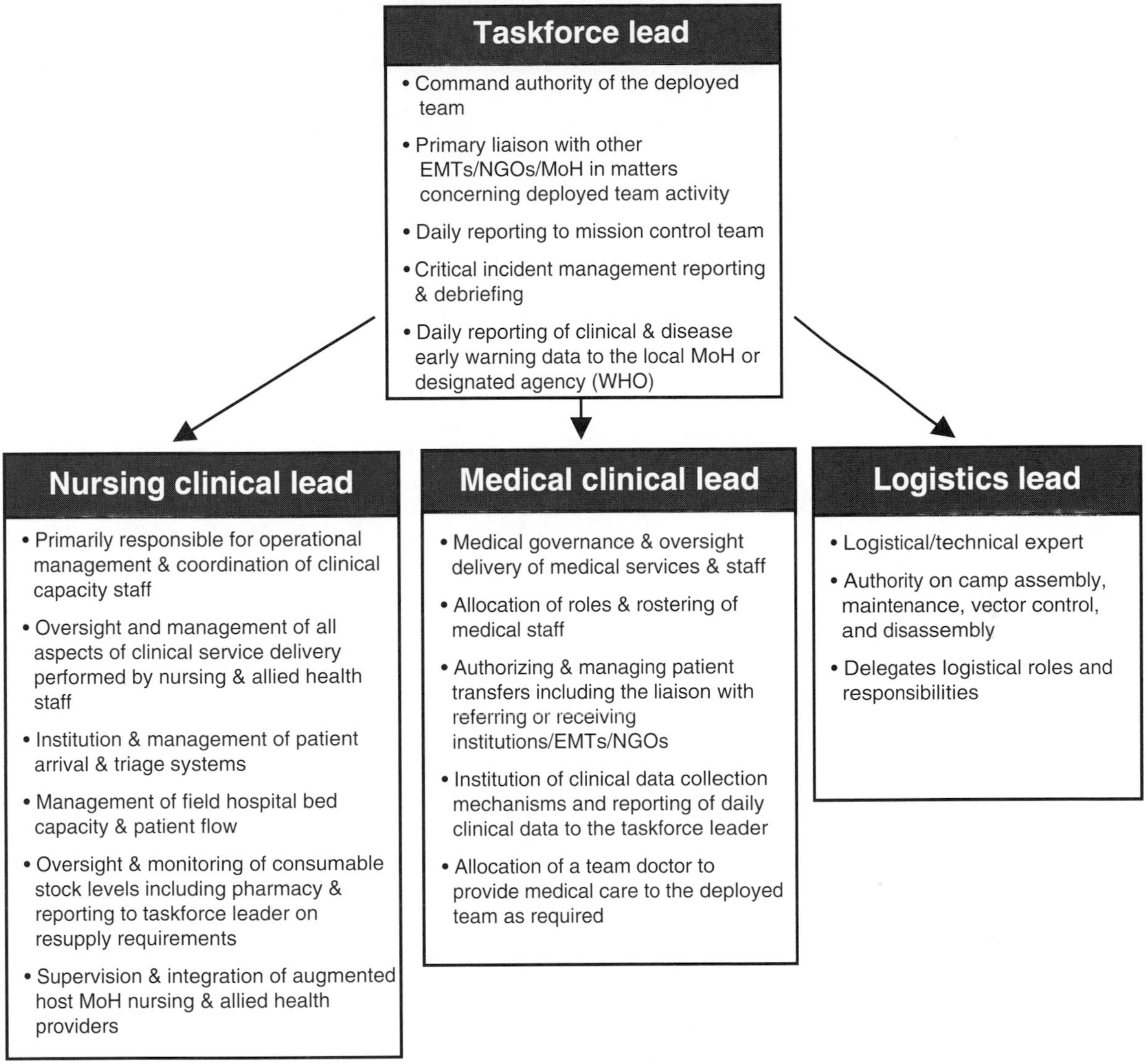

Figure 28.1 Example mission command team lead roles and responsibilities[1]

- external clinical agencies: nongovernmental organizations (NGOs), government organizations, and military
- local community representatives: police, social welfare, and pastoral care
- media and VIP guest visits
- EMT logistics' team leader and staff
- EMT clinical staff: medical, nursing, pharmacy, radiology, allied health, and paramedical
- family: patients and staff

Clinical Role

- member of the senior ethics group: decisions around limitations of care, palliation, and critical incidents
- expert/specialist advice and support to individual clinical areas
- monitoring and identifying clinical presentations with special needs: infectious, obstetric, palliative, and so on
- identifying and facilitating nursing care for high dependent or specialized-needs patients

- oversight care pathways/plans
- daily inpatient ward rounds (every 12 hours)
- clinical equipment management and troubleshooting

Operational Role

- clinical stores' consumable supply levels and resupply requirements
- identification of clinical infrastructure support requirements: water, power, lighting, and environmental control
- oversight of cleaning and maintenance for clinical areas
- oversight of inpatient kitchen and patient nutrition
- patient and family hygiene and sanitation

Administrative Role

- reporting births and deaths
- daily patient tracking and reporting
- daily field hospital activity situation report

While the breadth of responsibilities encountered as nursing team leader can be both arduous and highly challenging, many are not dissimilar to those potentially encountered in senior nursing management positions during the conduct of standard daily business in an acute-care hospital. Conversely, the predominate point of difference in the field-hospital setting, however, is the environment and context in which nursing leadership practice occurs. Extreme resource limitations (both human and physical) can significantly overwhelm or disintegrate local health systems, unprecedented patient volumes, acuity (across all age ranges and specialties), and the requirement to deliver clinical acute care services in temporary, standalone, fully self-sufficient, environmentally challenged, and isolated footprints.

Leadership and Governance Structure

Training and Education

The Sphere handbook states: "Health care is a critical determinant for survival in the initial stages of a disaster [2]." Without qualified nurses to address the health-care needs of disaster-affected communities and people, the ability to alleviate human suffering is severely limited.

Considerable collaborative work has been undertaken by the World Health Organization (WHO) and

International Council of Nurses (ICN) following specific recognition of the need for core competencies identified in Disaster Nursing:

> Nurses, as the largest group of committed health personnel, often working in difficult situations with limited resources, play vital roles when disasters strike, serving as first responders, triage officers and care providers, coordinators of care and services, providers of information or education, and counsellors. However, health systems and health care delivery in disaster situations are only successful when nurses have the fundamental disaster training.
>
> Nurses must be able to work internationally, in a variety of settings with nurses and health care providers from all parts of the world. To assure a global nursing workforce ready to respond in the event of a disaster, competencies are essential[3].

ICN subsequently developed and established a supporting competency framework for disaster nursing, which is organized under four main thematic areas:

- mitigation and prevention
- preparedness
- response
- recovery and rehabilitation

Within these four areas, a further 10 domains were identified and subclassified as illustrated in Figure 28.2.

The ICN disaster nursing competencies assume the generalist nurse possesses the basic skills in emergency and trauma care, including respiratory and airway assessment, pain management, cardiovascular assessment, management of hypovolemia and fluid replacement, burn assessment, hemorrhage management, mental status assessment, eye lavage, and management of crush injuries and fractures[4].

More specifically relevant to the EMT field-hospital environment, recommendations for a global operational learning framework[5] outline a foundation three-stage approach, which has been identified to assist in the optimal preparation, education, and training of EMT clinicians:

1. Professional competence and license to practice
2. Supported adaptation of technical and nontechnical professional capacities into low-resource emergency context
3. Preparation for an effective team performance in the field

In summary, therefore, to enable nurses to excel in their role while deployed into a field hospital, it is essential that they are not only first and foremost

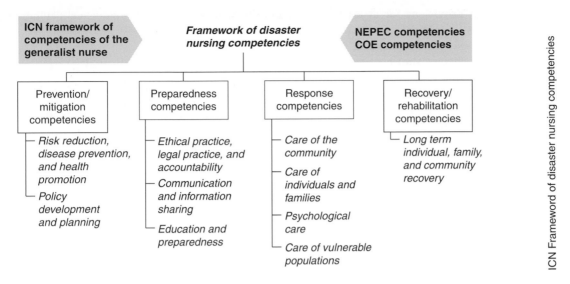

*COE: center of excellence; ICN, international council of nurses; NEPEC, nursing emergency preparedness education coalition.

Figure 28.2 ICN framework disaster nursing competencies

appropriately skilled and trained, but also secondly, and most importantly, *supported in the translation and adaptation of their nursing practice* into the context of limited resources in an austere and environmentally challenging setting.

Nursing Scope of Practice and Transdisciplinary Role Augmentation

The context and environment in which nursing care is delivered in a field-hospital setting in itself mandates the delivery of flexible and adaptive nursing and interdisciplinary care models, facilitating and supporting the ability of all clinicians to work to their respective optimal scopes of practice. When enabled, this approach will maximize not only the efficiency of field hospital service delivery but also its clinical efficacy, ultimately improving care outcomes and timely access to appropriate services for patients.

Caution must also be taken, however, in considering substitution (as opposed to augmentation) of nursing roles by less qualified/unlicensed nursing-support staff (nursing aides, patient care assistants, and so on) given the strong evidence and association demonstrated with higher mortality rates, increased adverse events, and poorer patient outcomes[10].

Substitution of core nursing roles by nonnursing disciplines that represent service delivery outside of and beyond their normal scope of practice, such as midlevel providers (physician assistants, paramedics, and medical technicians) is not an acceptable safe practice in the field-hospital setting given its known limitations in terms of personnel, skill mix, and supervision capacity. Such disciplines should be augmented into clinical areas where their foundation skills and knowledge are directly applicable and transferrable as complementary to the multidisciplinary team, not in replacement of other core nursing or medical roles/functions in these areas[10].

Minimum nurse to nonnursing staffing safety threshold ratios must be identified for all areas delivering patient care to ensure appropriate clinical governance, supervision, and oversight is both achievable and maintained[10].

Organization

Specific, detailed clinical care service delivery technical guidelines are outlined in WHO's *Classification and Minimum Standards for Foreign Medical Teams in Sudden Onset Disasters*[6]. Part of the preplanning phase for all EMTs is to ensure that the provision of basic needs, for both patients and staff, can be met for a minimum of two weeks of a deployment. For example, an EMT type 2 classified field hospital needs to ensure enough provisions for at least 20 inpatients and 100-plus outpatient presentations daily: this encompasses everything including beds, linen, toileting, and hygiene (showers, running water, and toilets). It is the responsibility of the nursing team leader to liaise with the logistical team to prioritize the setup and provision of these essential services to support the effective functioning of the field hospital.

Principles of Care in the Austere Environment

The primary goal in humanitarian response to humanitarian crisis is to prevent or reduce excess morbidity and mortality. The way health interventions are planned, organized, and delivered in response to a disaster can either enhance or undermine the existing health systems and their future recovery.

The philosophical approach to the treatment of the patient in the austere environment focuses on rapid triage, evaluation, stabilization, and transfer as appropriate, rather than definitive evaluation and care in the early phases following a sudden-onset disaster (SOD). Use of simple procedures and processes will assist in the evaluation and stabilization of the patient. Triage in the austere environment functionally does not change, but the allocation of categories such as expectant may be considered in this resource-poor environment.

An acceptable minimum level of care is reliant on the type of disaster, distance to definitive care, restoration of local infrastructure, and available resources. Initial management includes stabilization, prevention of further deterioration, therapeutic interventions in line with available resources, monitoring, reassessment, and reassurance[7].

Host Governments and Health Systems

An international EMT deployment can only occur following the request for assistance from the host nation. The local MoH/department of health will operate in the same manner to be expected in any other national department of health: setting the clinical/geographical/ functional or operating boundaries under which international EMTs within their country are permitted to operate, and, in addition, often issuing a formal "authority to practice" to individual clinicians within I-EMTs. While the MoH has no authority for the direct clinical management within international EMT field hospitals, it does retain the right to stop any I-EMT operating within

country, as well as removal of an individual's authority to practice[6].

Embedding Host Nation Clinical Staff

Levels of health services vary across the world, ranging from the very basic to the very sophisticated. The nursing team leader must be astute to the local health standard of care and models, particularly when considering embedding host nation national staff. It is essential that a good rapport is established early and maintained in any interactions, which can be varied and specific to type of deployment, including:

- MoH officials
- managerial and clinical staff of local health facilities
- host nation clinical staff embedding into the international EMT field facility (disciplines may include nursing, medical, allied health, and support services)
- logistical support: EMT field facility cleaning, catering, and security

The nursing team leader needs to have an awareness of the host nation's health and societal culture, language, and potential for dialect barriers, which may affect the abilities of both deployed and embedded staff to deliver clinical care. The nursing team leader must ascertain the embedded staff's clinical scope of practice and ensure alignment with allocated duties and integration with EMT nursing workforce.

Ethics and Cultural Considerations

The austere field hospital environment can present many ethical challenges. Clinical scenarios that may undergo relatively straightforward management in a referral hospital may present significant ethical dilemmas in the field. Such illnesses can be a major cause of stress to clinicians and the team as a whole.

A senior ethics group structure can be used to address difficult clinical decision-making (such as end-of-life and difficult ethical decisions) and is generally comprised of[1]:

- team leader (one or both CTLs)
- treating clinician (nurse or doctor)
- another member of clinical staff not involved in the patient's care

When approaching difficult clinical decision-making, practitioners may find it useful to consider the following questions:

- What is the current gold standard of care in the high-resource environment?
- What is the standard of care locally?
- What are the patient's/family's wishes?
- What can be reasonably achieved with the resources at hand?

"Resource limitations + operational environment = limitations of care"

Informed Consent

It is a standard of care that all patients undergoing any treatment give informed consent in their native language at all times where possible[6]. Achieving informed consent may therefore require the use of an interpreter. Where possible, an independent, qualified person should be used as a translator, but in the austere environment this may not always be possible.

For minor procedures (such as intravenous cannula insertion, indwelling catheter, and so on), verbal consent is considered to be appropriate and sufficient. For more invasive procedures, a written consent should be obtained and either documented in the notes or on a designated consent form[1]. Practitioners and clinicians need to be aware that, although persons may speak English as a second language, they are likely to best understand complex medical terminology/explanations in their native language. In addition, it should be noted, apart from native language translation needs, persons from other cultures may have significant different world/religious/health views and beliefs, which should be taken into account when planning care and seeking consent.

Operations

Nursing Workforce Considerations

The many constraints encountered in the coordination and delivery of clinical acute care services in temporary, standalone, fully self-sufficient, environmentally demanding, and often isolated footprints are extremely challenging and arduous. Such challenges can lead to extreme human and physical resource limitations, which, in combination with unprecedented patient volumes and acuity (across all age ranges and specialties), demand constant and active management through highly developed, dedicated nurse leadership to ensure effective maintenance and delivery of clinical services.

Commonly, nursing scope of practice may be more limited in the developed countries where EMTs originate, and nurse to patient ratios are conversely very high in comparison in contrast to the deployed field hospital setting. Minimum nurse staffing ratios and skills are defined in WHO's *Classification and Minimum Standards for Foreign Medical Teams in Sudden Onset Disasters*[6] to ensure safe delivery of nursing care in the austere, resource-limited setting, and are clearly defined for international EMT field facilities.

Nurse staffing ratios:

- nurse/ward beds 1:8
- nurse/intensive care beds 1:2
- nurse/operating table 5:1
- nurse/medical staff 3:1

Specialist nursing skills:

- emergency and trauma care
- primary and endemic health
- maternal and child health
- perioperative care
- intensive care (EMT 3 only)
- inpatient surgical/medical care
- inpatient pediatric care

Nursing specific considerations such as specialized competencies, seniority to maintain a skill mix, balanced with active fatigue management and monitoring, along with the need to provide minimum staffing ratios continuously across a 24-hour period, collectively highlight the need for constant flexibility and adaptation when planning, allocating, and maintaining a deployed operational clinical workforce roster.

Essentials of Nursing Care

The delivery and provision of essential nursing care is imperative in the field hospital setting. Ensuring that a patient's *basic needs such as food, water, shelter, warmth, and safety* are met is critical to enable patients to recover and begin the healing process after a SOD or event of significance.

It is important to note that, following disasters, *fresh food and water supplies are often limited* or nonexistent. The host country will rely on the EMT being self-sufficient and resourced to provide sufficient food and water for patients, next of kin, and all staff in the field hospital. Dehydrated/prepackaged food is often utilized in the first instance and, as the local community begins to recover and international aid is distributed, local markets may resume, providing opportunity for fresh local food to be purchased in the weeks following a SOD. The sourcing and provision of local cooks will ensure that culturally appropriate food is being provided for patients and improve their nutritional requirements to aid wound healing and patient recovery.

Patient positioning and mobility can be compromised in the field hospital as many patients are initially treated in chairs or on stretchers on the ground. Ideally positioning the patient in a semirecumbent position would be preferable, but this may be limited to the type of beds/stretchers available in the field hospital environment. Therefore, the nurse will need to *prioritize and be highly flexible* in the utilization of beds/stretchers and, at times, will need to rationalize the use of certain types of beds/stretchers depending on patient needs.

Physical space is often limited and the room between beds/stretchers can be compromised by family being in attendance and the footprint of the shelters available, thus making it difficult to encourage mobility of patients. Physical aids such as crutches, walking aids, and wheelchairs may be limited, but need to be considered to enable patients *safe access to toilets and showers*, as well as providing opportunity to mobilize outside.

Infection control/hand hygiene is imperative in the austere field-hospital setting. Easy access to running water within clinical-care areas wherever possible is preferential; alternatively, sanitizing hand gels/rubs may be used (note contents of the specific agents for transport requirements as these are often classed as dangerous goods due to contents). *Patient linen* should be changed a minimum of daily and remain individual to individual patients.

Clinical waste management when delivering acute care services in temporary/standalone, self-sufficient austere field-hospital sites is one of the most challenging and confronting contrasts to standard nursing practice. In general, there are two types of waste generated during the deployment of a field hospital: general household and medical hazardous waste. Basic principles of good waste management include methodical separation and minimization wherever possible of both

general and biohazard waste in the austere field setting. Specifically, *sharps and body fluids/waste* handling management procedures need particularly close attention in the field setting: logistical staff guidance for nursing staff in relation to host nation guidelines and legislative requirements is essential.

The same *principles of medication management* should apply in a field hospital as they do in the deploying organization's home country. However, additional consideration and review is often required to ensure practice is in accordance with the host nation legislation. Care should be taken to ensure that standard nursing practice adheres and complies with local host nation and home country legislation for the prescribing, administration, dispensing, supply, and storage of medications.

Allied health is an integral part of the EMT, but *access to all allied health disciplines is often severely limited* in the immediate aftermath of a disaster and therefore many allied health duties provided in a conventional hospital environment will need to be incorporated into the nursing role in the field.

Communication with patients and family for international EMT field hospital staff can be challenging particularly when the host country is non-English speaking or the EMT staff do not speak the language. Access to interpreters is necessary and should be considered prior to deployment and sourced in the early stage of the deployment.

The issue of risk management associated with *patient falls and pressure injury* is still relevant in the field hospital environment due to the unconventional, temporary nature of patient beds and clinical-care areas. The risk of patients developing pressure injuries is high; nursing staff therefore need to be vigilant in ensuring regular pressure care is provided and patients are assessed each shift for signs of pressure injury. Nursing staff need to be conscientious and diligent in identifying fall risks and escalating concerns to the nursing team leader.

Clinical Handover

Clinical handover between shifts is vital, as is documentation, assessment findings, emerging patient needs, and care delivered: these are all paramount in the austere setting. Extreme resource limitations (human and physical), unprecedented patient volumes and acuity (across all age ranges and specialties), and the requirement to deliver clinical acute care

Table 28.2 Handover checklist

Hand hygiene	
Introductions ID band check	I
Condition/diagnosis Immediate concerns	S
History Allergies Social concerns	B
Observation chart Medication chart Fluid balance chart Risks: falls/pressure ulcer prevention strategy/ lines Dressings Oxygen and suction Environment check	A
Clinical upcoming events Patient care boards updated Staff questions Patient questions Give/accept handover	R
Hand hygiene	

services in temporary, standalone, fully self-sufficient, environmentally challenged, and isolated footprints can overwhelm clinical staff, all of which collectively can represent *significant additional risk to patient safety and standards of clinical care.*

The aim of handover in all circumstances is to ensure a seamless exchange of information between care providers. The ability to communicate effectively between and with health professionals is imperative to ensure the transfer of information, accountability, and responsibility for patients. Using a communication tool and standardizing key principles for clinical handover will aid *effective, concise and complete communication in all clinical situations* and facilitate care delivery and improve patient safety. The ISBAR mnemonic (identify, situation, background, assessment, recommendation) is a useful clinical handover tool, which can be utilized to communicate effectively between health professionals and nursing shift handovers (Table 28.2).

Patient Tracking and Identification

Each patient should be given a unique identification number, which stays with them throughout their treatment by the EMT facility, including any subsequent occasions of treatment. In addition, all patients admitted to the inpatient wards of the field hospital must have an identification band applied. The band should include: patient name, age, date of birth, gender, patient unique identification number, and allergies[6].

Patients who are transferred to another facility must have an identification band in situ, medical records, and a transfer referral letter accompany them. On discharge from the hospital, patients should be provided with a discharge summary.

It is essential that the local MoH, who will be responsible for the ongoing care of the patients seen throughout the field facility mission, are given a copy of all medical notes. In addition, they should also be provided a copy of all births, deaths, and patient transfer activities which occur within the field hospital. For this reason, cumulative field facility patient registers should be maintained and completed for all incoming and outgoing patients to the field facility[1]:

- emergency clinic consults (includes review consults)
- admissions
- discharges
- births and deaths
- transfers
- operating theater activity
- bed occupancy at the time of day mandated by the local MoH/EMTCC
- surveillance data, as required by MoH/WHO/EMTCC

Daily Routine

It is vitally important to set and maintain a regular routine for field-hospital environments as soon as possible after arrival and facilities are established. Without structure and common reference points provided through leadership among the chaos, staff can become overwhelmed, lacking direction and cohesive, prioritized coordination to their efforts.

As a general rule, most outpatient and primary-care clinic areas are only operational during daylight hours in the deployed field hospital setting (08:00–18:00 hours) while emergency resuscitation and all inpatient clinical areas are required to sustain 24-hour operational capability[6].

Clinical areas will therefore function most efficiently on a 12-hour rotational roster system, enabling effective staff fatigue management with minimal disruption to patient care. In addition, this also facilitates the opportunity for clinical leadership to brief and update the entire clinical staff on current issues/considerations twice daily, immediately following shift handover.

277

Staff Huddles[1]

1. Mission command team:

    a. twice per day: ideally immediately prior to start and at completion of main daily activities

    b. brief update of each area hot topics/needs: taskforce, log, and clinical

2. All staff:

    a. twice per day: ideally immediately prior to start and at completion of main daily activities

    b. individual clinical staff allocations

    c. clinical topics/information of relevance

    d. summary of relevant mission hot topics/needs: taskforce and log

Clinical Rounds[1]

3. Joint clinical team leaders:

    a. twice per day: ideally immediately prior to shift changes

    b. patient care coordination, referral, and discharge planning

    c. scouting for problems and finding solutions

    d. bed occupancy in each area

    e. clinical liaison with local MoH facilities/referral providers

    f. overall hospital daily activity (total number of presentations, operating theater cases, and ward occupancy) noted on evening round

4. Surgical team:

    a. twice per day: immediately prior to operating theater list start and after completion

    b. preoperative/postoperative care coordination

    c. new outpatient reviews/referrals

    d. operating theater list daily scheduling

5. Allied health and rehabilitation team:

    a. daily: immediately following morning shift change and surgical round

    b. interdisciplinary patient care, referral, and discharge planning

    c. liaison with local/community/referral providers

6. Nurse team leader:

    a. rotating through all clinical areas at three-hourly intervals: 06:00–23:00 hours

    b. patient flow and bed occupancy management

    c. communication between inpatient/outpatient/operating theater clinical shift teams

    d. clinical equipment/consumables oversight

    e. scouting for problems and finding solutions

Summary

- The absence of high-tech, modern diagnostic tools in the disaster setting necessitates a return and emphasis on the basic clinical skills as the foundation principles of nursing care.

- Nurses should not only be appropriately skilled and trained but most importantly also supported in the translation and adaptation of their nursing practice into the context of an austere and environmentally challenging setting.

- Nursing staff need to have an awareness of the host nation's health and societal culture, language, and potential barriers, which may impact on the ability to effectively deliver clinical care.

- Nursing specific considerations collectively highlight the need for constant flexibility and adaptation when planning, allocating, and maintaining a deployed operational clinical workforce roster.

- Strong nursing leadership is pivotal in ensuring effective and efficient running of a deployed field hospital with limited resources in an austere and environmentally challenging setting.

References

1. Australian Medical Assistance Teams (AUSMAT). Clinical service delivery guide for clinical leaders. 2016: National Critical Care Trauma Response Centre. Australian Government.

2. Young H, Harvey P. The sphere project: the humanitarian charter and minimum standards in disaster response: introduction. *Disasters* 2004: **28**(2): 99.

3. World Health Organization and International Council of Nurses (2009). ICN framework of disaster nursing competencies. http://www.wpro.who.int/hrh/docu ments/icn_framework.pdf?ua=1competencies%20or%2 0abilities%20to%20rapidly%20and%20effectively

4. Veenema, T. Managing emergencies outside the hospital: Special events, Mass gatherings, and mass casualty incidents, in Veenema T (ed.) *Disaster nursing and emergency preparedness for chemical, biological, and radiological terrorism and other hazards.* New York: Springer Publishing Company; 2007: 205–19.

5. Amat-Camacho N, Hughes A, Burkle FM, et al. Education and training of emergency medical teams: recommendations for a global operational learning framework. *PLOS Currents Disasters* 2016: 1.

6. Norton I, von Schreeb J, Aitken P, Herard P, Lajolo C. *Classification and minimum standards for foreign medical teams in sudden onset disasters.* Geneva: World Health Organization; 2013.

7. Hogan D, Burstein JL. *Disaster medicine.* Second edn. 2007.

8. Australian Commission on Safety and Quality in Health Care (2012). Standard 6 clinical handover, safety and quality improvement guide. https://safetyandquality .gov.au/wp-content/uploads/2012/10/Standard6_ Oct_2012_WEB.pdf

9. Curtis K and Ramsden C. *Emergency and trauma care.* Second edn. Australia: Elsevier; 2016.

10. International Council of Nurses. Position statement – evidence-based safe nurse staffing. 2018.

Chapter

29
Forensic Medicine and Victim Identification in the Field Hospital Setting

S David Gertz, Chen Kugel, Ladd A Tremaine, and Louis N Finelli

Introduction

In addition to the essential medical and technical specialties, the field hospital is incomplete without capabilities in the fields of *forensic medicine* (FM) and *victim identification* (VI). The specifics of what constitutes appropriate or necessary circumstances and what are the indications and required capabilities for deployment of FM and VI services in the field-hospital setting is the subject of this chapter.

For operational purposes, field hospitals can be divided into two major types: (1) those deployed *within the borders of the parent jurisdiction* of the care provider, and (2) those deployed, per official request, *within another jurisdiction* such as within the context of remote *humanitarian missions*. In the former, deployment of FM and victim identification services, with all the associated complexities, is both impractical and counterproductive when these activities remain fully operational and easily accessible in facilities not compromised by the effects of the disaster. An exception to this would be circumstances, natural or hostile, that resulted in neutralization of the local, permanent facilities. In such cases, field deployment of these essential services may be necessary.

Field hospitals are usually erected in areas where the available functional resources are insufficient to meet basic medical needs from the standpoint of personnel and equipment. It has been argued by some that, under such emergency circumstances, FM should not be a priority. However, proper mortality management cannot be avoided. Absence of definitive identification prevents closure for the bereaved family and is a well-recognized source of unrest and friction between the affected population and the authorities. Pressure from public officials to identify the decedents can be tremendous. For these reasons, identification of human remains has been recognized by WHO as one of the major required tasks of medical agencies[1]. FM is also needed to assist in reconstructing factors leading up to the disaster, establishing the cause and mechanism of

death, and presenting detailed explanations to the bereaved relatives. Other essential functions of FM include documentation of medical treatment and discussing this with the providers, evaluation of the effectiveness of protective gear, documentation of distribution of wounds, and, in the case of hostilities, correlation of mechanisms of injury with weapons specifications.

Mortality Management in the Field-Hospital Setting

FM and VI require a multidisciplinary team of different professions from different agencies, as will be explained later in this chapter. The responsibility for identification of human remains usually rests with the local governmental jurisdiction.

A major challenge, worldwide, for those responsible for VI is *preparedness for circumstances when the number of casualties exceeds the capabilities of the responsible jurisdiction to perform the task within an acceptable period of time.*

The success of the identification and the investigation process depends on the efficiency of organization, level of experience, and the accuracy of interpretation of findings. Communication between staff members from different agencies and different fields of expertise can be difficult. Because of the complex nature of the tasks related to management of the dead and VI, application of international protocols for disaster victim identification (DVI) operations such as Interpol, WHO, and the International Committee of the Red Cross (ICRC) provides important standardization[2,3]. Intactness of the functional integrity of the responsible local jurisdiction and its operational divisions is of major importance for the success of such efforts.

Major Steps in Victim Identification

Regardless of whether the task is performed within a permanent facility or in a field hospital setting, VI involves many, if not all, of the steps listed below. Each of these steps requires adequate professional staffing. Moreover, VI procedures must be closely coordinated with, and usually follow, an examination by a forensic pathologist or FM specialist (see "Postmortem Procedures in the Field Hospital" later in the chapter) so as not to disturb critical physical evidence.

1. Preparation of site for arrival of victims and remains: close coordination with remains retrieval units
2. Ordinance screening: close coordination with explosive ordinance disposal (EOD) units
3. Assigning a unique identifier for all victims and detached remains
4. Description and labeling of personal effects without disturbing forensic evidence
5. Antemortem data collection or access to previously collected antemortem records
6. Postmortem CT scan, if available
7. External forensic survey (general, wounds, treatments, and photography)
8. Fingerprints
9. Dental evaluation and crossmatching
10. DNA specimen collection and management
11. DNA laboratory processing and analysis
12. Transfer of body to the medical examiner for advanced postmortem identification if needed
13. Data evaluation by senior forensic committee
14. Temporary or final burial

Teams at the Scene

An advanced team from the FM department of the field hospital should visit the disaster site as early as possible before items and bodies are removed. This is necessary to evaluate the terrain, the extent of the damage, the number and state of the deceased (e.g., degree of dismemberment and fragmentation or advanced decomposition), suspicion of contamination of remains, the need for any special equipment for recovery, and the optimal method for transporting the bodies.

According to the information gathered by the advanced team, a second search/recovery and evidence-collection team (not necessarily from the intrinsic forensic team of the field hospital) should be sent to the scene. This team should have at least one forensic pathologist whose job

it is to provide the necessary medical experience regarding management of the bodies and to ensure preservation of means of identification and other medical evidence important for the investigation. A forensic anthropologist, operating under the authority of a medical examiner, can fill this role if he or she has adequate recovery experience.

It is the job of the advanced team to provide technical advice for the search and recovery team. The specific location of each body (or body part) should be recorded. Other pieces of evidence (documents, belongings, and so on) should also be recorded and collected by the accompanying nonmedical personnel. The objects found on the scene could be crucial for identification and subsequent investigation of the event; hence, the location of each item should be registered individually and accurately recorded in relation to the body. This emphasizes the need for meticulous documentation of the recovery site (description, photographs, or sketch of the position of the body and location on a grid or map). Nevertheless, the extent of advance detail collected may need to be modified by the officer in charge in circumstances requiring hasty recovery.

It should be emphasized that determining the original association of detached body parts should be done only at the FM department of the field hospital itself and not at the scene. Only authorized forensic medical experts can do this; not recovery personnel. Many times, the matching can be performed only by genetic methods (DNA) and not anatomically. This is the reason why each detached body part should be labeled by a separate distinct number and be treated as a separate body.

The state of preservation of the bodies is a major component of successful identification and investigation. Since the condition of bodies can deteriorate very quickly depending in large part on exposure to environmental conditions, effort should be made to move the body to a proper storage facility as soon as possible. In cases of significant delay, it may be advisable to collect a DNA sample from the human remains (from blood or muscle tissue) before commencement of the recovery operation provided trackable identification (body and sample) is assured.

It is essential that the field-hospital management staff make sure that communication routes are established to ensure flow of information from the scene of disaster and with all relevant authorities and relevant agencies.

Postmortem Procedures in the Field Hospital

Identification of human remains can be divided into three types:

1. Visual recognition
2. Definitive, positive, scientific identification
3. Circumstantial identification

In a multicasualty event, it is highly recommended to refrain from visual identification. Disfigurement of bodies, changes due to decomposition, and the general psychological atmosphere of stress and urgency can lead to mistakes in identification. It is always most advisable to use scientific methods of identification. Most of the scientific identification methods are based on comparison of postmortem data (from the body) with antemortem data from the same person while he or she was alive. The comparison is based on stable and unique characteristics: stable, that do not change during life, and will be comparable regardless of when they were taken and when death occurred; unique, that have sufficient power of differentiation and resolution between individuals.

The antemortem data regarding the individual are usually still unavailable when the body arrives at the field hospital. Thus, all relevant biometric parameters (fingerprints, dental examination, X-ray and/or CT scan, and genetic markers such as DNA) should be collected on arrival.

The external forensic examination is an essential tool for the investigation of the event (see below). Complete autopsy is an excellent and recommended tool for investigation of the cause of death and collection of other forensic data. However, it is seldom necessary for the purposes of identification. Considering that autopsy is a time- and effort-consuming procedure, and taking into account the heavy workload in the setup of a field hospital, the chapter authors recommend, in contrast to most existing comprehensive protocols, to save the resources and perform autopsy for the purpose of identification only when all other means of identification have failed.

Regarding *work flow*, in the case of multiple decedents arriving at the field hospital, one efficiently run line has been determined to be preferable, resulting in fewer mistakes and less chance of "bottlenecks." However, in mass-casualty events with a large number of fatalities, it may be necessary to work in multiple separate lines as depicted in Figure 29.1. This will reduce hold-ups on the line such as those caused by complicated cases. It should be stressed that all findings should be photographed and documented, and the process as a whole should be supervised and quality controlled.

The postmortem team at the field hospital should include forensic pathologists, mortuary technicians, forensic odontologists, forensic anthropologists, photographers, trace-evidence officers (for fingerprinting and data collection), and secretarial workers to document all retrieved data. A team manager should be appointed to direct and identify problems in the work flow.

Fingerprints should be taken by forensic officers (e.g., law-enforcement officers, death investigators, or forensic pathologists). In the setup of a field hospital, fingerprints will usually be taken as ink prints. In a jurisdictional framework where there is a reservoir of fingerprint data, a scan can be used such as in the case of an automatic fingerprint identification system (AFIS)[4]. Fingerprinting is one of the first steps in the data collection process because of its efficiency and promptness of results.

All *personal items* and clothing that accompany the body must be described, photographed, and kept for further investigation since they can provide valuable information of relevance to the identity of the individual and circumstances of his or her death. These include identification cards, jewelry, watches, credit and bank cards, notes, wallets, and so on. Clothing should be described for size, color, brand, and so on. Clothing is important not only for support of identification but also for signs of penetration or impact, since many times it can preserve the evidence of the impacting object better than the skin. Clothing is also important for detection of gunpowder residue, explosive material, cuts and tears, thermal effects, and so on.

Collection of medical data by *external examination* is very important for the investigation and assessment of injuries, and is not less important for the process of identification. The external examination can point to scars of surgical procedures or healed injuries. It can reveal tattoos, birth marks, anatomical variations, and even simple differentiating data (e.g., color of the eyes, color of the hair, hair length, age, ethnic group, weight). All findings of the external examination should be described and photographed with inclusion of a ruler in each frame.

Photography is used not only for body marks but also for documenting jewelry, clothes, general features

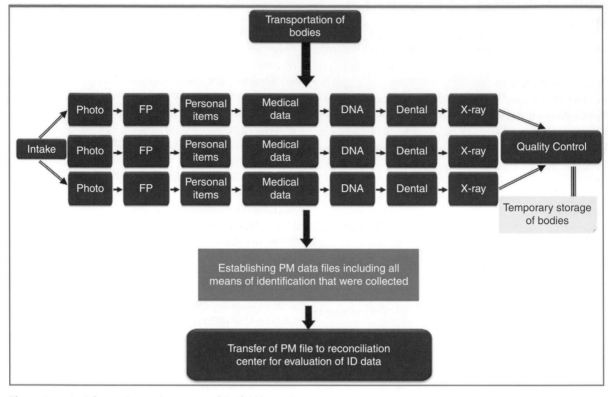

Figure 29.1 Work flow in the FM department of the field hospital

of the body, and documentation of wounds, injuries, scars, and so on. Photography is important not only for maintenance of the chain of evidence but also for relatives who would like to see the body as it was when it arrived at the field hospital.

Samples for DNA can be obtained from blood, muscle, mucosa, and sometimes from bones where soft tissues are missing or decomposed. In case of fragmentation of bodies, samples must be taken from each body part. However, in cases where the fragmentation is severe (explosions, airplane crashes, and so on), the number of tissue fragments can be very high, exceeding the practical processing capacity of the DNA lab. In such circumstances, a managerial decision must be taken to determine the minimal size of tissue fragment to be sampled. It is impractical to sample every piece of tissue the size of few cubic centimeters. However, meticulous sampling can be necessary for determining the number of casualties in cases of severe fragmentation of bodies. Establishment of the number of deceased is accomplished not by counting anatomic structures (this can be grossly inaccurate) but by counting genetic

profiles. In many multicasualty events there are individuals represented only by one, or a few, body parts.

No field hospital is equipped with a forensic molecular biology laboratory. This means that the tissue samples must be preserved in accordance with the requirements of the laboratory that will process the samples. Constant communication must be maintained between the FM department of the field hospital and the *DNA processing laboratory* regarding quality of tissue, need for resampling, and feedback regarding profile analysis.

Dental examination should be performed on all bodies where possible. In some cases, it can be difficult due to rigor mortis or decomposition. One might ask why perform this time-consuming examination when usually just a small percentage of the bodies are identified by dental means. One may argue that only bodies that are not identifiable by other means should undergo dental examination. However, dental examination (including dental X-ray) can provide important unique morphological information of relevance to identification even when antemortem dental records are unavailable. It can also reveal valuable morphological and pathological data that can provide clues of direct relevance to the death investigation.

Comparison of *postmortem radiographs* to antemortem radiographs taken at the same view can be a very important tool for identification. X-rays can reveal prostheses, evidence of previous surgical procedures including their locations, positioning of indwelling catheters or other devices, anatomical variations, presence of jewelry in case of burned bodies, and location and characteristics of penetrating projectiles such as bullets, and so on. When there is no hint or indication regarding identity, X-ray can assist in estimating the age, sex, and sometimes even race of an individual.

If there is a possibility to obtain a CT scan it is highly recommended. *Mobile CT units* are available and can be deployed to the field-hospital area when possible and practical. Although most mobile CT units, if deployed to the field-hospital setting, will be used for the injured, total-body CT is a matter of few minutes, and the relevant information can be available in a few more minutes. This can provide valuable forensic data and save extremely time-consuming and invasive postmortem surgical procedures. On the other hand, total body X-ray takes approximately 45 minutes and much more effort is involved. A postmortem CT scan can create a three-dimensional reconstruction of the body with its skeleton and also produce dental panoramic radiographs at the same session, thereby also eliminating the need for dental X-rays.

Antemortem Data

As mentioned earlier, most of the identification methods are based on comparison of postmortem and antemortem data. The antemortem data can be collected from military or police identification reservoirs, from medical facilities, or from next of kin, and so on. The members of the antemortem data collection teams should be experienced in investigations and liaison. Their primary mission is to create a list of missing persons who may be victims of the disaster and gather their records necessary for comparison.

Populations for identification are divided into two groups: an *open group* and a *closed* group. A closed group refers to unidentified persons who belong to a fixed group of people whose names are known; for example, passengers of a crashed commercial airplane or inmates of a prison destroyed by fire. The names of the victims are actually known, and the task of the identification team is to "attach a name to a body." An open group relates to unidentified people who have no records or available indication of their names (e.g., earthquake). The FM staff of a field hospital might be called on to deal with either of these kinds of group. Naturally, an open group will be much more difficult to deal with. Gathering antemortem data related to unidentified bodies with minimal indication of their identity can be difficult or impossible. Nevertheless, the better the indication regarding the identity of the missing person, the easier it is and the greater the likelihood of collecting relevant antemortem data.

To reach a positive identification of an individual there must be *some hint* directing us toward his or her identity. Clearly, even if one has a detailed dental description with X-rays, it is impossible to compare these to all the dental X-rays in the state. However, if a *fingerprint repository* and *AFIS system* are available, such as for military personnel and individuals with criminal records, identification can be made with relative ease even in the situation of an "open population." Antemortem fingerprints can be obtained from where they were taken intentionally (e.g., police, army, workplace, immigration) or where they were left unintentionally (e.g., car mirrors, glasses, CDs, travel documents). *Antemortem DNA* samples can be obtained from repositories (usually military), from previous medical examinations (e.g., biopsies or blood samples), or from personal items (e.g., toothbrushes, combs, underwear). DNA can be also obtained from first-degree relatives. *Dental records* can be obtained from private clinics, medical insurance companies, school dental services or from reservoirs (e.g., military or correctional facilities). *Medical data* can be obtained from hospitals, clinics, insurance companies, next of kin, and so on. Information gathered from relatives or friends can also be relevant for identifying jewelry, personal belongings, clothing, and so on. The latter are not primary means of identification but can give an indication and point toward the presumed identity of the individual.

Beside the investigators, the antemortem team should be accompanied by medical personnel (forensic pathologist and dentist), who can ascertain if any item or medical record has any relevance for purposes of identification.

After finalizing the process of data gathering, and creating the postmortem and antemortem files, comes the process of evaluating the quality and comparing the data. The legally responsible official, be it the medical examiner in charge of the jurisdiction, the forensic pathologist, or other legally responsible civilian or military official, may, at his or her discretion, use a *reconciliation and identification board*. The latter, when convened, is a multidisciplinary team, which usually includes a forensic pathologist, an odontologist, forensic anthropologist, fingerprint identification expert, the physician in charge, and an investigator. The board gives its recommendation as to whether the collected data are sufficient for definitive, positive identification or if additional evidence/studies are deemed necessary. Considerable time is saved when data collection, processing, and interrogation-enabled evaluation software is used.

The Death Investigation Process

Apart from VI, it is the responsibility of the FM department of a field hospital to provide information regarding the *cause, manner, and mechanism of death.* This includes searching for evidence of missiles, projectiles, tool marks, explosive devices, and so on. In addition, the forensic team documents the *distribution of wounds* and attempts correlation with weapons specifications. The team also searches for specific injury pattern characteristics (e.g., of injuries of suicide bombers or those found on airplane pilots after ejection) and estimates *survival time.* This is a multidisciplinary team approach in which the forensic pathologist provides objective postmortem findings to care providers.

Unlike for identification purposes, a proper, scrutinized investigation of the cause, manner, and mechanisms of death requires a full autopsy covering the entire body. The information gathered for purposes of identification is largely "target oriented." The examiner is looking for specific characteristics or parameters. By contrast, information necessary to be retrieved from the body for the death investigation process is not just that which is based on a priori assumptions; rather, it is frequently not anticipated, and data obtained can be of great importance for future inquiries. In some cases, even a second autopsy or examination is necessary if new information or evidence of relevance is discovered. When hostile acts are suspected as the cause for a mass-casualty event such as a terrorist act, forensic investigation involving full autopsy is often unavoidable to identify key elements related to the investigation. The data obtained at autopsy are compared with evidence

collected by the scene investigation team at the site of the disaster such as location of the victims, nature of the attached debris, blood spatter, trace evidence, and so on.

As mentioned before, autopsy is a time- and resource-consuming procedure. Hence, when the caseload is heavy, a decision must be made regarding which bodies are of top priority. Frequently, the cause of death can be determined using surrogates such as postmortem CT scan.

If a criminal investigation is taking place, it is even more crucial to preserve the evidence and its chain of custody. This can create a situation that is at odds with the usual atmosphere of a field hospital: disposing of any object that is unnecessary for treatment or disturbing the general cleanliness and speed of work flow. As repeatedly stressed in the Interpol protocol[2], body fluids, remains of explosives, ammunition, pieces of equipment, and so on are important pieces of forensic evidence. These items and samples must be collected by trained forensic experts and should not be contaminated, altered, or destroyed. This re-emphasizes the importance of deployment of the FM/VI department of the field hospital compound within a separate structure, which permits independent, unobstructed work flow with free and independent access to recovery vehicles, adequate waiting and cold storage areas, and direct access to a mobile imaging unit.

To avoid entrance of previously undetected contaminated human remains or other contaminated forensic evidence to the area of the FM department and the field hospital compound in general, *access to the area should be restricted* and heavily monitored.

Examination by EOD and, if the circumstances dictate, chemical, biological, radiological, and nuclear (CBRN) investigators, must occur in an area away from the field hospital to preserve safety of all. Approved personnel should enter the forensic identification department only for authorized operational reasons. No exhibit or specimen should be altered or removed from the body or its proximity before it is examined, described, and photographed. All items should be registered and documented, and a chain of custody should be established for items that need to be transferred to another investigative authority. Again, as phrased by Interpol and others, avoid being a "member of the evidence eradication team[2,3]."

Decisions to omit, shorten, or modify any of the steps in the forensic investigation and VI process, be it in the field hospital setting, or in a permanent parent facility, must be made on site by the physician in charge of FM. These decisions by the physician in charge should be made in consultation with the chief or commander of the field hospital, as appropriate, and other national and/or military officials as required. The decisions must be based on consideration of the entirety of circumstances and specifics of the event in question from professional, logistic, strategic, and tactical aspects, as well as other issues such as national, local, and individual security.

Factors that Affect Priorities, Caseload, and Time Required for VI in the Field-Hospital Setting

The *nature of the incident* profoundly influences the decision of whether to deploy assistance in VI and/or forensics to another jurisdiction in general and to a field-hospital setting in particular. *Each incident has its own unique characteristics*, which can modify decision-making for deployment.

1. Driving force of incident: natural disaster or hostile forces
2. Mediating mode of the disaster (wind, fire, water, geologic)
3. Magnitude of the disaster (e.g., category 3 or more storm [national; US National Weather Service classification] or high Richter earthquake of dangerous proximity and depth)
4. Location of the disaster (e.g., geographical complexities, access, communications): helicopter landing areas, proximity to airfield
5. Accessibility of antemortem data: functional integrity of the local government (domestic or foreign)
6. Language barrier
7. Presence of military and/or civilian victims
8. Presence of foreign nationals among the victims
9. Religion of victims
10. Degree of body fragmentation
11. Presence of comingled remains
12. Availability of trained personnel for each task
13. Time and level of detail required for external forensic survey
14. Presence of contaminated remains: CBRN
15. Safety: presence of hostile forces
16. Local public health concerns
17. Availability and time required for postmortem CT scan
18. Time for dental evaluation
19. Availability of adequate DNA laboratory facilities and time for processing
20. Availability of on-site refrigerated storage facilities
21. Accessibility (administrative or geographical) of sufficient temporary burial sites

Mobilization and Deployment

As indicated earlier, successful deployment of VI services within a field-hospital setting, be it within the parent or remote jurisdiction, is dependent on careful advance assessment by an advance expert expeditionary delegation, which evaluates the magnitude and nature of the event and assesses the potential site of deployment based on the 21 items listed above. If field-hospital deployment of VI and FM services is within a foreign jurisdiction, advance assessment must also include early contact with the local or regional emergency incident commander to gather specific information related to integrity of facilities and capabilities for performing each of the required tasks related to VI and forensic investigation detailed above.

Efforts to Improve Preparedness for VI

Preparedness for VI in circumstances where the magnitude of the disaster exceeds the capabilities of the local, responsible jurisdiction remains a worldwide concern. This stems from widespread, chronic shortages of dedicated, trained personnel and equipment. These shortages traverse military as well as civilian agencies and jurisdictions. Efforts to improve DVI preparedness must focus on three fronts: (1) improving local jurisdictional level readiness, (2) combining forces at the national level (civilian with military), and (3) forging agreements for international cooperation. Major ongoing efforts for assistance and improvement of preparedness for VI and fatality management with multiagency cooperation at the national and international levels have been undertaken by the following groups/organizations:

- International Criminal Police Organization (Interpol); based in Lyon, France[2].
- The ICRC; Geneva, Switzerland[3].
- The USA National Disaster Medical System (NDMS). The NDMS Division of the Office of Emergency Management under the authority of the US Assistant Secretary of Health and Human

Services (HHS) for Preparedness and Response (ASPR) is the primary agency responsible for providing federal assistance of medical services to local jurisdictions when summoned[5].

- Disaster Mortuary Operational Response Teams (DMORT). Aid from the NDMS includes deployment of several (± 10) regional DMORT units, which are now part of the HHS/NDMS framework. When summoned and activated, they are deployed either within the permanent facilities of the local jurisdiction or in the field within preexisting, largely self-contained, morgue facilities termed disaster portable morgue units[6].

- The Armed Forces Medical Examiner System via subordinate divisions of The Office of the Armed Forces Medical Examiner (OAFME) Department of Defense DNA Operations – Current Day Operations (AKA Armed Forces DNA Identification Laboratory [AFDIL]). The Director of Military Support (DOMS) of the DoD and the Joint Task Force-Civil Support (JTF-CS) coordinate military support to civil authorities. When local jurisdictions are overloaded and unable to handle the DNA processing, by special interagency agreement emergency federal assistance may be summoned from the AFDIL in Dover, Delaware[7]. In such cases, DMORT may assist AFDIL in DNA sample collection for processing and analysis.

- US Army Research Development and Engineering Command, Military Improved Response Program and Department of Justice, Office of Justice Programs, Office for Domestic Preparedness, spearheading preparation of Capstone Document[8].

- Interagency Mass Fatality Management Working Group (MFMWG). The MFMWG has been established to assist the NMDS/OEM/HHS in providing for comprehensive assistance to local jurisdictions in times of need. This working group includes over 50 participants from several federal and regional agencies (including two of the chapter authors [Ladd A Tremaine and Louis N Finelli]) as well as several international participants (including one of the chapter authors [S David Gertz]). Its charge is to develop standard operating procedures (SOPs) for assessing jurisdictional capabilities and development of procedures, protocols, and assistance packages for federal assistance when summoned[9].

- Regional Mass Fatality Management Response System and Regional Catastrophic Preparedness

Team, supported in part by the Department of Homeland Security, development of cooperative interjurisdictional framework to manage mass fatality events[10].

- Identification of Victims of Mass-Casualty Events (IVMCE) Working Group. Established by signed agreement between the US DoD, Office of the US Assistant Secretary of Defense for Health Affairs for the US Armed Forces Medical Examiner System and the Israel Ministry of Defense for the Israel Defense Forces (IDF) Medical Corps and IDF Forensic Identification Unit. The IVMCE agreement permits engagement in the sharing of information, training and readiness, technologies, forensics, equipment, and other tactics, techniques, and procedures for the identification of victims of mass-casualty events. This effort has been ruled to be consistent with the Homeland Defense Cooperation Terms of Reference (HDC TOR) signed between the two departments of defense on September 1, 2006, and updated on December 3, 2009, and has become an official section in the data exchange agreement between the two countries and the Bilateral Shoresh Conference since 2010. This agreement reflects the continued commitment for academic and operational collaboration including mutual, hands-on support and assistance for fatality management in times of need.

Moral Responsibility

It is a generally accepted guiding principle in virtually all western-oriented countries that each of the fallen should have definitive identification and be brought to an individual, marked site of burial. It therefore behooves all capable governments to lend assistance, whenever and wherever possible, to any jurisdiction, worldwide, who turns to them for this purpose. However, it is also generally agreed that achievement of this noble goal should not supersede protection of the living, and that body retrieval and VI should not involve endangering the living unless doing so is a key element in a rare, strategic national security issue.

In situations of extreme mass disasters, where the integrity of the local jurisdictional government is severely compromised, VI efforts may be severely hampered and of low priority. In the 7.0 magnitude earthquake of 2010 in Haiti, over 220 000 people died (some estimates reach over 300 000)[8]. The local government ceased to function, and its buildings were in ruins. Antemortem data were virtually inaccessible. Residents were without shelter, without food, and without drinking water. Identification of the dead became a low priority. The dead, in some cases, were seen being transported in dump trucks along with broken furniture into mass graves. VI efforts within the field hospital framework were, in this case, largely limited to specific requests such as identification of foreign nationals where there were available antemortem data.

No country or jurisdiction on the planet has the capability to reach definitive identification of this many victims within an acceptable period of time. It should be noted that, even at the time of writing of this chapter, years after the September 11, 2001 World Trade Center Attack in which 2,606 people died, approximately 40% of the victims remain unidentified despite the extensive resources available to the Office of the Chief Medical Examiner of the City of New York and its special operations response team[11].

It is our view that all countries must realize the need to prepare contingency plans for combining civilian and military resources for mobilization and deployment for VI in mass-casualty events. These unified contingency plans should be rehearsed with joint exercises for the rare, but harsh, eventuality of failure to cope during a severe national disaster. Failure to improve preparedness by avoiding planning, preparing, and rehearsing such combined efforts because of stubborn refusal to transgress the principal of "separation of military and civilian efforts," or fear that individual, personal authority, or professional thunder will be usurped, is no longer acceptable and will almost certainly result in serious questions being raised, and consequences demanded by bereaved citizens who cannot reach ultimate closure with their fallen loved ones.

References

1. World Health Organization, Pan American Health Organization (2004). Management of dead bodies in disaster situations disaster manuals and guidelines series, No 5. http://www.who.int/hac/techguidance/management_of_dead_bodies.pdf (See also updated editions, reference 3, below.)

2. International Criminal Police Organization (Interpol) (1997). Disaster victim identification guide. http://vistinomer.mk/wp-content/uploads/2016/08/INTERPOL-angliski.pdf

3. Cordner S, Coninx R, Kim HJ, et al. (eds.) (2016). Management of dead bodies after disasters: a field manual for first responders. https://www.icrc.org/en/publication/0880-management-dead-bodies-after-disasters-field-manual-first-responders

4. Federal Bureau of Investigation, Criminal Justice Information Services (2008). Privacy impact assessment for the fingerprint identification records system (FIRS) integrated automated fingerprint identification system (IAFIS) outsourcing for noncriminal justice purposes – channeling. Website. https://www.fbi.gov/services/records-management/foipa/privacy-impact-assessments/firs-iafis

5. The National Disaster Medical System (NDMS), Division of the Office of Emergency Management, Office of the US Assistant Secretary of Health and Human Services (HHS) for Preparedness and Response (ASPR), Emergency Support Functions, including ESF #8 (2015). Website. http://www.phe.gov/Preparedness/support/esf8/Pages/default.aspx#8

6. Disaster Mortuary Operational Response Teams (DMORT), National Disaster Medical System (NDMS), Office of the US Assistant Secretary of Health and Human Services (HHS) for Preparedness and Response (ASPR) (2017). https://www.phe.gov/Preparedness/responders/ndms/ndms-teams/Pages/dmort.aspx

7. Health.mil (2016). US Armed Forces medical examiner system. Online article. http://www.health.mil/afmes

8. Capstone Document: Mass fatality management for incidents involving weapons of mass destruction (2005). http://www.ecbc.army.mil/hld/dl/MFM_

9. United States Department of Health & Human Services (2015). Fatality management, federal perspective. https://asprtracie.hhs.gov/documents/Fatality-Mgt-Federal-Perspectives.pdf

10. Regional mass fatality management response system, and regional catastrophic preparedness team (2015). http://www.regionalcatplanning.org/plans_mfm.shtml

11. New York Daily News (Friday, September 9, 2016). "This has defined my career": New York medical examiners still working to identify more than 1,000 World Trade Centre victims, 17 years later. https://www.independent.co.uk/news/world/americas/9-11-victims-remains-identify-office-of-chief-medical-examiner-new-york-a8532921.html

Prehospital Care in the Disaster Setting

Chapter 30

Dan Hanfling

Introduction

The delivery of health and medical services occurs across a continuum, which includes prehospital, ambulatory based, facility-based, and rehabilitative care. When a disaster event occurs, disruption to any one of these integrated levels of care can have tremendous impact on the ability to meet fundamental health and medical needs of the affected community. When considering the effects of a "catastrophic disaster," defined by Quarantelli to have key characteristics including the loss of governance, the loss of mutual aid, and the loss of key municipal services[1], it can be assumed that the prehospital phase of health-care services will barely be functioning, if at all. Furthermore, it is under these conditions that national capacities in the health-care delivery sector are anticipated to be overwhelmed, thus requiring the support of the international medical and humanitarian response community.

The intent of this chapter is to explore the types of prehospital care that can be expected to be provided under catastrophic disaster conditions. The chapter will review the role of the International Red Cross and Red Crescent Movement, particularly as it relates to the delivery of emergency medical services (EMS). It will explore the role of type I emergency medical team (EMT), defined by WHO as those teams capable of providing initial, stabilizing emergency care in the outpatient environment[2,3] in response to the health and medical needs of an acute phase response (Box 3). In addition, the chapter will highlight the complementary role that the urban search and rescue (USAR) response system provides with regards to both the focused delivery of stabilizing emergency care to rescued victims, as well as the fundamentally important public health support role that medical staff is available to provide in the acute phase of a disaster response.

Models of Prehospital Health-Care Service Delivery

It is important to understand the existing models of prehospital services that are likely to be encountered in the host country, recognizing that, in many cases, the prevailing system may represent a hybrid or combination of multiple approaches. It is important also to note that the degree of prehospital service capability will likely vary depending on the existing social and economic constructs of the host county. High- and middle-income countries are more likely to have functioning prehospital care systems, whereas in the case of low-income countries, prehospital services may be entirely un-resourced and essentially nonfunctioning.

There are two models of prehospital care that are largely recognized, and often emulated, based on sociopolitical, historical, and geographic precedents. In the case of low-middle and low-income countries, these precedents may be less important given the absence of resources that inhibits the ability to develop such capabilities. The Franco-German model of care emphasizes the utilization of ambulance-based physicians who provide care to patients directly in the field, thus limiting the number of patients transferred for evaluation to the hospital emergency department[4]. This emphasizes a "stay, play, and stabilize" approach, which intends to bring a level of sophisticated hospital services to the patient. The attending emergency physician, who deploys along with paramedical assistance, is authorized to make complex and difficult decisions in the field setting, as well as to conduct an advanced array of physician-level services, which may include intubation, central-line placement, diagnostic evaluation with portable ultrasound, and other advanced techniques. With respect to the disaster response teams that deploy to support field medical operations, this model is similar to the approach taken by the medical

---

Box 3

Type 1 Fixed EMT
Provide outpatient initial emergency care of injuries and other significant health-care needs. Teams must be capable of treating at least 100 outpatients per day and function during daytime. Key services include triage, first aid, patient stabilization, referral of severe trauma, nontrauma emergencies, and care for minor trauma injuries. These teams can work from suitable existing structures or supply their own fixed or mobile outpatient facilities, such as tents or special equipped vehicles.

Type 1 Mobile EMT
Provide outpatient initial emergency care of injuries and other significant health-care needs. Teams must be capable of treating at least 50 outpatients per day and function during the daytime. Key services include triage, first aid, patient stabilization, referral of severe trauma, nontrauma emergencies, and care for minor trauma injuries. These teams do not work out of a fixed structure and the team, including all equipment, can be easily moved throughout the mission deployment.

---

component of USAR elements, but may also be used by the type 1 mobile EMTs. In the case of the USAR response, this is mostly due to the longevity and complexity of field-based rescue efforts, which require a component of medical support to the patient over a prolonged course of the rescue effort. It presupposes self-sufficiency and a high degree of clinical competence required to manage complex patients in a field setting prior to being able to get them to the more definitive field hospital for ongoing stabilization, definitive diagnosis, and therapeutic interventions, including surgery, if warranted.

In contrast, the Anglo-American model emphasizes a "scoop-and-run" approach, in which paramedics or emergency medical technicians are responsible for the initial stabilization of patients in the field, and they facilitate rapid patient transport to the emergency department, where definitive patient management can commence[5,6]. With regards to the dispatch of EMTs to support a host nation disaster response, this approach is exemplified by responding type 1 fixed EMTs. They are designated to establish prehospital services chiefly focused on providing initial stabilization and basic treatment, with referral to a type 2 or 3 fixed field hospital made for those patients requiring definitive interventions and ongoing care.

In addition to describing the approach to prehospital care, as noted above, it is also useful to place these efforts within the context of the Red Cross and Red Crescent Movement. The movement promotes the delivery of humanitarian assistance and medical care in the setting of armed conflict and large-scale emergencies, and has an important role in coordinating the delivery of health-care services under adherence to humanitarian principles and the rule of law. In that context, they help to promote the integration of emergency responders into an existing emergency response system "adapted to local needs and realities[7]." Thus, many prehospital transport units in the country affected by disaster will be marked by the Red Cross, Red Crescent, or Red Star of David (Magen David Adom) and are tightly linked to the existing national health-care system providing EMS.

Levels of Service in the Prehospital Environment

It is undisputed that, in the initial hours, and perhaps days, of a sudden-onset disaster (SOD) event, the vast majority of lives saved, including rescues made from collapsed structures, are those undertaken by citizen first responders[8,9,10]. Most victims of disaster who can provide assistance to fellow victims do so spontaneously and without specific training or background in medical or rescue experience. Given that prehospital services are likely disrupted in the initial phase of such an event, not to mention overwhelmed by the surge response required, the initial response in the field setting will be largely spontaneous, including the likely coalescence of field triage sites, which arise in areas of common purpose or buildings of opportunity (for example, a school gymnasium or a shopping center parking lot)[11,12]. There are a variety of disaster threat events that can disrupt prehospital services, including conventional, large-scale attack (e.g., sustained military action) and SOD due to natural (e.g., earthquake) or terrorist activity (e.g., including the use of unconventional weapons such as chemical or radiological contaminants). Regardless of the type of event, and despite variation in the social and cultural context in which such events occur, the role of the citizen first responder, often overlooked and underappreciated by the humanitarian response community, will be critical to saving lives and affecting an initial response to a disaster event.

When existing prehospital resources can mobilize in the initial response, they will do so within the context of the prehospital environment that exists in their region. The standard division of EMS is based on the level of training and experience, along with the availability of accompanying resources matched to the level of training of prehospital providers. This ranges from basic (basic life support) to advanced (advanced life support), although in areas with a sophisticated system of health-care service delivery, this may also include the delivery of ground- or rotor-wing-based critical-care services in the out-of-hospital setting. However, in many disaster events, particularly those in low-middle and low-income countries that have not had the opportunity to develop strong prehospital capabilities, the availability of resources may be limited to a van with a stretcher and a vehicle driver. Trained medical personnel, let alone the availability of medications or basic lifesaving medical supplies, may not be present.

Regardless of the model of service delivery in practice, the diligent and consistent application of field triage principles is paramount to the timely and effective utilization of prehospital services. Although beyond the scope of this chapter, suffice it to say that the triage process requires a consistent application of clinical and ethical considerations based both on physiological parameters and ethical decisions made in the context of the situation at hand (see Chapter 32 on medical ethics).

The Role of the Type 1 EMT

The type 1 EMT is a team that is primarily focused on the delivery of outpatient based medical services and interventions, concentrating on the delivery of healthcare services needed to address the initial emergent care of injuries, illnesses, and other time-dependent healthcare needs[2]. Basic services that are rendered include the delivery of first-aid care, initial patient assessments, and the triage and identification of patients who will require more advanced, definitive medical interventions. This includes the ability to provide stabilizing care to victims of disaster prior to their retriage and transport for additional medical, critical care, or surgical services. Type 1 teams need to be prepared to manage both trauma and nontraumatic medical emergencies, much like those capabilities inherent in

traditional prehospital and emergency-department service offerings. Therefore, these teams should be capable of providing definitive care and treatment to minor, less complex injuries or illnesses, with a good referral mechanism provided to patients who might need to seek additional care if circumstances of patient recovery are not straightforward, or injuries or illness develop in a time frame beyond the initial evaluation and management of patient needs. These teams are expected to be able to manage at least 100 patients per day, with services provided during daytime hours, and it is the expectation that they will be staffed and equipped to manage patients of all ages[2].

Type 1 EMTs can work from suitable existing structures, or supply their own fixed or mobile outpatient facilities, such as tents or special equipped vehicles. They should be available to arrive in the fastest possible time, ideally within 24–48 hours, and be considered light and portable. Their staff should be experienced in those elements of initial trauma care that relate to triage on a mass scale, wound and basic fracture management, and basic emergency care of pediatric, obstetric, mental health, and medical presentations[2].

Therefore, type 1 teams can be categorized as being either "fixed" or "mobile," depending on their configuration and ability to move locations. Some teams may have both capabilities simultaneously. In addition, the basic minimal requirements for these teams are focused on the provision of initial, stabilizing treatment and provision of basic medical and surgical care. The full array of expected minimal standards is described in Table 30.1.

The staffing requirements for a type 1 EMT include provision for at least three doctors trained in emergency and primary care, with the remainder of the team comprised of nurses, paramedics, and logistics and administrative support staff. The WHO classification calls for a doctor to nurse ratio of one doctor and three nurses[2]. Specific capabilities include knowledge and experience in the delivery of emergency and trauma care, maternal and child health, and working familiarity with the management of endemic diseases. It is fundamentally important that type 1 EMTs be able to recognize patients that exceed their capability or experience to be able to manage, and refer them to type 2 or 3 teams, if not to local health-care delivery assets, as soon as possible. This requires the capability to communicate in real time with those advanced medical assets, with plans for urgent transport of patients between facilities worked out ahead of time.

Table 30.1 Minimal requirements for type 1 EMT[2]

Initial assessment and triage	Initial and field triage
Resuscitation	Basic first aid and life support
Patient stabilization and referral	Basic stabilization and referral
Wound care	Initial wound care
Fracture management	Basic fracture management
Anesthesia	General anesthesia not provided
Surgery	Not provided
Intensive care	Not provided
Communicable disease care	Basic outpatient care
Emergency obstetric care	Basic emergency obstetric care
Emergency pediatric care	Basic outpatient chronic disease care for minor exacerbations
Rehabilitation	Outpatient or mobile services provided or referred
Laboratory and blood transfusion	Basic rapid detection test, no blood transfusion
Pharmacy and drug supply	Outpatient drug supply to treat for the foreign medical team's (FMT) declared capacity for two weeks, the WHO EML or equivalent tetanus prophylaxis
Radiology	No diagnostic imaging

The Role of the Medical Component of Urban Search-and-Rescue Teams

While the WHO EMT registration and classification system is overwhelmingly geared toward the development of a tiered approach to delivery of health and medical needs in a SOD, it is recognized that certain aspects of the international USAR response system also meet a number of the type 1 classification requirements. In fact, it is most common to have both search and rescue and EMTs deployed simultaneously to SOD events. Therefore, it is important to understand the basic capabilities and mission focus of deployed USAR teams, which serve in a complementary fashion to national and international type 1 EMT resources. However, although related by mission and capabilities, it is important to note that the medical component of a USAR team should not be mistaken for a type 1 EMT.

The medical components of USAR teams are primarily configured to manage the day-to-day health and medical requirements of the deployed team members, whose work is by its very nature dangerous and fraught with the potential for minor or more significant traumatic injury. Medical team staffing includes three doctors and at least six paramedics, although in fire-service-based team composition, there may be many more emergency medical technicians and paramedic trained providers serving in other disciplines

(i.e., search, rescue, administration) on the team. The medical team is geared to manage basic oversight of team deployment safe practices, including promotion of routine health-care activities and basic public-health measures such as appropriate hand hygiene, compliance with oral hydration and nutrition, and the provision of basic mental-health support, if required. In addition to having the basic medical supply and equipment to manage team-based issues or injuries, the USAR medical component is designated to provide initial stabilizing medical management of victims rescued in the field, including individuals entrapped in a collapsed environment. It is by this metric that the greatest distinction from type 1 EMTs must be drawn. Whereas the type 1 EMT is focused on providing basic emergency care to large numbers of patients, the focus of the medical component of USAR is much narrower, described better as "high capability, low capacity[15]."

Medical capabilities focused on patient management in the field setting include the medical care delivered to patients entrapped in debris or encumbered within a "void space" created by falling debris allowing a pocket of protection from further immediate injury. The delivery of care under such conditions is referred to as confined-space medicine, given the austere conditions under which such care is rendered. This often requires the evaluation, care, and management of trapped individuals over long periods of time,

293

and necessitates close coordination with other elements of the USAR team, including structural engineers, canine handlers, and rescue specialists. In the direst circumstances, field amputation or joint disarticulation may be required as a lifesaving measure when all other rescue options have been exhausted or the risk to the patient is too great to sustain prolonged extrication efforts[16]. Successful rescue should be followed immediately by a patient "hand off" to local EMS, if such capabilities exist, or to existing type 1, 2, or 3 EMTs. This necessitates close coordination and an established communications channel to ensure an appropriate "handoff" can be made without jeopardizing patient care. Often, USAR medical team members will augment the field transport of a patient to definitive care, particularly in the low-middle and low-income countries where the prehospital services are expected to be minimal, at best.

Other medical activities provided by the medical component of USAR include interactions that occur with patients encountered during the reconnaissance phase of USAR operations, when victims of disaster may actively seek medical attention. This may occur during the initial response phase of a SOD event, when the team first arrives in the disaster zone. Or it may be a function of having to respond to secondary events such as may occur with severe aftershocks in an earthquake response, or additional building collapse due to inherent instability. Whereas initial medical evaluation and very basic care may be offered, patients identified in this setting should ideally be referred for definitive management at available type 1, 2, or 3 EMTs, depending on the triage assessment and determined patient requirements.

Finally, there are recovery efforts that the USAR medical team will engage in, including providing assistance with the recovery of deceased victims in the collapsed environment. As the pace of rescues begins to wane in the days following a sudden-onset disaster, provision of input regarding the "time-to-rescue" discussion with local emergency management authorities becomes very important[17,18]. This is an opportunity to provide input into the decision to cease rescue operations and initiate the transition to a recovery operation, suggesting the likelihood of survivability in an entrapped environment is considered beyond possible due to chronological and physiological considerations.

At the request of local emergency management authorities, additional health-care activities and support of fundamental public health efforts may be requested. This includes undertaking assessments of existing health-care capabilities in the affected disaster zone, including evaluation of the structural integrity of key health-care institutions, and input on the viability of building reoccupancy (this is done in concert with USAR structural engineers). Medical team members may be asked to assist in the conduct of health needs assessments, including providing input regarding fundamental water and sanitation needs. Related focus on infectious-disease management and vector-borne diseases is also often requested. Finally, as the acute response phase transitions toward recovery, medical team leadership will play a role in facilitating donations of pharmaceuticals, medical supplies, and other equipment, which may be turned over to host nation health-care entities.

Summary and Future Trends

As the EMT initiative continues to proliferate and draw in additional supporters and participants, it is important to consider what future trends are likely to develop. There are a few considerations to contemplate in this regard. Firstly, future global needs for EMTs must consider not just the development of international capacities that may be required but perhaps more importantly support for the national capacities on which international response will be based. In other words, a strong national capacity to be able to manage medical and health crises suggests a lower likelihood for the need for external resources. Because the "burden of disease" in SODs is clearly a time-dependent phenomenon, the ability to mount a rapid response is critically important[19].

With regards to type 1 teams, it is important to emphasize the need to proliferate and broaden availability and accessibility to national-based mobile or fixed type 1 assets. This is based on the premise that every country requires rapid-response mechanisms which are already in place to respond to a domestic emergency. In keeping with this philosophy, countries that are planning on offering bilateral assistance are likely to want to concentrate their efforts on the development of more type 2 and 3 teams, assuming that type 1 teams become prioritized for national capacity building. Of course, there is still going to be the need to support the full array of health and medical response requirements, but with regards to future planning, this underlying premise should be given weighted consideration.

Another key issue for future planning relates to the long-term consequences of EMT interactions with the communities that they serve. There is a delicate balance that must be established between meeting the acute resource needs of a community after disaster impact, and simultaneously setting in motion the appropriate steps that lead to successful recovery. The long-term vibrancy of a community will only be assured with adequate attention to this transition. EMTs that have been selected to serve in remote, significantly impacted communities have an extraordinary opportunity to contribute to both the acute and the long-term needs of the local community. While EMT personnel provide a valuable service during the short-term recovery phase following a disaster, it is important to remember that they will not remain in the communities they are serving forever. In addition, responding agencies must remember that many communities will have providers who are not able to practice due to shortages in supplies and/or physical disruption to their facilities. This is particularly true of outpatient-based practitioners, for whom the type 1 teams may be providing temporary support. Such disasters are likely to impact the personal and economic viability of these same practitioners. Therefore, whenever possible, type 1 EMTs should work to integrate local health and medical providers into their operations as early as possible and in a sustained fashion. This attention to local integration ensures the provided assistance is not a short-term reaction but a long-term commitment. In addition, there is the potential for capacity building as EMTs work with local providers in an instructional manner.

Finally, with regards to the coordination of responsibilities between EMTs and the medical component of USAR, it is worth exploring how USAR medical team members might be able to further contribute to the ongoing health and medical activities needed to support the host nation, particularly as rescue operations come to a halt and the transition toward recovery begins. This might include having USAR medical personnel take on support responsibilities with the Emergency Medical Team Coordination Cell (EMTCC), and suggests the need for further education and training to support this and other humanitarian response-oriented activities.

References

1. Quarantelli EL (2000). Emergencies, disasters and catastrophes are different phenomena. Preliminary Paper #304, University of Delaware Disaster Research Center. http://udspace.udel.edu/bitstream/handle/197 16/674/PP304.pdf

2. Norton I, von Schreeb J, Aitken P, Herard P, Lajolo C. *Classification and minimum standards for foreign medical teams in sudden onset disasters.* Geneva: World Health Organization; 2013.

3. World Health Organization (2018). Humanitarian health action. Emergency medical teams. Online article. http://www.who.int/hac/techguidance/prepa redness/emergency_medical_teams/en

4. Dick, WF. Anglo-American vs. Franco-German emergency medical services system. *Prehospital and Disaster Medicine* 2003: **18**(1): 29–35; discussion 35–7.

5. Sasser S, Varghese M, Kellermann A, Lormand J. Prehospital trauma care systems. World Health Organization; 2005.

6. Pan American Health Organization. Emergency medical services systems. Lessons learned from the United States of America for developing countries. Holtermann K (ed.) Washington DC: PAHO HQ Library Cataloguing-in-publication; 2003.

7. International Committee of the Red Cross (2013). Ambulance and pre-hospital services in risk situations. Website. https://www.icrc.org/en/publication/4173-a mbulance-and-pre-hospital-services-risk-situations

8. Crippen D. The World Trade Center attack. Similarities to the 1988 earthquake in Armenia: time to teach the public life supporting first aid? *Critical Care* 2001: **5**(6): 312–14.

9. Graham DA (August 28, 2017). Why ordinary citizens are acting as first responders in Houston. The Atlantic. https://www.theatlantic.com/politics/archive/2017/08/ ordinary-citizens-are-first-responders/538233

10. Nicogossian AN, Metscher K, Zimmerman T, Hanfling D, Wise R. Community training in bioterror response. *Journal of Homeland Security and Emergency Management* 2007: **4**(3).

11. Hrdina CM, Coleman CN, Bogucki S, et al. The 'RTR' medical response system for nuclear and radiological mass casualty incidents: a function triage-treatment-transport medical response model. *Prehospital and Disaster Medicine* 2009: **24**(3): 167–78.

12. Cantrill SV, Pons PT, Bonnett CJ, Eisert S Moore S. Disaster alternate care facilities: selection and operation. 2009: AHRQ Publication No. 09–0062.

13. Barbera JA, Macintyre AG. Urban search and rescue. *Emergency Medicine Clinics of North America* 1996: **14**(2): 399–412.

14. Petinaux B, Macintyre AG, Barbera JA. Confined space medicine and the medical management of complex rescues: a case series. *Disaster Medicine and Public Health Preparedness.* 2014: **8**(1): 20–9.

15. INSARAG Medical Working Group. Defining USAR medicine and the role of USAR medical personnel. http://www.insarag.org/images/WG_Bali_2017/MWG/Attachment_C_Defining_USAR_medicine_INSARAG_MWG_Final_agreed.pdf

16. Macintyre AG, Kramer E, Petinaux B, Glass T, Tate CM. Extreme measures: field amputation on the living and dismemberment of the deceased to extricate individuals entrapped in collapsed structures. *Disaster Medicine and Public Health Preparedness* 2012: **6**(4): 428–35.

17. Macintyre AG, Barbera J, Petinaux B. Survival interval in earthquake entrapments: research findings reinforced during the 2010 Haiti earthquake response. *Disaster Medicine and Public Health Preparedness* 2011: **5**(1): 13–22.

18. Macintyre AG, Barbera J, Smith ER. Surviving collapsed structure entrapment after earthquakes: a "time-to-rescue" analysis. *Prehospital and Disaster Medicine* 2006: **21**(1): 4–17.

19. Von Schreeb J, Riddez L, Samnegård H, Rosling H. Foreign field hospitals in the recent sudden-onset disasters in Iran, Haiti, Indonesia and Pakistan, *Prehospital and Disaster Medicine* 2008: **23**(2): 144–51.

Long-term Deployment and Continuity of Care

Seema Biswas, Harald Veen, and Inga Osmers

Extending Deployments

Emergency humanitarian assistance and long-term deployment would, at first glance, appear to be contradictory concepts in emergency medical response. However, in armed conflict and/or in low-income countries, extending the provision of emergency care into the long term may become an unavoidable necessity and logical consequence of the context. Poverty, inequality, and a lack of functioning political structures typically result in inadequate health infrastructure, poor health indices, and a lack of public and social services[1,2]. This may lead to political instability, conflict, the further destruction of health and social infrastructure, halted or reversed economic development [3], inadequate disaster preparedness, and poor disaster response – completing the vicious circle of the underprivileged. Quoting Didier Cherpitel, as head of the Federation of the Red Cross and Crescent Societies: "Disaster seeks out the poor and ensure they stay poor [4]." Long-term deployments, therefore, are not simply a protracted response to a single emergency, but must serve to build capacity in environments with long-standing deficiencies in health provision or where existing health structures have been decimated by war or disaster. Thus, depending on the context, deployments may substitute or support existing institutions initially, but as far as possible, and as the deployment progresses, long-term deployments should support local health-care services and assist the development of local expertise. Working relationships with local partners and existing ministries of health take on an enduring importance.

Chronic Emergencies

While disaster is usually characterized by a sudden onset and a slow, but constant recovery phase, armed conflict often has a protracted beginning, followed by a steady increase in medical need, which is paired with a progressive deterioration of infrastructure and

health care resources[5,6]. Medical teams embarking on mission in areas where there is armed conflict should be prepared for long-term deployment in a constantly changing environment. Equally, after disaster in low-income countries, medical needs are usually insufficiently met by local stakeholders, even when the acute phase is over. A field hospital deployed to help trauma patients after an earthquake will quickly become a care provider for patients with other emergencies, including patients in need of cesarean section, patients injured in road traffic crashes, and those presenting with acute abdominal conditions[7]. Field hospitals will also need to address the chronic health needs of populations to whom regular follow-up and medication is no longer accessible, with surgical centers taking on patients with complications of chronic medical conditions. Patients who received initial lifesaving surgery will require longer-term treatment plans for reconstructive surgery and rehabilitation. With time, the number of patients with disaster-related injuries will decrease while the nondisaster-related emergencies will increase.

The term "chronic emergency" was coined to reflect this and similar situations. As outlined in Office for the Coordination of Humanitarian Affairs' (OCHA) brief on slow-onset emergencies[8]:

There is a widespread recognition that the nature of humanitarian emergencies is changing. Although catastrophic, sudden-onset events like tropical storms, earthquakes and tsunamis will continue to happen, and will require rapid and well-coordinated humanitarian interventions, many more humanitarian crises emerge over time based on a combination of complex and interrelated circumstances. A slow-onset emergency is defined as one that does not emerge from a single, distinct event but one that emerges gradually over time, often based on a confluence of different events . . . Human suffering, when measured by the most agreed indicators such as acute malnutrition (wasting) or excess mortality is often higher in situations of chronic vulnerability than in situations in which there is a clear trigger for humanitarian action.

The Changing Emphasis of an Extended Mission

In chronic emergencies it becomes difficult for an emergency medical team (EMT) to define the time point at which to end the emergency mission. Once the decision has been made to extend the deployment beyond the acute phase, attention should turn to the training of local staff and other measures to increase sustainability, which may include the development of working partnerships with local health-care and rehabilitation providers, expanding the roles of local staff, and increasing the capacity of local health services through long-term investment in the development of health-care infrastructure. Emphasis, therefore, turns to long-term planning and development.

Nevertheless, long-term deployment must have defined goals and an end date. Handing over the delivery of health-care services should be built into the planning of long-term deployments from the outset. Positions initially covered by international staff should be increasingly handed over to trained local staff, in preparation for a smooth transition phase, which will eventually lead to the handover of the project. Knowledge and skills should be passed on, together with equipment and hospital infrastructure, to maintain the continuity of medical care after the international team leaves.

Even with the best planning and intent, successful transition and continuity of care may not be guaranteed. Electricity, water, and rent payments must be continued. The retention of medical, administrative, and maintenance staff will depend not simply on the regular payment of salaries at the same level but on working conditions and security. Although these aspects go well beyond the sphere of influence of intervening teams and their organizations, they should be taken into consideration when planning a long-term deployment.

Dilemmas in Long-Term Deployments

Medical teams on long-term deployments face difficult choices from the outset. According to context and needs, admission criteria may be exclusive or inclusive, but they need to be defined from the very beginning

because they determine the requirements for staff, equipment, and infrastructure. Although this is essential to the planning, running, and eventual withdrawal from a project, the exclusion of patients with particular conditions will spark ethical discussion within the team. Admission criteria may be difficult to adhere to. Limiting the admission criteria to disaster or war-wounded patients only is ethically and practically difficult to realize. Even the limitation of admissions to emergency cases only will eventually transform a field hospital into a district hospital, as disaster-related emergencies decrease and nondisaster-related emergencies increase over time. Limitations in primary care mean that the majority of patients seen are emergency and not elective cases[9].

Another pitfall to consider is the impact of a long-term humanitarian assistance program on local health-care providers. Health care is not free of charge in many low-income countries. International teams, providing free health care, may present prohibitive competition for local practitioners. While the negative effects of competition may become apparent only after the decision to withdraw from a program has been made, the potential for problems should be mitigated from the very beginning of deployment.

In 2009, the International Committee of the Red Cross (ICRC) set up an independent hospital in Peshawar, Pakistan, close to the border of Afghanistan. Before the program was started, an agreement was signed with the authorities in Pakistan that only wounded from inside Afghanistan be treated so there would be no competition with local health-care providers. As always, treatment provided in the ICRC hospital was free of charge.

Case Study: Médecins Sans Frontières (MSF) Long-Term Deployment in Haiti in Response to the 2010 Earthquake

MSF provided emergency medical assistance after the 2010 earthquake in Haiti. Multiple immediate and long-term population health needs were targeted with a number of different projects serving different medical needs (e.g., trauma, maternity, and primary health care). The main focus was on trauma. During the peak of the emergency intervention, MSF was running 14 operation rooms in 9 surgical centers. Haiti was already in a state of serious health-care crisis prior to the disaster and had no resilience in response to the earthquake. Given the context (a chronic emergency) all MSF emergency interventions were started with the anticipated option to transform them into long-term projects. Having an entire network of MSF surgical centers enabled the establishment of specialized units for the treatment of obstetrics, burns and orthopedics.

One MSF hospital with surgical, obstetric, and orthopedic services was located in Léogâne, close to the epicenter of the earthquake. After a successful emergency intervention that was transformed into a long-term project, MSF made the decision to withdraw in 2015. During these five years, the hospital had admitted 45 400 patients, performed 17 000 surgical interventions and assisted 25 000 deliveries. The hospital provided services in primary health care, surgery, gynecology, pediatrics, neonatology, and mental health. By 2015, the hospital was known and frequented well beyond the city of Léogâne and its surrounding area. National and international staff provided a free and reliable service to patients on a 24-hours-a-day, 7-days-a-week basis without supply ruptures or other noticeable shortcomings. The hospital was filling a significant health-care gap. Closing the project would have left the population of Léogâne without adequate health care. To maintain the service, MSF was looking for possible partners to continue health-care provision. It was difficult to find an organization that was able and willing to take over a hospital of this size. The administrative and financial obligations of such a project are significant and exceeded the capacity of many local organizations, private and public.

Prior to the planned handover, MSF learned that a local orthopedic surgeon had run a private practice in the area before the earthquake. With MSF providing a free orthopedic service, the local surgeon would have clearly faced a tough competitor. Although a single orthopedic surgeon with a private practice could have never cared for the number of patients MSF has taken care of, this example should highlight possible conflicts and underline the clear message of actively searching for possible local health partners from the very beginning of any emergency project.

The ICRC Experience

In addition to short-term programs in response to emergencies, there have been long-term ICRC deployments, lasting up to five years, albeit with a smaller range of specialties. The assortment of deployments illustrates the flexibility in planning necessary to respond effectively to local needs, share

responsibility, and build capacity. Some of these hospital projects entailed the deployment of medical and surgical teams; some were purely surgical.

The ICRC has temporarily moved away from the substitution model, as described in Chapter 2, and focused increasingly on clinical support and training, including on-the-job bedside training and theoretical seminars such as the emergency-room training course for acute trauma care, the war surgery seminar, university teaching modules, accredited online training courses, workshops in hospital management, biomedical engineering, and the management of relief operations.

It may be argued that there are only three justifiable situations for the establishment of an independent ICRC hospital today:

1. Protection of the ICRC medical mission and access of patients to adequate health care.
2. A complete lack of local human resources.
3. No other acceptable alternative in service provision due to a total lack of acceptable local partners.

Through these adaptations the ICRC has been able to maintain hospital services particularly important in long-term deployments:

1. Develop and maintain a recognized level of competency in specific fields: surgery, hospital administration, and the overall management of war wounded patients.
2. Deliver care in favor of a target population that is easily identified and accepted as of prime concern to the ICRC: the casualties of war – the wounded and sick.
3. Diversify programs – upstream and downstream – in favor of this target population (prehospital care, amputation stump-revision surgery in conjunction with ICRC prosthetic workshops).
4. Diversify programs – with greater specialization – in favor of this target population: training for maxillofacial reconstructive surgery, vascular surgery, neurotraumatology, vesico-vaginal fistula repair programs.
5. Increase local capacity based on the recognized ICRC competencies: seminars in war surgery and hospital management and systems analysis for hospital finance and administration. Improve prehospital care.
6. Accept the ultimate lesson: there is no single model that fits all situations where the ICRC is called on to intervene.

Pitfalls: Scenario

The context is an ongoing surgical mission in a country neighboring a war zone. Civil war across the border has continued for years. There is no real health-care program in the country, aside from a couple of government military hospitals struggling to cope with casualties among the military corps. The treatment of casualties from opposing forces is ad hoc. There are no organized health-care facilities for the opposition. Nor is there health-care provision for the civilian population, repeatedly displaced, suffering years of famine, setbacks in farming and agriculture, without work or education, and with no prospect of an end to hostilities in sight.

A hospital substitution program was set up close to the border. Initially launched with generous admission criteria for adults and children of a large displaced population, there were problems in the host country from the outset. These problems entailed import delays of equipment, renegotiations around the memorandum of understanding for the project, rental of the land on which the hospital was located, and the licenses required for expatriate staff to practice.

Within the first weeks that the hospital was set up and treating patients, security threats were received, and the program had to close down. Only at this stage did it become clear to the humanitarian organization running the hospital that they were not welcome. The generous admission criteria at the hospital were perceived by local medical colleagues as a threat to their practice as financial competition. Patients fleeing the conflict and able to pay for medical treatment were expected by local clinicians to boost their practice revenues.

These delays and difficult negotiations at the beginning were not interpreted correctly by the humanitarian organization, and, ultimately, the message was delivered and understood in terms of security threats. This is not a rare scenario.

Working toward Successful Outcomes

We have much to learn from a wealth of organizations that have carried out successful long-term missions overseas[10] (Table 31.1).

As we learn best from our mistakes, the following account sets out the pitfalls we must avoid and principles we should adhere to when planning and implementing missions that produce the best and most sustainable long-term projects.

In 2010, Welling summarized the main mistakes in overseas missions as the "seven sins of humanitarian medicine[11]:"

1. leaving a mess behind
2. failing to match technology to local needs and abilities
3. failure of NGOs to cooperate
4. failing to have a follow-up plan
5. allowing politics, training, or other distracting goals to trump service, while representing the mission as "service"
6. going where we are not wanted or needed/being poor guests
7. doing the right thing for the wrong reason

Using these "seven sins", let us follow the process chronologically, and recognize the pitfalls at each stage.

Extending the Emergency Response to Disaster or Conflict

Before embarking on a long-term plan for assistance, a reliable assessment of continuing needs and the recovery or establishment of functioning local services must be performed. The assistance program needs to be based on health needs that are not already covered and encourage local health partners to strengthen their provision of services.

Continuing an emergency deployment is not possible without the approval of the hosting country and not feasible without the acceptance of the local community, already familiar with the successes and failures of the initial emergency response. The local ministry of health (MoH) remains in charge (this is often forgotten by NGOs). It is the MoH that is the best coordinating body, knowing the local capacities, needs, and priorities in the development of lasting health services for the future.

Running a Long-Term Program

As discussed above, the nature of medical assistance required changes over time. The nature of the mission itself also changes, however. Large contingencies of expatriate staff are increasingly conspicuous in local communities. Large missions occupy space, property, and influence small local economies[12]. The effects are not always beneficial. Organizations require staff to adhere to codes of conduct that include appropriate interaction with members of the local community.

Table 31.1 Recommendations for long-term educational programs adapted from the survey of nongovernmental organizations (NGOs) providing pediatric and congenital cardiac surgery educational training programs[10]

Preparation	• ensure the possibility of maintaining real-time communications with headquarters when in the field • be certain that there is local interest among partners for obtaining assistance • identify specific needs and priorities • establish that there is a real desire among all stakeholders and donors to develop a long-term program
Site selection	• identify important demographic characteristics of the local and regional population • ensure means for air and ground transport, secure access for patients, means for the transfer of patients • choose a site in a region with political stability and security • ensure adequate patient referral and access • ensure structural soundness, building, repair, and maintenance of the site for the hospital program • ensure access to essential infrastructure (water, sanitation, electricity) • ensure protection from hazards: flooding, earthquakes • avoid proximity to active military conflict while ensuring that vulnerable communities have access to care • explore prevailing cultural attitudes toward medical treatment, especially attitudes toward western medicine • check the proximity of already established and functioning health services
Medical work	• work with local staff • carefully triage and select cases for surgery; accept that not every patient can be treated and that not every patient will experience an ideal outcome • establish a rapport with local staff and community so that there is an understanding of the challenges of treating advanced disease and complications • ensure that the patients understand the purpose of the field hospital and the mission/goals of the hospital • ensure that patients are well consented for surgery, speaking, if necessary, to family members and local community leaders • monitor, record, and evaluate surgical outcomes and evaluate the program continuously • ensure that the case mix adheres to mission goals, but be prepared to adjust the program to local needs and program evaluation in liaison with headquarters • train local staff at every opportunity (hands-on training is always the most effective means to learn skills) • work to maintain standards; rotating and recruiting staff when appropriate • choose the right operation for the right patient at the right time
Continuing deployment	• maintain a steady source of funding • ensure a steady supply stream • readjust the goals of the program as appropriate • assist rather than undermine the recovery or development of local health services • adapt training methods as local capabilities change
Leaving	• plan well in advance an exit strategy that does not, as far as organizationally possible, leave the local population compromised in terms of health and protection • liaise with local and national government on handing over and continuing support

Aid organizations not only offer free medical treatment, which may be perceived by patients as superior to local alternatives, local staff working long term with these organizations may earn higher salaries, receive more training, and enjoy more work-related benefits in terms of health care, leave, and pensions. Local businesses find it hard to compete with well-funded aid organizations.

Managing Human Resources and Personnel

As in all working environments, fresh busy teams actively engaged in meaningful work from which immediate outcomes are readily perceptible are always the most efficient, harmonious, and successful in terms of outcomes for the patients. Guarding against fatigue, periods of inactivity, and monitoring and evaluating outcomes are essential to running successful long-term deployments. Dealing with negative outcomes quickly and within a culture that is supportive, educational, and focused on patient benefit is also essential. An inclusive surgical hierarchy, regular rest and recuperation periods, and a built-in empathetic culture that factors real-time experience of team members into program planning is essential. An understanding administrative hierarchy is also essential: leave, clinical rotation, professional development, and job-planning are increasingly embraced by human resources departments of large organizations to facilitate the retention of high-quality staff deployed on long missions to austere environments.

Handing Over at the End of Long-term Deployments

Handing over a project is a real phase that should be planned and implemented as early as possible. Crucial to the process of handover is the engagement of local staff. There are different options for the employment of staff. A long-term project planned to be handed over should be run mostly with local staff (category 3 and 4 as listed below). A situation in which patients are handed over from doctor to doctor and nurse to nurse should be avoided.

MSF employs the following criteria for the staffing of long-term projects:

1. Expatriate staff flying in and out for their mission
2. Local staff on the MSF payroll
3. Local staff on MoH payroll, receiving incentives from MSF when dealing with MSF patients
4. MoH staff

Special Considerations in Conflict: Handing Over Data

Although conflict and disaster have very similar challenges, a few aspects should be highlighted that are of special consideration when providing aid in a war zone. As a principle, the ICRC and MSF always try to stay in contact with all sides of the conflict. However, the authorities in an area might change and stable structures, such as MoHs, are not always present. When handing over a project to the authorities, overseas organizations should also ask themselves whether handing over sensitive patient data is safe, especially in a situation where tensions remain between factions in the country and various stakeholders.

Special Considerations in Conflict: Staying On

The mandate of individual organizations directs the opportunities for humanitarian intervention. NGOs have freedom, so long as they are transparent to their donors, to follow their own organization's mission. The ICRC, through its mandate to assist all victims of armed conflict and insist on the observance of international humanitarian law (IHL) in war, should have access to all sides in conflict, to assist all populations affected, with transparency and agreement of warring parties.

Unlike the tail-end of a disaster response scenario where local conditions improve over time, people recover their livelihoods and national infrastructure is repaired, in conflict, the local situation usually deteriorates over time, with increasing supply ruptures, further destruction of infrastructure, and fewer available and qualified local staff. Project planning for long-term deployments needs to compensate for these challenges often over long time periods. Added to the security challenge, which is increasingly the main determinant of access to and provision of health-care services[13,14], conflict deployments need to factor in mechanisms for continued care.

Providing aid to all sides of the conflict is also likely to raise tensions inside the health-care facility, both between patients from different sides of the conflict and between caregivers and patients from different ethnic or political backgrounds. Working through these issues requires experience and skill in project management from the outset.

Summary

The world's most fragile states contain 38% of the world's population and are among the world's poorest. In these states, up to 10% of all deaths and 20% of deaths among young adults may be attributed to untreated surgical disease[15,16]. International aid organizations have a notable presence in fragile states; the potential of these organizations to address disparities in access to surgical care through long-term deployments should be optimized. Priorities include acute trauma, surgical, and obstetric care. Every opportunity for training and support of local health-care staff is to be valued. The success of long-term deployments rests on sound planning before the implementation of programs and honest appraisal of ongoing programs. While effective disaster response may lead to recovery and re-establishment of local health services, deployments in conflict situations tend to last much longer and require careful consideration of the ongoing supply of equipment and employment of trained staff. Security threats in both conflict and disaster scenarios are a considerable impediment to the delivery of continued effective assistance to some of the world's poorest and vulnerable communities.

Take-Home Messages

- Correct planning of long-term deployments is crucial to the effectiveness of assistance programs.

- Programs of assistance should be appraised in real time and adjustments made to prioritize the delivery of care to patients most in need.
- Security threats are an unfortunate reality of deployments. These threats may prohibit the delivery of care and planning should incorporate mitigation strategies from the outset.
- Every effort should be made to train and support local health-care providers.
- Long-term deployments may serve as useful adjuncts for the recovery and development of local health-care services. This is to be encouraged.

References

1. Braithwaite A, Dasandil N, Hudson D. Does poverty cause conflict? Isolating the causal origins of the conflict trap. *Conflict Management and Peace Science* 2014: **33** (1): 45–66.

2. Miller M. Poverty as a cause of wars? *Interdisciplinary Science Reviews* 2013: **25**(4): 273–97.

3. Collier P, Hoeffler A. Resource rents, governance and conflict. *Journal of Conflict Resolution* 2016: **49**(4): 625–33.

4. International Federation of the Red Cross and Red Crescent Societies (2002). World disasters report 2002: focus on reducing risk. Website. http://www.ifrc.org/Global/Publications/disasters/WDR/32600-WDR2002.pdf

5. Hayari L, Shir On E, Fedorenko A, Szvalb S, Zidan J, Solomonov E. Complications of dysgerminoma: meeting the health needs of patients in conflict zones. *BMJ Case Reports* 2017.

6. Stewart F, C Huang, Wang M. War and underdevelopment, in *Internal wars in developing countries: an empirical overview of economic and social consequences.* Volume 1. Oxford: Oxford University Press; 2001.

7. Cartwright C, Hall M, Lee ACK. The changing health priorities of earthquake response and implications for preparedness: a scoping review. *Public Health* 2017: **150**: 60–70.

8. OCHA occasional policy briefing series brief No. 6: OCHA and slow-onset emergencies (2011). https://www.unocha.org/sites/unocha/files/OCHA%20and%20Slow%20Onset%20Emergencies.pdf

9. Kang P, Tang B, Liu Y, et al. Medical efforts and injury patterns of military hospital patients following the 2013 Lushan earthquake in China: a retrospective study. *International Journal of Environmental Research and Public Health* 2015: **12** 10723–38.

10. Corno AF. Paediatric and congenital cardiac surgery in emergency economies: surgical 'safari' versus educational programmes. *Interactive Cardiovascular and Thoracic Surgery* 2016: **23**: 163–7

11. Welling DR, Ryan JM, Burris DG, Rich NM. Seven sins of humanitarian medicine. *World Journal of Surgery* 2010: **34**(3): 466–70.

12. International Committee of the Red Cross. The impact of humanitarian aid on conflict development. Online article. https://www.icrc.org/eng/resources/documents/article/other/57jpcj.htm

13. Coupland R. Security of health care and global health. *The New England Journal of Medicine* 2013: **368**(12): 1075–6.

14. International Committee of the Red Cross (2011). Health care in danger: sixteen-country study. https://www.icrc.org/en/doc/resources/documents/report/hcid-report-2011-08-10.htm

15. Meo G, Andreone D, DeBonis, Cometto G, et al. Rural surgery in southern Sudan. *World Journal of Surgery* 2006: **30**: 495–504.

16. King M, Bewes P, Cairns J, Thornton J. Background to surgery, in *Primary surgery*. Volume 1. Oxford: Oxford University Press; 2003.

17. Gosselin RA, Gyamfi YA, Contini S. Challenges of meeting surgical needs in the developing world. *World Journal of Surgery* 2011: **35**: 258–61.

Ethical Dilemmas in Field Hospital Deployments

Ofer Merin, Avraham Steinberg, and Dan Hanfling

Introduction

A field hospital can be deployed under different scenarios including response to natural disasters (e.g., earthquakes, typhoons), infectious disease outbreak, war/conflict zones, and in support of health and medical needs of developing nations. Each circumstance brings with it a set of different and unique ethical challenges.

The ethical framework that governs the deployment of these resources under these various settings will require a variety of different considerations. These range from the macro-level of organizational support (budget allocation, personnel recruitment, supply, equipment acquisition and maintenance, travel, and so on) to the micro-level (how health care will be provided to patients at the bedside)[1].

Ethical codes and expectations in disaster response are well described in the literature, and are considered a part of the expected practice of medicine under such conditions. The large international organizations – World Medical Association [2], International Committee of the Red Cross (ICRC) and Red Crescent[1,3], American Medical Association[4] – all have documents relating to ethical codes in disasters.

Commonalities across these ethical "position statements" that relate to the expectations of victims of disaster can be found centered on the importance of distributive justice. These include the following: transparency in decision-making and consistency in the application of decisions, especially as it relates to triage decisions and the access to care; accountability of decision makers; and the notion that access to health care ought to be considered a "human right." Conventional medical ethical tenets highlighted earlier in this chapter may not always apply in the context of disasters, and they may present certain tensions. For example, can patient autonomy be maintained when there is a need to share information for the public good? Can an individual patient's medical

needs be met, when the decision to support one may adversely impact the ability to support many?

Tenets of medical ethics including the Hippocratic oath, Geneva conventions (GCs), and human research protections may have within them certain inconsistencies when examined in the context of managing large numbers of victims of disaster events. For example, in the Hippocratic oath, and the Geneva Declarations that are its modern equivalent, the centrality of a health-care provider's adherence to ethical principles is highlighted. After so many examples of horrors perpetrated under genocidal regimes (Nazi Germany, Cambodia, and Rwanda) to victims of war in the twentieth century, it was clear that a renewed focus on the centrality of ethics in the context of managing victims of disaster was required. Yet, under the duress of a disaster response, regardless of whether this is due to a natural event or an industrial accident, is it possible to achieve ethical clarity? How will the rights of the individual and principles of autonomy be balanced against the decisions taken that may result in more widespread benefit to society? In the allocation of scarce resources, are certain population groups to be promoted for access to such resources over others? Is the refusal to provide care – for example, to terrorist perpetrators of acts of mass violence – permissible? What about the withdrawal of care? Or the withholding of information from patients, their families, and the public at large?

A common framework used in the analysis of medical ethics is the "four principles" approach postulated by the philosophers Tom Beauchamp and Jim Childress[5]. It recognizes four basic moral principles, which are to be judged and weighed against each other, with attention given to the scope of their application. The four principles are:

1. Respect for autonomy: Acknowledge a person's right to make choices, to hold views, and to take actions based on personal values and beliefs. The patient has the right to refuse or choose his or her treatment.

2. Justice: Treat others equitably, distribute benefits/burdens fairly. Concerns the distribution of scarce health resources, and the decision of who gets what treatment (fairness and equality).
3. Nonmaleficence: Obligation not to inflict harm intentionally: "First, do no harm" (primum non nocere).
4. Beneficence (do good): Provide benefits to persons and contribute to their welfare. Refers to an action done for the benefit of others. A practitioner should act in the best interest of the patient.

The need to establish international standards to protect the dignity of disaster victims has been raised in the international community. One of the commonly used approaches developed for and by the international humanitarian assistance community are the "Sphere standards" contained in the Sphere handbook: Humanitarian charter and minimum standards in humanitarian response[6]. The Sphere standards are a set of minimum standards and guidelines based on human rights and developed to guide the aid and assistance community during humanitarian crisis. This project is a joint effort by the ICRC, Red Crescent, and NGOs. The Sphere principles are predicated on the notion that human actions and interactions should be based on a set of shared core values. In the context of humanitarian assistance to disaster areas, these include the importance of upholding certain ethical principles; chief among them accountability, transparency, and neutrality. One should acknowledge the fact that some of these values may conflict with each other. Humanitarian actors, therefore, might confront dilemmas which can lead to moral distress.

To alleviate some of these conflicts, adherence to a code of behavior and assurance of accountability are suggested strategies.

Code of Conduct

With the aim to establish common standards in disaster relief, the "code of conduct" for The International Red Cross and Red Crescent Movement and NGOs in Disaster Relief, was developed and agreed on by eight of the world's largest disaster response agencies in the summer of 1994[7]. This identifies the alleviation of human suffering as the prime motivation for humanitarian assistance, which must be provided on the basis of need alone and not as an instrument of government or foreign policy.

This code seeks to safeguard high standards of behavior and maintain independence and effectiveness

in disaster relief. It lays down ten points of principle, which all humanitarian actors should adhere to in their disaster response work, and goes on to describe the relationships that agencies working in disasters should seek with donor governments, host governments, and the UN system. The principles are as follows:

1. The humanitarian imperative comes first.
2. Aid is given regardless of the race, creed, or nationality of the recipients, and without adverse distinction of any kind. Aid priorities are calculated based on need alone.
3. Aid will not be used to further a particular political or religious standpoint.
4. Humanitarian responders should endeavor not to act as instruments of government foreign policy.
5. Humanitarian responders should respect culture and custom. (We suggest adding respect of religion as this might have direct impact on patient treatment.)
6. Humanitarian response agencies should attempt to build disaster response on local capacities.
7. Ways shall be found to involve program beneficiaries in the management of relief aid.
8. Relief aid must strive to reduce future vulnerabilities to disaster, as well as meeting basic needs.
9. Humanitarian organizations should hold themselves accountable to both those we seek to assist and those from whom we accept resources.
10. In our information, publicity, and advertising activities, humanitarian organizations shall recognize disaster victims as dignified human beings; not hopeless objects.

Accountability

Accountability of disaster responders is part of the ethical framework they are obligated to follow. When responding to a disaster, providers must follow international standards and protect the dignity of the victims. Examples of this include consent for treatment, proper documentation for continuity of treatment, and feedback from the beneficiaries.

The number of foreign field hospitals (FFHs) and international medical teams mobilized in SODs has increased. While they have been beneficial in many situations, they have also been frequently questioned regarding their timeliness, self-sufficiency, ability to adapt to the local system, or even the quality of service provided[8].

Much has been written about the international response to the Haiti 2010 earthquake. In that case, personnel and equipment that were mobilized and utilized in the response were not necessarily matched to the true needs[9,10,11].

Recognition of these issues gave rise to an initiative in creation of the Foreign Medical Teams (FMT) Working Group, and now referred to as the Emergency Medical Teams (EMT) initiative, under the auspices of the global health cluster (GHC) and the World Health Organization (WHO). They commissioned a document, *Classification and Minimum Standards for Foreign Medical Teams in Sudden Onset Disasters*, which provides trauma and surgical care in the first month following a sudden-onset disaster (SOD)[12].

To promote accountability, teams should follow well-established international standards, such as those of WHO. Other important codes that teams are urged to follow are those set by the Core Humanitarian Standard on Quality and Accountability. This is an initiative in which the Humanitarian Accountability Partnership International, People In Aid, and the Sphere project joined forces to seek greater coherence for users of humanitarian standards[13].

Ethics in the Predisaster Phase

Developing a preventive ethics approach in the pre-disaster phase helps to reduce conflicts during the disaster phase.

One reality is clear. Communities that have not planned and prepared for such an eventuality will be less well-equipped to face its complexities than communities that have. The noted political scientist, Richard Neustadt, wrote, "Crises are a bad time to do planning. Only if plans are developed in advance, and then critiqued, rehearsed, and refined, will various agencies and actors be able to respond effectively to a disaster[14]."

Development of clinical practice guidelines in the predisaster phase and use of guidelines-based criteria in health resource allocation in the response phase may minimize potential ethical conflicts that arise during decision-making in disasters.

Once disaster strikes, teams preparing to deploy must take some practical decisions, which will have a direct impact on the ethical dilemmas they will encounter: notably the type of medical equipment and types of personnel, and numbers of responders,

that will deploy. These decisions will significantly influence the type and level of care that can be delivered. An example of an ethical dilemma an EMT might confront is treatment of preterm labor. If a team has both the right personnel and equipment to treat such cases, the ethical dilemma that will arise in the context of a deployment will center around the many resources that would be required to manage a single patient. Deciding beforehand not to take part in the treatment of neonates, for example, explicitly relieves the response team from having to encounter such a dilemma, although the urge and instinct to provide care, no matter how basic, will likely still exist.

We need to expect that planning will be imperfect. Unexpected events will occur, necessitating making on-the-spot ethical decisions during deployment. For this reason, it is important that ethical considerations are made explicit during the planning process so when ethical and clinical judgment is required in the field, it will be consistent with the spirit that guided the planning process.

Dilemmas During Deployment in Disaster Zones

Ethical issues are inherent in humanitarian action. Confronting a large number of patients in a disaster zone mandates adjusting medical care. Not all can be treated, and for those who will receive medical care the standard of care might need to be adjusted.

These two major dilemmas – resource allocation and standard of care – will be discussed from the ethical perspective.

Triage Ethics

Mass-casualty triage needs to be implemented when available resources are insufficient to meet the needs of all patients in a disaster situation. The basic principle is to do the maximum good for the most casualties with the least amount of resources. Disasters require physicians to shift to "utilitarian-based ethics" in which medical decisions are based on available resources, much in the way that a triage system prioritizes victims who are predicted to have the best chance of survival[15]. The World Medical Association (WMA) statement on medical ethics in disasters recognizes these unique situations and notes, "The physician must act according to the needs of patients and the resources available. He/she should attempt to set an order of priorities for treatment that will save the greatest number of lives and restrict morbidity to a minimum[2]." Such situations will inevitably lead to serious ethical dilemmas. Efforts will be needed to achieve a balance between individual and collective rights. There is generally a conflict between autonomy of the individual and the desire to protect and promote public health. This "dual loyalty" also exists in many disaster situations. It is necessary to develop a system that identifies patients by their medical/surgical needs and the likelihood of benefit, especially in the context of disaster response, but also during short-term initiatives.

Because of the complexity of triage in such conditions, the basic concept underlying the process should be decided before departure. In addition, the process must be fair, transparent, and meet the principles of distributive justice[16]. Triage can conflict with human rights legislation, and even with humanitarian laws, but "accountability for reasonableness" can temper the disagreements on the setting of priorities. Triage in a disaster setting, however, requires a basic change in thinking. Of necessity, this adjustment includes dealing with ethical dilemmas for which most medical personnel are not adequately prepared[17,18].

Two fundamental goals guide triage decisions:

1. Utilitarianism: To do the greater good for the most. One can argue whether the meaning of this principle is chiefly intended to maximize the number of lives saved, or the "life years" saved. If we measure the likelihood of years of life that would be saved, then an approach that favors the young may take precedence over providing care to the elderly. However, such an approach requires a discussion regarding what constitutes "old." Another approach would be to consider the quality of life saved and then prioritize treatment for patients who will have better life quality. In practical terms, this suggests that patients with nonreversible injuries (for example, spinal cord injuries) should not be prioritized in a setting of scarce resources. However, this may raise another moral difficulty specifically pertaining to those with chronic diseases: should we deprive such patients of lifesaving treatment under scarce resource conditions? At any given age, the healthy would be saved before the sick, since the former are expected to have a longer life expectancy. While it does sound reasonable to advocate for the preferential treatment of a young, otherwise healthy person as compared to an elderly patient with a terminal disease, this may open a Pandora's box

of ethical challenges: what are the boundaries to this? One cannot "computerize" the various factors: disability expected, quality of life expected, and life-years saved. These are distinctly "unknowable" outcomes, which are not easily determined. The imperfections of decision-making, even with the best intentions in mind, are likely to be exposed.

Balancing all these goals is nearly impossible. There is an inherent conflict between efforts intended to save the maximum number of patients as compared with the decisions required to save patients based on preserving the maximum quality of life. Therefore, the process will inevitably involve judgment and compromise.

In the setting of disaster response, more factors can be brought into this "equation" while trying to implement the utilitarianism principle. These factors include decisions taken to help prioritize patients. If age and prognosis are not used, should decisions simply be based on a first come, first served approach?

Moreover, if a patient, within limited resources, is triaged to treatment, but then along his or her treatment course he deteriorates, does the patient warrant reevaluation and reconsideration under existing triage criteria? Meaning, should one reconsider again and again who should get the limited resources at that point in time? Can a patient who was previously allotted for treatment lose this entitlement? Treating physicians are accustomed and culturally educated to give patients the best possible treatment once that treatment is initiated. The implication of retriage and potential withdrawal of care may be very hard for caregivers and families to accept. Teams must find a way, in a deteriorating patient who reaches a point of extremely limited survival chances, to consider withdrawal of treatment, aiming to save other patients.

Is it ethically permissible to withdraw care from one patient to provide that care to another patient who may be more likely to survive? This ethical dilemma is certainly a debatable issue: there are opinions that one can never hasten death of a person by an act, even if it is done to save someone else. For example, is it unacceptable to withdraw life-support measures from a dying patient with very poor prognosis to obtain his or her organs to save someone whose prognosis with the transplant might be much enhanced? Nevertheless, one can argue that, in the unique situation of two people in front of our eyes –

one with close to zero chances to survive even with the available – however limited – resources, and another one with much greater chances to survive provided he or she would receive the lifesaving measures given to the first one – it would be morally justified to do so.

The chapter authors' opinion is that, given the complexity of issues raised along religious, political, and ethical lines, such decisions must be contemplated by medical, legal, and ethics experts in the local community/host country.

2. **Egalitarianism:** Equality among patients. Again, the question is how to implement this: does it mean that elderly and young should be treated in a similar fashion? Does it mean that the chronically diseased or terminally ill should be treated like people with no medical issues? It is clear to all that we cannot discriminate on the base of gender, race, religion, economic status, and other social attributes. But it is less clear whether this prohibition rules out consideration of age or disability status. Some believe age may be considered only as it relates to underlying organ function and prognosis[19]. These philosophical questions arise when the medical benefits following survival are unequal, and some consideration of this question should guide medical prioritization.

Moral goals might contradict each other, and adherence to a strict policy may be impossible. Clear guidelines will be difficult to decide before arriving in a disaster zone, although the process by which they may be discussed and adjudicated should be put in place prior to arrival in the field setting.

Once deployed, triage guidelines should be set. These should be based on legitimate factors, relevant to the conditions, and as transparent as possible.

Resource allocation strategy needs structure and transparency, this is important both to the receiver and provider. The chapter authors' experience, from many deployments to large-scale disaster events, with responsibility for a large number of health, medical, and rescue providers, is that in disaster deployments not all caregivers are aware of the "big picture." Therefore, these dilemmas must be discussed and shared. Having a defined procedural process can improve the transparency, accountability, and quality of decisions. Dealing with ethical and triage issues while responding to the Haiti earthquake taught us how imperative it is to establish and strictly follow clear-cut guidelines[18].

Standard of Care

We should differentiate between medical decisions related to limited resources, and the issue of standard of care.

Are physicians allowed to give substandard care? If so: substandard related to what? To the standard of care in their home country, the standard of care in the receiving country, or the standard of care that is available at that point in time in the disaster setting?

Disasters do dictate changes. Reaching the point of surge of medical needs, a choice must be made: "Conventional" standard of care for some or an adjustment in the type and level of care provided to many? The ethical code of conduct suggests emphasis on the latter. Responders, seeking to assist more patients, will provide less intense care per patient than is standard in normal time. The term "crisis standard of care" is defined in this context as "substantial change in usual health care operations and the level of care it is possible to deliver, which is necessary . . . by a catastrophic disaster[20]." It was developed to help promote the notion that under catastrophic conditions, in which resources are significantly depleted or not available, the delivery of care will likely transition from a conventional standard to something significantly impacted by the lack of resources. Although it is often understood that the level of care is always going to be influenced by the availability of resources, one additional concept described within the transition to "crisis standards" is the recognition that care may have to be withdrawn from one patient in order to provide for another patient more likely to survive.

One might frame these standards in clear minimum standards as suggested by the Sphere project[6] and WHO[12].

The National Academies (US) Institute of Medicine acknowledges the need to establish guidelines in crisis, and issued three reports focused on this complex set of issues. The second of these documents is entitled: *Crisis standards of care: a system framework for catastrophic disaster response*[20]. It describes the full breadth of concepts around scarce resource allocation decision-making and highlights that crisis standard of care should be planned and implemented in accordance with ethical values, which are necessary for the allocation of scarce resources. "Health care professionals must adhere to ethical norms even in conditions of overwhelming scarcity that limit practitioner and patient choices. As a starting point for

Crisis standard of care planning deliberations, ethical values should include the concept of fairness, together with professional duties to care for patients and steward resources. The Crisis standard of care development process should be guided by key ethical values, including transparency, consistency, proportionality, and accountability."

The 2009 letter report of the Institute of Medicine states: "... in an important ethical sense, entering a crisis standard of care mode is not optional – it is a forced choice, based on the emerging situation. Under such circumstances, failing to make substantive adjustments to care operations – i.e., not to adopt crisis standards of care – is very likely to result in greater death, injury or illness[21]."

An argument countering the Institute of Medicine approach elucidating the need for establishing crisis standards of care noted that "altering the standard of care in disasters (would be) unnecessary and dangerous[22]." The authors of this paper acknowledge that creating algorithms to equitably and rationally allocate scarce resources is necessary and appropriate. But they raise concerns that adoption of a lower legal care standard would encourage implementation of less effective approaches and could undermine the impetus to constantly improve the care of disaster victims. They are worried that making the standard less rigorous in effect might permit physicians to be less accountable.

The chapter authors' experience is that, in disaster scenarios, standard of care must be adjusted, but altogether accountability can and must be kept.

The legitimacy of a change in the standard of care does raise the question whether there is any minimum to the quality of care that is provided. The strict answer, in our view, is yes: there are some universally minimum "rules" to be kept. Teams must set, in every operation, what are the standards that fit this specific event.

The question is, what is permissible, what is legitimate, and what is mandatory?

Mandatory: We believe that it is imperative that field-hospital providers keep human dignity and patients' rights at the forefront of all decision-making. Always get the patient's consent for treatment. According to the WMA: "The most appropriate treatment available should be administered with patient consent. However, it should be recognized that in disaster response there may not be enough time for informed consent to be realistic possibility

[2]." Our experience is that unless the patient is dimensionally incapacitated, even given the time constraints, some consent is always possible, and mandatory in our view. (Do not amputate, for example, without the full awareness of the patient about the long-term sequelae of such actions). Certain patients' rights should always be safeguarded.

Teams should acknowledge that in some cases there will be a need for immediate consent from the patient, but this is no different than how urgent cases in non-disaster areas are managed.

Legitimate: In our view, it is legitimate and expected to have to adapt the level of care based on the availability of resources and the demand for health-care services. Although it is difficult to set clear guidelines, some rules should apply: Teams should be obligated to deliver at least an equivalent level of care that is available at that time. An EMT should not, for example, operate under substandard conditions.

An example of this approach is exemplified by two missions conducted by the Israel Defense Forces (IDF) field hospital to earthquake-struck areas: Haiti (2010) and Nepal (2015). In both missions, the team confronted many orthopedic injuries. Unlike the situation after the 2010 earthquake in Haiti, which completely engulfed an already weak medical infrastructure that was barely functioning prior to the onset of the disaster, the medical system in Nepal, although overwhelmed, was still able to provide some degree of care. Under such circumstances, the chapter authors believe outside teams should be obligated to deliver at least an equivalent level of care. In Nepal, the local hospital that was adjacent to the placement of the IDF field hospital was equipped with fluoroscopy. Although this is a modality that was not immediately available in the tent-based field hospital, its availability in proximity meant that this should be the standard of care by which cases should be managed. In this case, EMTs should not operate in surgeries that mandate fluoroscopy without it, as its availability set the existing standard of care. In Haiti, the level of care that could be provided was much lower, given the absence of basic capabilities, such that a lower standard of care turned out to be acceptable. Another example the IDF confronted while operating in the Haiti disaster zone was that there were no ventilators available even in the conventional, nondisaster setting. Once the field hospital ventilators were all used, the team confronted uncertainty on how legitimate it is to ventilate patients for a prolonged period using just an ambu bag. This is considered a substandard approach in developed countries, but in some developing regions such an approach is the standard. Would it be considered acceptable to use such practices while providing humanitarian aid during disasters in these regions? A clear answer does not exist, but in our view if the alternative is no treatment, it is probably acceptable.

The second issue: even if "allowed" to deliver care under a lower standard, to what extent is it acceptable to compromise quality standards in a mass-casualty event?

Teams may confront, due to limited resources, issues they do not deal with in their routine care giving. Is it acceptable to declare "early" do-not-resuscitate decisions in patients who need many resources and have only a slight chance to survive? Can you stop ventilating a patient who has almost no chance of survival to ventilate someone else?

It seems difficult to have clear guidelines to every possibility, yet still some overarching rules must apply. The chapter authors believe one cannot stop treatment in one patient to allocate this resource to another, even if he or she has better chances. However, as mentioned earlier, this might be a debatable issue in some cultures.

Another issue to be contemplated has to do with an exploration of what constitutes the delivery of substandard care: is it acceptable for medical personnel to work beyond their abilities? For example, should clinicians be permitted to perform procedures for which they have limited experience and for which they are not qualified if they are the only personnel available?

The list is endless. While it is accepted that standards of care can and should be adjusted[20], teams still ought to have clear policies and standards.

The chapter authors' recommendations dealing with the difficult issues of the standard of care in the field setting are as follows:

1. It is acceptable to adjust the standard of care.
2. Some guidelines should be kept: transparency, consistency, proportionality, and accountability.
3. The level of care can be adapted while keeping the minimum, which is the level that is provided at that time in those circumstances. One cannot give standard of care below that.
4. As mentioned, in situations of crisis and urgency, some modifications may need to be taken while receiving informed consent. Still, human dignity cannot be compromised. The patient's autonomy rights should be maintained at all costs and whenever possible: the patient should be able to decide in an informed manner the treatments, among those possible, he or she will receive.

Operating in War Zones

The challenges to operating medical field hospitals in a conflict setting are particularly vexing. There are many issues at play; chief among them the struggle to balance the "duty to care" with the responsibility for saving oneself and one's colleagues from harm. Thus, the value of saving lives might conflict with personal security. In these cases, aid workers may choose to refrain from engaging in assisting needy patients[23].

The "humanitarian imperative," the ethical basis of most humanitarian organizations, declares that there is an obligation to provide assistance unconditionally, wherever and whenever it is needed.

The American Medical Association medical code states: "Individual physicians have an obligation to provide urgent medical care during disasters. This ethical obligation holds even in the face of greater than usual risks to their own safety, health or life [24]."

The ethical issues arising from operating in war zones while risking one's own safety and those dealing with treatment of enemies are beyond the scope of this chapter.

Similar considerations might arise while deploying to geographical regions requiring assistance in the context of an emerging infectious disease event, particularly those with highly transmissible disease entities. WHO, in a statement, acknowledges that the duty of health-care workers to work in the setting of health risks is not unlimited. They encourage governments to develop policies regarding professional obligations during epidemics[25].

Summary

Disasters are inevitable. Treatment decisions made under disaster conditions must reflect available resources. Confronting difficult ethical issues before deployment, such as triage decision-making issues, forces EMTs to set clear ethical/moral codes to be accountable to the care they are delivering. Human rights law operates during both peaceful and disaster times, and is founded on the principle that all humans are equal in dignity and must be treated equally.

Health-care providers operating in disaster zones must make decisions that are unique and different from those encountered in their routine health-care work environment. Examples include decisions such as not to treat patients, secondary to limited resources, who otherwise could be saved, or declaring a do-not-resuscitate status for a patient who might still have a slight chance of survival, again secondary to limited resources. These decisions can be justified for the benefit of the population but contradict individual rights.

Clinical practice is mainly concerned with individuals, while the focus of humanitarian aid is on populations. In the context of disasters with limited resources, there might be a conflict between individual rights and community benefit.

Teams operating in devastated zones should be aware that their health-care providers will become fully engaged with such dilemmas. Ethical issues should be identified, and individuals should be prepared to confront them.

Preparedness to deal with these will allow better medical care, higher ethical standards, and better accountability to patients. Awareness and identification of ethical issues will help health-care personnel to alleviate some of the burden of confrontation with these expected issues.

It is strongly recommended that organizations involved in humanitarian assistance set clear international standards such as those by Sphere and WHO, and train personnel to deal with these issues.

Debriefing after every deployment is a well-established method. Teams usually discuss key issues from the deployment experience. These include issues related to logistics challenges, medical interventions that were performed and the medical cases that were managed. But on top of that, the chapter authors believe it is essential to review the difficult cases in which the team confronted ethical issues. The process of decision-making made in these cases should be discussed. This may help build an ethical guidelines framework for future missions. The other key benefit of undertaking these debriefings is to help alleviate the difficult mental burden that is likely to weigh heavily on the minds of team members.

References

1. Clarinval C, Biller-Andorno N. Challenging operations: an ethical framework to assist humanitarian aid workers in their decision-making processes. *PLOS Currents* 2014: **23**: 6.

2. World Medical Association. Statement on medical ethics in the event of disasters adopted by the forty-sixth World Medical Association general assembly. https://www.wma.net/policies-post/wma-statement-on-medical-ethics-in-the-event-of-disasters/

3. International Federation of Red Cross and Red Crescent Societies (IFRC). Strategy. http://www.ifrc.org/Global/Publications/general/strategy-2020.pdf

4. American Medical Association. The AMA code of medical ethics. Online article. https://www.ama-assn.org/about-us/code-medical-ethics

5. Beauchamp TL, Childress JF. *Principles of Biomedical Ethics*. Fifth edn. Oxford: Oxford University Press; 2001

6. Sphere. Minimum standards in health action. https://spherestandards.org/wp-content/uploads/Sphere-Handbook-2018-EN.pdf

7. Code of conduct for the International Red Cross and Red Crescent Movement and non-governmental organizations (NGOs) in disaster relief. http://www.ifrc.org/en/publications-and-reports/code-of-conduct/

8. Proceedings of the WHO/PAHO technical consultation on international foreign medical teams (FMTs) post sudden onset disasters (SODs). http://reliefweb.int/sites/reliefweb.int/files/resources/Cuba%20Meeting%20Proceedings_FMT.pdf

9. Gerdin M, Wladis A, von Schreeb J. Foreign field hospitals after the 2010 Haiti earthquake: how good were we? *Emergency Medicine Journal* 2013: **30**(1).

10. Redmond AD, Mardel S, Taithe B, et al. A qualitative and quantitative study of the surgical and rehabilitation response to the earthquake in Haiti, January 2010. *Prehospital and Disaster Medicine* 2011: 449–56.

11. Van Hoving DJ, Wallis LA, Docrat F, De Vries S. Haiti disaster tourism – a medical shame. *Prehospital and Disaster Medicine* 2010: **25**(3): 201–2.

12. Norton I, von Schreeb J, Aitken P, Herard P, Lajolo C. *Classification and minimum standards for foreign medical teams in sudden onset disasters*. Geneva: World Health Organization; 2013.

13. Core humanitarian standard on quality and accountability. https://corehumanitarianstandard.org/files/files/Core%20Humanitarian%20Standard%20-%20English.pdf

14. Roberts M, DeRenzo EG. Chapter 2. Ethical considerations in community disaster planning, in Phillips SJ, Knebel A. eds. *Providing mass medical care with scarce resources: a community planning guide.* Prepared by Health Systems Research, Inc., under contract No. 290-04-0010. AHRQ Publication No. 07-0001. Rockville, MD; Agency for Healthcare Research and Quality: 2006: 9–23.

15. Pesik N, Keim ME, Iserson KV. Terrorism and the ethics of emergency medical care. *Annals of Emergency Medicine* 2001: 37(6): 642–6.

16. O'Laughlin DT, Hick JL. Ethical issues in resource triage. *Respiratory Care* 2008: 53: 190–7.

17. Society of Critical Care Medicine Ethics Committee. Consensus statement on the triage of critically ill patients. *JAMA* 1994: 271: 1200–03.

18. Merin O, Ash N, Levy G, Schwaber MJ, Kreiss Y. The Israeli field hospital in Haiti – ethical dilemmas in early disaster response. *The New England Journal of Medicine* 2010: 362: e38.

19. Phillips SJ, Knebel A (eds.) Mass medical care with scarce resources: a community planning guide. https://archive.ahrq.gov/research/mce/mceguide.pdf

20. Hanfling D, Altevogt BM, Viswanathan K, Gostin LO. *Crisis standards of care: a systems framework for catastrophic disaster response.* Washington, DC: Institute of Medicine; 2012. http://www.americanbar.org/content/dam/aba/events/health_law/2015_Meetings/DocLaw/Papers/01_crisis_stds_of_care_iom_01.authcheckdam.pdf

21. Altevogt BM, Stroud C, Hanson SL, et al. (eds.) (2009). Guidance for establishing crisis standards of care for use in disaster situations: a letter report. https://www.ncbi.nlm.nih.gov/books/NBK219954

22. Schultz CH, Annas GJ. Altering the standard of care in disasters – unnecessary and dangerous. *Annals of Emergency Medicine* 2012: 59(3): 191–5.

23. Iserson KV, Heine CE, Larkin GL, et al. Fight or flight: the ethics of emergency physician disaster response. *Annals of Emergency Medicine* 2008: 51(4): 345–53.

24. AMA code of medical ethics' opinion on physician duty to treat – physician obligation in disaster preparedness and response. https://journalofethics.ama-assn.org/article/ama-code-medical-ethics-opinion-physician-duty-treat/2010-06

25. World Health Organization. Ethical considerations in developing a public health response to pandemic influenza. http://www.who.int/csr/resources/publications/WHO_CDS_EPR_GIP_2007_2c.pdf

Legal Issues in Field Hospital Deployments

Chapter 33

Claire Clement

The deployment of field hospitals to meet the medical needs of the affected population is a common occurrence in the aftermath of many emergencies. Their use may give rise to a myriad of legal issues; from obtaining access to populations in need and protecting hospital staff and patients, to ensuring the suitability and standards of medical assistance provided. There is no single, comprehensive legal framework governing such matters. Instead, relevant rules, principles, and guidance may be found in a variety of national, regional, and international laws, as well as in nonbinding guidelines and standards (sometimes referred to as "soft law"). This chapter focuses primarily on the applicable international law, as well as on relevant soft-law instruments.[1] At present, relatively few of these sources address the use of field hospitals specifically. However, a number of laws and standards of a more general nature are relevant to the use of field hospitals, and should be taken into account by practitioners.

Legal considerations concerning the use of field hospitals will differ depending on whether the context of deployment is a situation of armed conflict, or that of natural or technological disaster.[2] Applicable standards may also depend on whether the field hospital and its associated personnel are military or civilian in nature, and whether the deployment is by a country's own health service and other national organizations responding to a domestic crisis, or alternatively by a foreign organization or foreign government assisting within the affected state. This chapter addresses, first, the relevant framework governing situations of armed conflict, and second, the rules and standards regulating the deployment of field hospitals in emergencies outside of armed conflict.

Use of Field Hospitals in Situations of Armed Conflict

Protection of Medical Units and Personnel

In situations of armed conflict, international rules concerning medical units, including field hospitals, are long established and well developed. Forming part of the body of law known as IHL,[3] such rules are primarily concerned with the protection of medical units from the effects of war. Medical units must be protected and respected in all[4] circumstances,[5] and only lose their protection if they are used to commit acts harmful to the enemy, outside of their humanitarian function.[6]

The rules of IHL also set out, in broad terms, the level of care owed to the sick and wounded in armed conflicts. In particular, they must be treated humanely, on the basis of medical need alone, and must receive the medical care required by their condition, to the fullest extent possible and with the least possible delay.[7] In treating the wounded and sick, medical personnel must not be compelled to carry out work that is contrary to the rules of medical ethics, and may not be punished for carrying out activities compatible with medical ethics.[8] Further, medical personnel may not be forced to share information about patients where this would be harmful to the patients or their families.[9]

Facilitation of Humanitarian Assistance

In addition to medical units belonging to or authorized by the parties to the conflict, field hospitals may be deployed in conflict situations as part of wider international humanitarian assistance efforts, including by the UN, international NGOs, governments, and other bodies. IHL contains a number of provisions regulating the delivery and control of humanitarian relief, which vary depending upon whether a territory is under occupation, is affected by an international armed conflict, or by a noninternational armed conflict.

In occupied territory, it is the primary responsibility of the state in control of the territory (also known as the occupying power) to ensure that the civilian population is adequately supplied and that its material needs are met.[10] Where unable to do so, it has the duty to

313

agree to relief schemes, which may include the provision of medical supplies.[11] Such assistance must be humanitarian in nature (that is, it must meet the sole aim of alleviating suffering) and must be provided without adverse distinction.[12] The occupying power must not hamper the delivery of assistance, but may implement necessary measures of control.

In international armed conflicts (those involving two or more states), parties to the conflict shall agree to assistance that is humanitarian and impartial in nature, where the needs of the civilian population are not met. While this obligation is qualified by the need to secure the consent of the affected state, such consent may only be withheld for valid reasons[1]. Starvation of the civilian population as a method of warfare is strictly prohibited.[13] Relief personnel may take part in assistance schemes subject to the approval of the controlling state, and must be respected and protected.[14]

The situation in noninternational armed conflicts depends on, first of all, the nature of the conflict, and second, the relevant treaties agreed by the state upon whose territory the conflict is taking place. According to the treaty law, in most situations of noninternational armed conflict, while relevant organizations may offer their services, there is no explicit obligation on the affected state to accept such an offer.[15]

There is growing support for the application of a general rule in all types of conflicts that consent to humanitarian assistance may not be refused on arbitrary grounds.[16] However, the parameters of what may be considered as arbitrary reasons for refusal are not necessarily settled, and there may be considerable discretion afforded to the affected party.[17] In addition, even if a basis for intervention could be found in law, in practical terms invoking such a rule would not necessarily ensure the safety of relief operations or of populations in need. For organizations providing humanitarian assistance, the consent of all parties concerned is normally vital to ensuring the safety of their operations[2].

Use of Field Hospitals in Emergencies Outside of Armed Conflict

It is possible that armed conflicts may coincide with the onset of natural or human-made disasters within the same area.[18] In such situations, often referred to as "complex emergencies," the abovementioned rules of IHL will be broadly applicable, providing an essential framework for the delivery of humanitarian relief,

including the provision of medical assistance. Elements of the disaster response that are not covered by IHL may be regulated by other bodies of law, including human rights law and the country's domestic laws, as well as other applicable principles and standards.

In emergencies occurring outside of armed conflict, while the affected state may choose to use field hospitals as part of its own domestic response (should it have the capacity to do so), relevant legal issues arise primarily in the deployment of field hospitals by third states and foreign organizations and bodies, including national government ministries, national militaries, intergovernmental bodies such as the UN and NATO, the organizations of the International Red Cross and Red Crescent Movement, international NGOs, and private organizations. The provision of medical assistance is a key component of international disaster relief more generally. The scale of such international assistance has increased enormously over the past couple of decades.[19]

In spite of their recurring use in the aftermath of disasters, there is a lack of existing international law regulating the use of foreign field hospitals (FFHs), or the use of foreign medical teams [FMTs] in general. This reflects a wider absence of binding international obligations on states in relation to cross-border disaster management[3]. While a limited number of international rules have been developed regarding specific types of incidents and certain methods of response, typically many states view this area as being subject to the principle of voluntariness, rather than governed by legal obligations.[20] To fill this gap, a large number of "soft" or nonbinding guidelines, codes of conduct, and sector-specific guidance have emerged, some of which are set out below.

Consent to Offers of Disaster Relief and Access to Those in Need

Timely access to medical care in the immediate aftermath of a disaster can be critical to saving large numbers of lives, depending upon the nature of the event. However, such access may be hampered by both practical and political factors. Practical obstacles may include damage to infrastructure, communication, and supply routes, leading to delays in the delivery and distribution of assistance. In terms of political challenges, an affected state may be unwilling to give its consent to the provision of external relief even where the impact of a disaster on its population is severe, if such assistance is perceived as interference in its domestic affairs.

In simple terms, in the provision of international disaster relief, the consent of the affected state to such actions is vital. Such consent is viewed as a necessary corollary of the corresponding responsibility on states to respond to disasters occurring on their own territory, within the overriding framework of state sovereignty. This position is also compounded by the absence of an existing explicit right of individuals to receive humanitarian assistance under international law[4].[21]

There have been periodic attempts to establish a positive duty on states to allow external assistance where their domestic capacity is overwhelmed, in particular in circumstances where such refusal may result in violations of existing international obligations, such as those under international human rights law. One such approach has advocated for the invocation of the "responsibility to protect" doctrine in the aftermath of a disaster causing serious harm to the affected population.[22] However, this assertion is subject to significant controversy. Seeking to provide relief in the absence of express consent by the affected state will give rise to a host of practical and operational difficulties. Assistance delivered in such a way may also no longer fulfill the requirements of generally accepted principles governing humanitarian aid, in particular that the assistance be impartial and neutral.[23]

More recently, the issue has been addressed in a set of new draft articles on the protection of persons in the event of disasters, adopted by the International Law Commission[5].[24] The draft articles establish a duty on the affected state to seek assistance where domestic capacity is overwhelmed. While state consent to international assistance is required, the draft articles maintain that such consent should not be withheld arbitrarily.[25] However, these clauses have received criticism from some states insofar as they attempt to develop what are perceived as new international obligations.[26] It is also worth noting that the need to obtain the consent of the affected state is reflected in nonbinding guidelines relating generally to disaster response,[27] as well as those specifically addressing the use of FFHs.[28]

Practical Issues in the Delivery of Assistance

International relief efforts may also be undermined by deficiencies in the aid provided. A great many

organizations and actors of varying abilities and experience will respond to large-scale disasters, in particular those that are sudden-onset in nature, and receive considerable global attention. Regarding FFHs, deficiencies that have been highlighted in previous response efforts include the following: a lack of registration of field hospital teams entering disaster zones; a lack of coordination with local authorities when on the ground; a lack of self-sufficiency; a lack of appropriately trained staff, appropriate equipment, and medicines; little understanding of or adherence to national and internationally acceptable medical practices; human rights violations and other criminal conduct. In addition, FFHs operating in post-disaster environments have been criticized for being too focused on emergency trauma care, while neglecting to address the secondary effects of such care, as well as the ongoing ordinary health-care needs of the affected population.[29] Similar to concerns raised about the effectiveness of humanitarian assistance more generally, the relevance, timing and cost effectiveness of some FFHs have also been questioned.[29]

To address the above challenges, a growing body of principles, guidelines, models of "good practice," and self-regulation frameworks have emerged, all of which are essentially nonbinding in nature. The growth of such soft-law instruments has advantages and disadvantages. On the one hand, the use of nonbinding guidelines can result in operational challenges being dealt with in a more timely manner. Further, self-regulation by the humanitarian sector may in turn foster greater willingness of affected states to allow international disaster relief[6]. However, it can be difficult to enforce the wide use of standards and criteria that are essentially voluntary. It may also be challenging for the affected state to ensure adherence by assisting actors to nonbinding guidelines, in particular if its institutions are weakened and resources stretched following an emergency. In such a situation there is a risk that international relief activities will be carried out in parallel: some within acceptable guidelines, and others potentially outside of them.

While an examination of all general guidelines, principles, and models applicable to disaster assistance is beyond the scope of this chapter, the Guidelines for the Domestic Facilitation and Regulation of International Disaster Relief, adopted in 2007, are of particular note. Informally known as the IDRL guidelines, their development was led by the International Federation of Red Cross and Red

Crescent Societies (IFRC).[30] The guidelines set out the responsibilities of "assisting actors," including the need to adhere to the humanitarian principles, the need to be adequate to meet anticipated needs and to be in line with international standards of quality, the need to coordinate with other actors, and to engage adequately trained personnel.[31] They also encourage states to adopt comprehensive legal, policy, and institutional frameworks to address disaster risk reduction and disaster response matters.[32] A growing number of states have reportedly made changes to their domestic disaster management frameworks in line with the IDRL guidelines.[33] However, progress is slow, and there are many states that still lack comprehensive laws and procedures for managing international disaster relief. Meanwhile, regulatory issues continue to impact the timeliness and effectiveness of international disaster response operations.[33]

Other guidelines that are of particular relevance to the use of FFHs include those aimed at managing the deployment of military assets in disaster response. A number of national militaries routinely deploy field hospitals and other medical units as part of international relief efforts.[34] From 1997 to 2006 it was reported that medical assistance, including field hospitals and personnel, constituted the second most commonly contributed military asset to international disaster relief operations, surpassed only by air transport[7]. The *Guidelines on the Use of Foreign Military and Civil Defence Assets in Disaster Relief* (Oslo guidelines), a revised version of which was published in 2007, aim to improve the effectiveness of the use of foreign military and civil defense assets in disasters occurring outside of armed conflicts[8]. Additional guidelines address the use of such assets in complex emergencies[9].

Specific issues relating to FFHs, as well as foreign medical teams in general, are addressed in two sets of guidelines and standards, both developed under the auspices of the World Health Organization (WHO) in collaboration with other bodies. The first of these, the WHO–PAHO's *Guidelines for the Use of Foreign Field Hospitals in the Aftermath of Sudden-Impact Disasters*, were published in 2003.[28] These guidelines set out essential requirements for FFHs, as well as additional optional criteria, to ensure that they benefit the affected population. Those elements considered essential include: that the hospital is operational on site within 24 hours following the impact of the disaster; that the hospital be entirely self-sufficient; that

the hospital offer comparable or higher standards of medical care than were available in the affected country to the precipitating event.[28]

In spite of the adoption of the WHO–PAHO guidelines, difficulties in ensuring professional and principled medical assistance in disaster response continued to be experienced.[35] Following a consultation process again established under WHO and coordinated with the global health cluster (GHC), a new framework, the *Classification and Minimum Standards for Foreign Medical Teams in Sudden Onset Disasters*, was adopted in 2013. The minimum standards build on the WHO–PAHO guidelines, but focus on the services provided by medical personnel (that is, FMTs), rather than the physical structure in which they work.[35] They introduce a classification and registration system, as well as a set of minimum standards (including foundational principles and more technical criteria) for FMTs providing trauma and surgical care in the first month following a SOD.[36] The minimum standards also set out benchmarks that international teams should meet to provide more standardized services.

Similar to one of the key aims of the more generally applicable IDRL guidelines, the minimum standards are intended to enable states in need of international medical assistance to choose the most appropriate and effective services offered, and to be better able to regulate such services once operating in their territory. For FMTs, adherence to the minimum standards, including classification and registration, may potentially facilitate greater access to donor funding, a greater chance of being approved for deployment by the affected state, and greater access to support services once in country.[35] Although still in their infancy, the minimum standards were tested during the response to Typhoon Haiyan in 2013, when the Philippines government chose to adopt the new classification and registration form.[37] The results of the new system in that context appear to be somewhat mixed. The classification system reportedly facilitated a more efficient and appropriate deployment of FMTs, while helping to ensure a "coordinated, timely, and credible response to the disaster."[37] This being said, just under half of all FMTs responding to Typhoon Haiyan were not registered under the new system.[38] If the registration process is to fulfill its full potential, greater numbers of FMTs will need to take part.

Selected Domestic Legal Issues Applicable to Field Hospital Deployments

In addition to those international standards set out above, FMTs, including those assigned to FFHs, will be subject to and must abide by the local laws of the country in which they are operating. These will cover a range of activities, including immigration and visa requirements, the import of medicines and equipment, engaging local services and concluding contracts (unless the latter are agreed as being subject to the laws of the sending country), driving laws, and those covering criminal acts.[39] Field hospital staff will require sufficient support during their mission to ensure they operate at all times within the relevant domestic legal framework. While the central focus of this chapter is on international law matters, some issues relevant to field hospital deployments primarily covered by domestic laws are set out below.

Licensing of Medical Personnel

The licensing of international medical personnel in a situation of disaster is a matter regulated by domestic law.[40] States are under no international obligation to waive domestic licensing requirements for international personnel in such situations. The IDRL guidelines recommend the establishment of expedited procedures for temporary recognition of professional qualifications of foreign medical personnel, as well as other relevant professionals, such as engineers.[41] However, expedited procedures should not come at the expense of quality in response (as emphasized by the IDRL guidelines). For example, following Typhoon Haiyan, the Government of the Philippines waived requirements related to the existing licensing process for foreign professionals (including medical personnel) to facilitate their quick entry and deployment to the affected zones[10]. While positive in this sense, it was also reported that the waiver and an accompanying relaxation of visa and immigration regulations may have allowed for an influx of medical teams not registered under the new FMT system.[42]

Consent to Medical Treatment

The requirement of a medical practitioner to obtain the informed consent of the patient prior to carrying out any medical intervention or conducting medical research or clinical trials is enshrined in modern medical ethics,[43] and forms part of the domestic law in many countries.[44] In such jurisdictions, carrying out procedures or conducting research on patients in the absence of informed consent can lead to criminal charges being laid against the practitioner, as well as those related to professional negligence. The organization responsible for the practitioner may also find itself liable for such actions. Relevant domestic laws may make some exceptions to the need to obtain informed consent, such as for patients who are incapacitated, those suffering from communicable diseases (CDs), and those who have a mental illness.[45] While not all countries recognize informed consent as a legal right, it is a principle subject to increasing international acceptance. However, it may carry significant difficulties in application.[46]

The World Medical Association recognizes that a key condition for obtaining informed consent is good communication between the medical professional and his or her patient, and that major obstacles to such communication can be language and culture [11]. This may be particularly apparent in the contexts in which FFHs operate. In such situations, it is vital that every effort is made to ensure patients are fully aware of the reasons for and possible ramifications of any proposed treatment. This may involve engaging an interpreter and ensuring consent forms are translated into the appropriate language. In terms of culture, practitioners should be aware of any specific requirements regarding family or community involvement in the consent process. In all situations, it will be preferable for consent to be communicated in writing (applicable domestic laws may require written consent).[47] The WHO *Classification and Minimum Standards for Foreign Medical Teams in Sudden Onset Disasters* sets out in its guiding principles that all informed consent for medical procedures should be obtained in a language and culturally appropriate fashion[12].

Treatment of Unaccompanied Minors

Unaccompanied children or minors are those that have been separated from both parents and other relatives, and who are not being cared for by a responsible adult[13]. International law sets out various obligations on states to reduce the risk of family separation and, where such separation has occurred, to ensure reunification where possible. FMTs and their sending states or organizations should ensure that their systems and practices do not (even inadvertently) encourage family separation[13].

International legal standards require states generally to keep children from harm[14] and to grant then the highest attainable standard of health[13]. In addition, in all decisions concerning children (whether taken by public or private bodies), the best interests of the child shall be a primary consideration[13]. National laws and policies may set out a range of standards and requirements in relation to the care of unaccompanied minors.[48] There may also be tensions at the domestic level between the perceived need, on the one hand, to preserve a child's welfare and, on the other hand, the requirement to respect his or her rights.[49] While informed consent is, as set out above, important to establish,[50] the provision of, for example, lifesaving treatment may be deemed essential by the medical professional, even in the absence of consent.

Liability and Litigation

In the event of malpractice, negligence, or other wrongful acts committed by international health teams and their personnel, there is no overarching international framework governing such matters,[51] and no uniform approach among states or responding organizations. Compensation or other remedies may be available through private insurance, through insurance or other schemes provided by the sending organization of the individual or team, or through the tort system. Much will depend on the domestic laws of the affected state,[52] any insurance held by the health-care professional and his or her sending organization,[53] and any agreements made between the sending organization and the affected state which might govern such issues.

The risk of accident or malpractice will likely be greater in emergency contexts, owing to the extreme conditions, a potential lack of appropriate resources, language and cultural barriers, and the potential deployment of those without sufficient training. However, in general, there appears to be limited availability of suitable remedies or compensation for victims; in particular in developing countries, where legal institutions and processes may be weak and medical malpractice laws nonexistent.[54]

Summary

The legal framework governing the use of field hospitals differs depending on the context in which they are

deployed. If the emergency is one of armed conflict, the long-established body of rules comprising IHL sets out many specific rules regulating the protection and use of medical units, including as part of international relief efforts. In situations of disaster occurring outside of an armed conflict, there is no single applicable body of international law regulating the use of field hospitals (or of international disaster relief more generally). Rather, a fragmented collection of few international and regional rules, as well as a growing body of soft-law guidelines and standards (some of which have been developed specifically for FFHs and medical teams), serves as the applicable framework.

Summary Points

- There is no single, comprehensive legal framework governing the use of field hospitals in the aftermath of crises. Depending on the issue, a variety of national, regional, and international laws, as well as nonbinding standards and guidelines, may be relevant.
- In situations of armed conflict long-established rules of IHL provide for the protection of medical units and facilitate the provision of medical and humanitarian assistance to affected populations.
- In emergencies outside of armed conflicts, there is an absence of international rules regulating the deployment of FFHs. The consent of the affected state to such deployments is vital.
- Practical issues in the deployment of field hospitals, including the suitability and quality of the medical assistance provided, as well as the ability to secure the necessary legal facilities to operate at the disaster zone, are increasingly addressed through a growing body of principles, guidelines, models of "good practice," and self-regulation frameworks. While this can result in challenges being dealt with in a more timely manner, it may be difficult to ensure adherence to guidelines that are effectively voluntary in nature.
- Key nonbinding guidelines regulating the provision of assistance on disasters include the *Guidelines for the Domestic Facilitation and Regulation of International Disaster Relief*, adopted in 2007, originally developed by the IFRC.
- Guidelines and standards more directly relevant to the deployment of FFHs have also been developed in recent decades: these include the 2003 WHO–PAHO's *Guidelines for the Use of Foreign Field*

Hospitals in the Aftermath of Sudden-Impact Disasters, and, building on the former, the 2013 WHO *Classification and Minimum Standards for Foreign Medical Teams in Sudden Onset Disasters*. Operating as a classification and registration system for FMTs, the latter standards enable states in need of international medical assistance to choose the most appropriate and effective services offered, and to regulate such services in their territory.

- In addition to the above, a range of legal issues relating to field hospital deployments may arise which are primarily dealt with through domestic laws (usually of the country in which the hospital will be operating, unless subject to agreement with the sending country/organization). These include licensing requirements, consent by patients to medical treatment, treatment of unaccompanied minors, and medical liability issues. Some of the abovementioned standards may include limited guidance on these points.

Notes to the Text

1. In addition to relevant rules of international law, deployed field hospitals will normally be subject to all applicable domestic laws of the affected state. However, an examination of such domestic laws is beyond the scope of this chapter.

2. Armed conflicts may be international or noninternational in nature, but do not include situations of internal disturbances or tensions such as riots and isolated and sporadic acts of violence. The term "disaster" as used in this chapter may be defined as the following:

   > A serious disruption of the functioning of society, which poses a significant, widespread threat to human life, health, property, or the environment, whether arising from accident, nature, or human activity, whether developing suddenly or as the result of long-term processes, but excluding armed conflict[15].

3. Also known as the law of armed conflict. IHL sets out categories of persons and objects that must be respected and protected in armed conflicts, and limits the methods and means of warfare. Like all international law, IHL consists primarily of rules established by agreements between states (i.e., treaties) and rules established through the customary practice of states.

4. "Medical units" are defined as "establishments and other units, whether military or civilian, organized for medical purposes, be they fixed or mobile, permanent or temporary. The term includes, for example, hospitals and other similar units, blood transfusion centers, preventive medicine centers and institutes, medical depots, and the medical and pharmaceutical stores of such units[16]."

5. Such medical units must be exclusively assigned to medical purposes; civilian medical units must be recognized and authorized. Article 27, Convention (I) for the Amelioration of the Condition of the Wounded and Sick in Armed Forces in the Field, 12 August 1949 (First Geneva Convention) and Article 12(2) or 9(2), Protocol Additional to the GCs of 12 August 1949, and relating to the Protection of Victims of International Armed Conflicts, 8 June 1977 (Additional Protocol I).

6. Such acts may include, for example, the use of a hospital to launch an attack.

7. Article 10, Additional Protocol I.

8. Articles 16(1) and 16(2), Additional Protocol I.

9. Article 16(3), Additional Protocol I.

10. Articles 55 and 56, Fourth GC; Article 69(1), Additional Protocol I. Article 56 requires the occupying power to maintain hospital and medical establishments and services, public health, and public hygiene. The occupying power must meet these obligations "by the fullest extent of the means available" to it.

11. Article 59 of the Fourth GC allows for such schemes to be undertaken by states or by "impartial humanitarian organizations such as the International Committee of the Red Cross."

12. Article 70(1), Additional Protocol I. For humanitarian assistance to be accepted, it must be appropriate for the needs of the population, and must not favor any one group.

13. Article 54(1), Additional Protocol I. This prohibition is also a rule of customary law and equally applicable in noninternational armed conflicts[17].

14. Article 71(2), Additional Protocol I.

15. Article 3(2), common to the four Geneva conventions of 1949, states that, in noninternational armed conflicts: "An impartial humanitarian body, such as the International Committee of the Red Cross, may offer its services to the Parties to the conflict."

16. For example, Rule 55 of the Study on Customary IHL by the ICRC maintains that, in international and noninternational armed conflicts, consent to humanitarian operations must not be withheld on arbitrary grounds, while recognizing the right of warring parties to exercise control over the relief action[18].

17. One example of an arbitrary reason would be the refusal of medical assistance on the grounds that it could be used to treat enemy soldiers – such a decision would be contrary to the requirement that humanitarian relief be provided on the basis of need alone. For additional examples, see Akande and Gillard [19].

18. Examples of such emergencies include the effects of the Indian Ocean tsunami in Banda Aceh, Indonesia, in 2004, and flooding in parts of Pakistan in 2010.

19. For example, upwards of 10 000 NGOs were reportedly operating in Haiti following the earthquake in 2010.

20. One such example of a specific treaty is the Tampere Convention on the Provision of Telecommunication Resources for Disaster Mitigation and Relief Operations. Some binding agreements between states have also been adopted at the

regional level, for example, the ASEAN Agreement on Disaster Management and Emergency Response.

21. This being said, some organizations and experts have argued that such a right does exist, based on either the interpretation of the right to life, or alternatively as a result of the cumulative effect of other existing related rights. See for example Stoffels[20].

22. The responsibility to protect (R2P) doctrine was adopted by the World Summit in 2005 (it is therefore not a binding treaty obligation), and remains subject to debate in terms of its appropriate implementation. Its purpose is to compel the international community to address the most serious international crimes, including genocide, war crimes, ethnic cleansing, and crimes against humanity. In 2008, following the Government of Myanmar's refusal to allow international assistance in the aftermath of Cyclone Nargis, the R2P doctrine was raised by some as a possible means of forcibly providing aid. However, this proposal received considerable criticism. See Junk[21].

23. The humanitarian principles, namely humanity, impartiality, neutrality, and independence, emerged out of the original "fundamental principles" underpinning the work of the International Red Cross and Red Crescent Movement. They have since been adopted widely by the humanitarian sector through various guidance tools and codes of conduct (for example, the Code of Conduct for The International Red Cross and Red Crescent Movement and NGOs in Disaster Relief), as well as by a number of governments (one such example is the European Consensus on humanitarian aid), and are considered as governing the delivery of humanitarian assistance in all contexts.

24. Although currently nonbinding, the International Law Commission has recommended the elaboration of a convention based on the draft articles, which will be considered by the UN General Assembly in a future session.

25. Article 13, draft articles on the protection of persons in the event of disasters. This attempts to mirror developments in the parallel area of cross-border humanitarian assistance operations in situations of armed conflict.

26. See, for example, comments of the USA and Australia at the sixty-eighth session of the International Law Commission[22].

27. For example, the Guidelines for the Domestic Facilitation and Regulation of International Disaster Relief (hereafter the IDRL guidelines) recommend that an affected state seeks external assistance where its own capacity is overwhelmed, they also confirm that "[d]isaster relief or initial recovery assistance should be initiated only with the consent of the affected state" (paragraph 10.1).

28. The WHO–PAHO *Guidelines for the Use of Foreign Field Hospitals in the Aftermath of Sudden-Impact Disasters* (hereafter WHO–PAHO guidelines), adopted in 2003, confirm that field hospitals will be deployed only "following an appropriate declaration of emergency and a request from the health authorities of the affected country[23]."

29. These correspond to the major health-care needs following a sudden-onset disaster[24]. This study also found that, in a study of foreign field hospital use in four major SODs, of the facilities assessed, none were operational early enough to provide lifesaving, emergency trauma care. This renders the need to focus on secondary effects and general healthcare ever more important.

30. Although nonbinding, the IDRL guidelines were adopted by the International Conference of the Red Cross and Red Crescent, meaning that both states and the International Red Cross and Red Crescent Movement have endorsed them and agreed to endorse their use.

31. IDRL guidelines, para 4.

32. IDRL guidelines, para 8. The IFRC has developed a number of practical tools to assist states to make changes to their laws, where appropriate, in line with the IDRL guidelines. These include a model act and model emergency decree[25].

33. At the thirty-second International Conference of the Red Cross and Red Crescent in 2015, it was reported that 23 states have adopted new laws, rules, or procedures in line with the IDRL guidelines since 2007. Resolution 6, thirty-second International Conference of the Red Cross and Red Crescent, introductory paragraph 4[26].

34. For example, the Israel Defense Forces (IDF), the Canadian Forces, the USA military, and the British Armed Forces have all deployed field hospitals in the aftermath of various emergencies.

35. This was particularly evident in relation to the response following the earthquake in Haiti and flooding in Pakistan in 2010[12].

36. The *Classification and Minimum Standards* (p. 10) sets out six guiding principles and 13 core standards applicable to all FMTs. In addition, it establishes minimum technical standards for different categories of FMT and for each service.

37. This was the first time the form had been used in the context of a global disaster response[27].

38. Of 150 FMTs that provided health services during the response to Typhoon Haiyan, 67 were reportedly not registered[27].

39. United Nations' personnel and those of organizations such as the ICRC and International Federation of Red Cross and Red Crescent Societies may be subject to certain privileges and immunities recognized under international and/or national laws. See, for example, the Convention on the Privileges and Immunities of the United Nations, February 13, 1946[28]. However, such privileges still require relevant officials to abide by all applicable domestic laws.

40. This is the same in situations of armed conflict; IHL does not cover such matters.

41. Article 16(1)(c), IDRL guidelines. Article 16(3) of the guidelines also encourages states and assisting organizations to consider to what extent needs can be met by hiring local staff (who may already have appropriate licenses).

42. The government did, however, require all medical volunteers to purchase liability insurance in the Philippines, and for the individual and the sending organization to assume full responsibility for the outcome of the mission (including postoperative follow-up and any related financial costs)[29].

43. See, for example, the WMA Declaration on the Rights of the Patient.

44. For example, both the USA[30] and the UK[31] give effect to the right of informed consent in domestic regulations, as does the European Union[32].

45. In some such cases, the consent of the patient's legally entitled representative will be required.

46. This is especially so in emergency operations in developing countries, where FFHs are often deployed. For further practical discussion on informed consent in the context of recent foreign medical operations, see, for example, the debate concerning the use of experimental drugs in the 2014–2015 Ebola crisis in West Africa[33,34].

47. Where a patient is unable to write, oral consent may be given in the presence of one or more witnesses. Written or oral consent is that expressly given. Implied consent (indicated through patient behavior alone) may be deemed as given in limited circumstances.

48. For example, national laws may differ as to the age of consent for medical treatment (or may not establish a specific age). For those under the established age of consent (or where one is not provided), there may be criteria to determine the capacity of the child to provide informed consent to a procedure.

49. For example, at the international level, Article 12 of the Convention on the Rights of the Child recognizes the value of a child's views and the need to give them weight in accordance with the age and maturity of the child[14].

50. The ability of a child to consent or reject treatment of care may be based on a range of factors, aside from age; for example, psychological experience, maturity, and context. See, for example: "Age is Arbitrary: Setting Minimum Ages," Child Rights International Network discussion paper[35].

51. In situations of armed conflict, IHL does not cover such matters. While IHL prevents health-care professionals from being punished for acts carried out in compliance with medical ethics, it does not indemnify against liability for acts contrary to medical ethics, or accidents.

52. A small number of countries, including the USA, Australia, and South Africa, have enacted laws aimed at exempting from liability those assisting in an emergency, provided such acts were carried out "in good faith[36]."

53. Some larger organizations will provide professional liability coverage for all their staff, although it is reportedly more common for such coverage not to be provided (and for individuals to sign waivers acknowledging this fact). Individual coverage may be expensive and only be available through specialized policies, which can exclude certain contexts[37].

54. There is very little evidence available of malpractice suits against health-care professionals operating in response to international emergencies[38].

References

1. Akande D, Gillard EC. Arbitrary withholding of consent to humanitarian relief operations in armed conflict. *International Law Studies Series* 2016: **92**: 492.

2. Gillard EC. The law regulating cross-border relief operations. *International Review of the Red Cross* 2013: **95**(890): 351–82; 354.

3. Clement C. International disaster response laws, rules and principles: a pragmatic approach to strengthening international disaster response mechanisms, in Caron, D, Kelly M, Telesetsky A. eds. *The international law of disaster relief*. Cambridge: Cambridge University Press; 2014: 67–88; 69.

4. Spieker H. The right to give and receive humanitarian assistance, in Heintze HJ, Zwitter A. eds. *International law and humanitarian assistance*. Berlin Heidelberg; Springer-Verlag; 2011: 7–31.

5. United Nations. Draft articles on the protection of persons in the event of disasters. http://legal.un.org/docs/?path=../ilc/texts/instruments/english/draft_articles/6_3_2016.pdf&lang=EF

6. Bookmiller KN. Professional standards and legal standard setting: INSARAG, FMTs, and international disaster relief volunteers. *Vanderbilt Journal of Transnational Law* **48**; 957–84: 959.

7. Stockholm International Peace Research Institute. The effectiveness of foreign military assets in natural disaster response. http://reliefweb.int/sites/reliefweb.int/files/resources/236476A D3257088DC125741000474F20-sipri_mar2008.pdf

8. Office for the Coordination of Humanitarian Affairs. Guidelines on the use of foreign military and civil defence assets in disaster relief. https://docs.unocha.org/sites/dms/Documents/Oslo%20Guidelines%20ENGLISH%20(November%202007).pdf

9. Guidelines on the use of military and civil defence assets to support united nations humanitarian activities in complex emergencies. http://www.unocha.org/what-we-do/coordination-tools/UN-CMCoord/publications

10. http://www.gov.ph/2013/11/26/prc-waives-special-temporary-permit-for-foreign-professionals-assisting-in-typhoon-torn-areas/

11. WMA ethics manual, chapter two: 43. http://www.wma.net/en/30publications/30ethicsmanual/pdf/Chap_2_3rd_Nov2015_en.pdf

12. Norton I, von Schreeb J, Aitken P, Herard P, Lajolo C. *Classification and minimum standards for foreign medical teams in sudden onset disasters*. Geneva: World Health Organization; 2013: 10, 13, 18, 31.

13. Inter-Agency guiding principles on unaccompanied and separated children (2004): 13, 23. https://www.unicef.org/protection/IAG_UASCs.pdf

14. Convention on the rights of the child. Article 3(1), Article 6, Article 19, Article 24. http://www.ohchr.org/EN/ProfessionalInterest/Pages/CRC.aspx

15. Guidelines for the domestic facilitation and regulation of international disaster relief, paragraph 2(1). http://www.ifrc.org/en/what-we-do/idrl/idrl-guidelines

16. International Committee of the Red Cross. Rule 28, Study on customary international humanitarian law. https://www.icrc.org/customary-ihl/eng/docs/v1_rul_rule28#Fn_89_2

17. International Committee of the Red Cross. Rule 53. https://ihl-databases.icrc.org/customary-ihl/eng/docs/v1_rul_rule53

18. International Committee of the Red Cross. Rule 55. https://ihl-databases.icrc.org/customary-ihl/eng/docs/v1_rul_rule55

19. Akande D, Gillard EC (2016). Oxford guidance on the law relating to humanitarian relief operations in armed conflict. Commissioned by UN OCHA. https://docs.unocha.org/sites/dms/Documents/Oxford%20Guidance%20pdf.pdf

20. Stoffels RA. Legal regulation of humanitarian assistance in armed conflict: Achievements and gaps. *International Review of the Red Cross* 2004: **86**(855); 515–46.

21. Junk J. Testing boundaries: Cyclone Nargis in Myanmar and the scope of R2P. *Global Society* 2016: **30**(1): 78–93.

22. Analytical guide to the work of the international law commission. http://legal.un.org/ilc/guide/6_3.shtml

23. WHO–PAHO. Guidelines for the use of foreign field hospitals in the aftermath of sudden-impact disasters. http://www.who.int/hac/techguidance/pht/FieldHospitalsFolleto.pdf

24. Von Schreeb J, Riddez L, Samnegård H, Rosling H. Foreign field hospitals in the recent sudden-onset disasters in Iran, Haiti, Indonesia and Pakistan. *Prehospital and Disaster Medicine* 2008: **23**(2): 144–51; 145.

25. IFRC. Disaster law. http://www.ifrc.org/en/what-we-do/disaster-law/

26. International Committee of the Red Cross. http://rcrcconference.org/wp-content/uploads/sites/3/2015/04/32IC-Res6-legal-frameworks-for-disaster_EN.pdf

27. Peiris S, Buenaventura J, Zagaria N. Is registration of foreign medical teams needed for disaster response? Findings from the response to typhoon Haiyan. *Western Pacific Surveillance and Response Journal* 2015: **6**(1): 29–33.

28. The Convention on the privileges and immunities of the United Nations, 13 February 1946. http://www.un.org/en/ethics/pdf/convention.pdf

29. http://www.epijournal.com/articles/173/legal-liability-for-healthcare-volunteers

30. Office for Human Research Protections. https://www.hhs.gov/ohrp/regulations-and-policy/guidance/faq/informed-consent/index.html

31. General Medical Council. http://www.gmc-uk.org/guidance/ethical_guidance/consent_guidance_legal_framework.asp

32. Directive 2001/20/EC of the European Parliament and of the Council. http://ec.europa.eu/health//sites/health/files/files/eudralex/vol-1/dir_2001_20/dir_2001_20_en.pdf

33. http://www.ibanet.org/Article/NewDetail.aspx?ArticleUid=920c89de-c0de-4bbf-8c76-4d65d95be993; https://www.ncbi.nlm.nih.gov/pmc/articles/PMC4209768/

34. Forbes. Ebola, experimental drugs and informed consent: should those at risk simply take what the doctor orders? https://www.forbes.com/sites/elaineschattner/2014/08/31/ebola-experimental-drugs-and-informed-consent-should-those-at-risk-simply-take-what-the-doctor-orders/#7dc17ad21cb1

35. Child Rights International Network. https://www.crin.org/sites/default/files/discussion_paper_-_minimum_ages.pdf

36. http://www.epijournal.com/articles/173/legal-liability-for-healthcare-volunteers

37. http://www.epijournal.com/articles/173/legal-liability-for-healthcare-volunteers

38. Ueijima T. Medical missions and medical malpractice: current state of medical malpractice overseas. *ASA Newsletter* 2011: **75**(2): 22–24.

Index